Earl Mindell's

ANTI-AGING
BIBLE

Earl Mindell, R. Ph., Ph.D.

A FIRESIDE BOOK
Published by Simon & Schuster

New York   London   Toronto   Sydney   Tokyo   Singapore

FIRESIDE
Rockefeller Center
1230 Avenue of the Americas
New York, NY 10020

FIRESIDE and colophon are registered trademarks
of Simon & Schuster Inc.

Designed by Richard Oriolo

Manufactured in the United States of America

1   3   5   7   9   10   8   6   4   2

Library of Congress Cataloging-in-Publication Data

Mindell, Earl.
[Anti-aging bible]
Earl Mindell's anti-aging bible / Earl Mindell.
p.   cm.
Includes bibliographical references and index.
1. Longevity.
2. Longevity—Nutritional aspects.
3. Aging—Prevention. I. Title.
RA776.75.M55   1996
613—dc20   95-38420
CIP
ISBN 0-684-81106-5

Contents

Chapter 1

Maximum Maintenance, Maximum Health

Of all of the spectacular advances in medicine, science, and technology that have occurred during the past century, the ones that have had the most profound impact on our lives are those that have increased human life span. In 1900, the average life expectancy for an American citizen was forty-seven years of age. Today, as we approach the dawn of a new century, the average life span has increased by more than 50 percent to seventy-six. The fastest growing segment of the U.S. population consists of men and women aged seventy-five and older, a group referred to by gerontologists as the "old old." The number of octogenarians among us continues to grow, and some scientists say that humans may routinely achieve a life span of about one hundred fifteen years; still others contend that biological engineering will extend our life span to one hundred fifty years. A few scientists insist that humans could live to be as old four hundred!

The increase in life span that we have experienced during this century is primarily due to improved sanitation, the elimination of many lethal childhood diseases through vaccinations, and other medical advances such as the development of antibiotics. Rare today, death from infection during childbirth was a leading cause of mortality among women at the turn of the century. Thanks to penicillin and its "wonder drug" offspring, bacterial infections such as pneumonia and strep are no longer life threatening.

Although heart disease is still the leading cause of death in the United States, the mortality rate from heart disease is declining due to better prevention and more aggressive treatments. Although cancer continues to be the second leading cause of death in the United States, the prognosis for at least certain forms of the disease has vastly improved within the past century. We owe a debt of gratitude to the scientists and physicians who have taken us this far. But there are limits to what they have been able to do. Members of the medical establishment readily acknowledge that although we have managed to extend the length of life, in many cases we have done little to improve the quality of life. A recent editorial in a medical magazine lamented the fact that "the ratio of active life to disabled or functionally compromised life has not increased and may actually have diminished during the last quarter of a century" (*Patient Care*, February 28, 1994). In other words, people may be living longer, but they're not living better.

Despite the increase in life span, the perception of aging as a depressing downward spiral of growing wrinkled, growing senile, growing ill, and growing old persists. Indeed, for many of today's elderly, growing older is synonymous with illness. About half of all people over sixty-five are taking multiple medications for a wide variety of ailments. The average older person takes twelve doses of medication daily. For many older people, life is punctuated by visits to the doctor and the hospital. In addition to life-threatening diseases, life-diminishing diseases, such as arthritis, vision problems, memory loss, and sleep disorders, continue to plague the elderly.

This does not have to be the case. Sadly, and ironically, too many people suffer from ailments that are easily prevented or controlled through diet and lifestyle. According to the National Cancer Institute, as many as 35 percent of all cancers may be due to poor diet. Experts estimate that as many as 50 percent of all cases of heart disease might be averted by changes in diet and lifestyle, which themselves would greatly enhance both the quantity and quality of life.

Why and how we age is still very much a mystery. Serious research on aging is relatively new, and only a few scientists are doing concentrated work in this area. Until recently, scientists were disdainful of colleagues involved in aging research, likening it to alchemy or the pursuit of the mythical fountain of youth. However, as the U.S. population has begun to age, interest in the aging process and age-related illnesses has begun to attract greater attention.

Until recently, there was a fatalistic attitude about aging that was shared by both experts and laypeople alike. They believed that there was little they could do to prevent the ravages of aging. Today we know better. There is strong evidence that the downward spiral is not inevitable. For one thing, although they are still in the minority, there is a growing population of "old old" people who are aging well and who have managed to stay active and healthy. We see them on tennis courts, in adult education classes, in the gym, and sometimes still on the job. Researchers have begun to study the lives and lifestyles of these successful agers in the hope of discovering important information that will help us all age well. There is a growing body of research that suggests that with appropriate and timely intervention the downward spiral associated with aging need not happen. Researchers throughout the world are finding new and exciting ways to maintain health and vitality well into old age and innovative ways to prevent some of the common ailments associated with aging. Scientists all over the United States—at Boston's Tufts University, the University of California, Mount Sinai Medical Center in New York, and the University of Texas to name a few—are engaged in research that has generated important information on why and how we age. Here are some of their fascinating findings:

- Vitamins and supplements (antioxidants) may help to protect the body against compounds that may speed up the aging process.
- A handful of foods and supplements may substantially reduce the risk of developing cataracts and macular degeneration, the leading cause of blindness among the elderly.
- An ancient herb and other supplements may help to prevent memory loss and keep us smart and sharp.
- Vitamins and supplements may help to rejuvenate a "tired" immune system.
- Contrary to the popular belief that our muscles grow weaker as we age, it's actually possible, with the right kind of exercise, to build muscle and maintain strength well into our nineties and beyond.
- A supplement widely used in Japan as a treatment for heart disease (and available at natural food stores in the United States) may help to keep an aging heart pumping as strong as a younger one.
- Prostate problems (common among men over fifty) may be prevented or reversed by a combination of diet and supplements.
- The right combination of herbs and supplements can relieve the discomfort of menopause for many women.

Here is more good news: these tools are readily available to anyone who wants to use them. For the first time, we have the power and the knowledge to change our fate and make a real difference in both the quality and quantity of our lives. Although the sooner we start the better, positive changes can produce positive results at any stage of life.

This book will show you how to get started. I will examine the latest research on aging and show how you can use this information to help you live a longer, healthier life. I have compiled a list of the Hot 100 anti-aging substances—foods, vitamins, supplements, herbs, and other compounds—that can help you age successfully. With few exceptions, the vitamins, supplements, herbs, and foodstuffs that I discuss in this book are easily available in pharmacies and grocery and health food stores. I devote separate chapters to the unique aging issues that confront men and women and take a detailed look at the risks and side effects of prescription drugs. Perhaps most importantly, in the chapter "Staying Well: A Guide to Preventing the Common Ailments of Aging," I stress prevention and drug-free approaches to dealing with many problems that can seriously interfere with the quality of our lives.

Finally, I want to stress that the techniques I describe in this book are not a fountain of youth, although they can help us retain our youthfulness. An eighty-year-old who follows my suggestions is not going to look or feel the same as a twenty-year-old. What I am suggesting is that an eighty-year-old can be vigorous, strong, attractive, and full of life. My goal is not to turn back the clock, but to help you be the best fifty-, sixty-, seventy-, eighty-, and even one-hundred-year-old you can be.

Chapter 2

The Hot 100 Anti-Aging Arsenal from A to Z

The anti-aging Hot 100 contains a select group of vitamins, minerals, foods, herbs, and other supplements that can help us live longer, healthier lives. Except for the rare drug or supplement that may be available by prescription only, the anti-aging Hot 100 is available at natural food stores, pharmacies, herb shops, and, in some cases, your local supermarket.

Caution: If you are taking a prescription drug for a medical condition, do not discontinue the drug without first consulting with your physician or natural healer.

1. Acidolphilus
2. Allium vegetables
3. Aloe
4. Alpha-carotene
5. Alpha-hydroxy acids
6. L-Arginine
7. Ascorbic acid (vitamin C)
8. Ashwaganda
9. Aspirin

10. Astragalus
11. Beta-carotene
12. Bilberry
13. Bioflavonoids
14. Boron
15. Bromelain
16. Burdock
17. Butcher's broom
18. Calciferol (vitamin D)
19. Calcium
20. Capsaicin
21. L-Carnitine
22. Centella (Gotu Kola)
23. Choline
24. Chromium picolinate
25. Cinnamon
26. Citrus
27. Club moss
28. Cobalamin (vitamin B_{12})
29. Coenzyme Q_{10}
30. Cranberry
31. Cruciferous vegetables
32. Dandelion
33. Dong quai
34. Echinacea
35. Ellagic acid
36. Fenugreek
37. Fiber
38. Flax
39. Folic acid
40. Fo-ti
41. Gamma-linolenic acid
42. Genistein
43. Ginger
44. Ginkgo
45. Ginseng
46. Glutathione
47. Grapeseed extract
48. Green tea
49. Hawthorn
50. Horsetail
51. Legumes
52. Lemongrass
53. Licorice
54. Lignans
55. Ligusticum
56. Lutein
57. Lycopene
58. Magnesium
59. Melatonin
60. Menadione (vitamin K)
61. Milk thistle
62. Monounsaturated fat
63. Motherwort
64. Niacin (vitamin B_3)
65. Nitrosamine blockers
66. Nucleic acids (DNA and RNA)
67. Oat bran
68. Octacosanol
69. Omega-3 fatty acids
70. Papain
71. Pectin
72. Phytic acid
73. Potassium
74. Propolis
75. Protease inhibitors
76. Psyllium seed
77. Quercetin
78. Reishi mushroom
79. Resveratrol
80. Riboflavin (vitamin B_2)
81. Saw palmetto
82. Schizandra
83. Seaweed

84. Selenium
85. Sesame
86. Solanaceous foods
87. Soybeans
88. Sulforaphane
89. Thiamine (vitamin B_1)
90. Tocopherol (vitamin E)
91. Tretinoin
92. Turmeric
93. Umbelliferous vegetables
94. Vitex
95. Water
96. Wheat bran
97. White willow
98. Wild yam
99. Yohimbe
100. Zinc

Acidophilus

FACTS

Several years ago, a television commercial for a popular brand of yogurt contended that eating yogurt was the key to longevity. The commercial featured several centenarians from an obscure part of rural Russia who had one thing in common: they were all lifelong yogurt eaters. At the time, the premise of the commercial may have sounded a bit far-fetched, but scientists are now discovering that there might be something to it after all.

Yogurt contains *Lactobacillus acidophilus* (commonly known as acidophilus), a so-called friendly bacteria that is used to ferment milk into yogurt and is also present in the gastrointestinal tract. Acidophilus not only aids in digestion, but appears to help keep the growth of yeast, such as *Candida albicans,* in check. *Candida albicans* is the cause of many vaginal yeast infections. In fact, acidophilus is a common folk remedy for yeast infection, but more importantly, recent studies suggest that acidophilus may help the body ward off other infections as well.

Acidophilus is present in yogurt and is also available in capsules or granules.

THE RIGHT AMOUNT

Eat two 8-ounce cartons of nonfat yogurt with active cultures daily. (Be sure the carton specifies *active cultures*.)

Take 2 acidophilus capsules three times daily ½ hour before or after meals.

Mix 1 packet of acidophilus granules in 6 ounces of freshly squeezed juice one or two times daily.

POSSIBLE BENEFITS

Antifungal   •   Women who are menopausal should take note: the vaginal dryness that often accompanies the drop in estrogen can make you more prone to vaginal yeast infections. A carton or two of yogurt a day may be just what the doctor ordered. Those are the findings of a physician at Long Island Jewish Medical Center who recently studied whether acidophilus is effective against vaginal yeast infections. In her study, the physician instructed women with a history of chronic yeast infections to eat 8 ounces, or 1 carton, of yogurt with live acidophilus cultures each day and compared them to non-yogurt eaters. After 6 months, the women who ate the yogurt had far fewer yeast infections than those who did not.

Immune Booster   •   As we age, our immune system weakens, making us more vulnerable to infections of all kinds. Eating yogurt daily may help to maintain normal immune function. A researcher at the University of California studied the effects of yogurt with live cultures on the immune system. His findings: people who ate two 8-ounce cartons of yogurt daily had higher blood levels of gamma-interferon, a substance that helps the body to ward off infection. He also noticed that the people who ate yogurt with live cultures also had substantially fewer colds and allergy symptoms than those who did not.

PERSONAL ADVICE

I am frequently asked whether acidophilus capsules are as good as eating yogurt with live cultures. Actually, the capsules and granules provide a more potent form of acidophilus. Sometimes the capsules or granules are preferable, especially if you have a yeast problem or are taking an antibiotic that is wreaking havoc on your digestive system by killing off the friendly bacteria. (Erythromycin is a particular offender.) However, in normal circumstances, eating yogurt is probably good enough. In addition, yogurt offers the added benefit of a hefty boost of calcium, which is needed for strong bones and normal blood pressure and heart function.

Allium Vegetables

FACTS

There are five hundred plants belonging to the genus *Allium*, which include garlic, onions, chives, and scallions. The National Cancer Society is investigating many members of the allium family for their potential cancer-fighting properties. In addition, researchers have found that these special vegetables may be helpful in the prevention and treatment of a wide range of ailments including Alzheimer's disease and cardiovascular disease, two problems that are particularly prevalent among the older population.

THE RIGHT AMOUNT

Use these vegetables liberally in your cooking. Red and yellow onions and shallots have the highest flavonoid content of allium vegetables. (Flavonoids may protect against cancer.)

Fresh garlic should be eaten daily—I prefer to bake or stir-fry it. It has a milder flavor than eating it raw. If you can't stomach the stuff, try using odorless garlic capsules. Take 1 or 2 capsules after each meal daily. Try taking them with an internal breath freshener made from parsley seed oil or chlorella.

POSSIBLE BENEFITS

Alzheimer's Disease • At a 1994 meeting on medicinal foods organized by Rutgers University, French researchers reported on a study involving aged laboratory rats with an Alzheimer's-type disease. The researchers noted that garlic extract appeared to slow down brain deterioration. In addition, the garlic normalized the brain's serotonin system: if the serotonin system malfunctions, it can cause depression. Although this information is exciting, it is not yet known whether garlic would have the same effect on human brains.

Cancer Fighter • Hippocrates, the father of modern medicine, used garlic vapors to treat uterine cancer. Recent studies have shown that people who eat a diet high in allium vegetables—including garlic—have a lower rate of stomach cancer than those who don't. Researchers in China interviewed 564 patients with stomach cancer and more than 1100 people without cancer in a region where the risk for gastric cancer is high. Those with the highest intake of allium vegetables had a 40 percent reduction in risk for gastric cancer.

Garlic and onion are both rich in quercetin and selenium, two "hot" antioxidants that may play an important role in cancer prevention.

Garlic oil contains diallyl sulfide, which has been shown to deactivate potent carcinogens in animal studies. Garlic also stimulates the production of glutathione, a potent antioxidant found in the cells that helps to prevent cancerous changes.

Heart Disease • First-century physician Dioscorides prescribed garlic to treat atherosclerosis, a leading cause of heart disease. Indeed, numerous studies can attest to garlic's positive effects on blood lipids. In a recent study performed at the Clinical Research Center and Tulane University School of Medicine in New Orleans, forty-two healthy adults with total cholesterol levels over 200 milligrams per deciliter were given either 300 milligrams of standardized garlic powder in tablet form three times daily or a placebo. After 12 weeks, those who took the garlic experienced a 6 percent total drop in cholesterol versus a 1 percent decline among those on the placebo. Even better, those on the garlic had a 11 percent reduction in low-density lipoproteins, or "bad" cholesterol, versus a 3 percent drop in the untreated group.

Other studies have shown that people who eat an onion a day can raise their high-density lipoproteins, or "good" cholesterol.

Researcher Eric Block discovered a compound in garlic called *ajoene* that appears to be a natural blood thinner, which may prevent the formation of blood clots that can lead to a heart attack or stroke.

Natural Antibiotic and Antifungal • In the Middle Ages, monks used garlic to ward off plague. Before antibiotics, garlic poultices were used on wounds to prevent infection. In fact, garlic was dubbed "Russian penicillin," because during World War II, when antibiotics were scarce, Russian physicians used it to treat infections on the battlefield. Studies show that garlic has some antibiotic properties and is also one of the strongest natural antifungal compounds, especially against *Candida albicans* (yeast infection).

Anti-inflammatory • Eric Block recently discovered a sulfur compound in onion that in test tube studies blocked the chemical chain of events that lead to asthma and inflammatory reactions.

Food for Thought

Only 9 percent of all Americans eat five or more fruits and vegetables daily as recommended by the National Cancer Institute. According to experts at the National Cancer Institute, as many as 50 percent of all cancers could be prevented by eating the right foods.

Aloe

FACTS

There are more than three hundred species of the aloe plant, and several, including the famous aloe vera variety, have been used since ancient times to heal skin wounds. Aloe gel, derived from the leaf of the plant, is an excellent moisturizer and is a common ingredient in skin creams. Several studies confirm that used externally, aloe can promote healing of minor skin burns and abrasions. Recently, a study performed on animals at Texas A&M University showed that, taken internally, aloe may be a potent immune booster.

THE RIGHT AMOUNT

Aloe gel may be used liberally on the skin as needed. The leaf of the fresh plant is highly effective, but if you don't want to grow your own, aloe vera is available in many different forms at drug stores and natural food stores. Buy only products that are made from pure aloe and that list aloe as a primary ingredient. Many products that claim to contain aloe contain a watered-down version of aloe extract or reconstituted aloe vera.

Aloe, which is used as a treatment for constipation, can cause severe abdominal pain and cramps if taken in large amounts. One tablespoon one or two times daily is recommended. Aloe vera is also available in dry capsule form. Each capsule is equal to 1 tablespoon of the juice.

Caution: Aloe should not be ingested by pregnant women.

POSSIBLE BENEFITS

Wound Healing • Several studies have shown that aloe vera gel can help heal skin irritations and wounds due to radiation burns. At one time, researchers believed that aloe vera promoted healing by sealing in moisture, thus preventing the air from drying out the skin. However, scientists now suspect that there are specific chemicals in aloe vera gel that interact with the skin to speed up the healing process.

Wrinkles • Like other moisturizers, aloe gel may give the appearance of younger-looking skin by plumping out dry, fine lines. Thus, the wrinkles don't disappear, but they are less noticeable.

Immune Booster • This is one of the newest and most exciting uses of this ancient herb. Researchers at Texas A&M University tested aloe on mice implanted with sarcoma tumors. Mice who had been given aloe vera internally had a 40 percent survival rate. All of the untreated mice died. Interestingly enough, researchers found that it was impossible to implant tumors in mice who had been pretreated with aloe vera. Researchers say that the compound works by stimulating the release of *cytokines*, substances with activate the immune system. Aloe is now being tested on human patients.

Alpha-carotene

FACTS

The carotene family consists of about six hundred naturally occurring compounds found in dark, leafy vegetables and yellow and orange fruits and vegetables. Some of these compounds are potent antioxidants, such as beta-carotene and lycopene. However, only a handful of carotenes have actually been studied for their potential health benefits. Recently, researchers have focused on alpha-carotene, and their findings suggest that it may be as important a cancer fighter as any of its better-known cousins.

THE RIGHT AMOUNT

There is no recommended daily allowance for alpha-carotene. Fruits and vegetables are a rich source of many different carotenes, including alpha-carotenes. For example, about one-third of the carotene mixture in a carrot consists of alpha-carotene. Supplements containing alpha- and beta-carotene are available at natural food stores. Take between 10,000 and 25,000 international units daily.

POSSIBLE BENEFITS

Cancer Fighter • For more than a decade, studies have shown that people with diets rich in green and yellow vegetables have significantly lower rates of cancer than people who don't. Many scientists believe that carotenes are responsible for the reduced cancer risk.

A recent study compared the effects of alpha- and beta-carotene and no carotene on cancer cells in a culture medium. High levels of alpha-carotene stopped the growth of the cancer cells. An equal amount of beta-carotene produced a modest drop in cell growth. However, the cancer cells without any form of carotene experienced explosive growth.

In another study reported in *Cancer Research*, mice were fed a known carcinogen and then divided into three groups. One group of the mice was fed a beta-carotene supplement, a second group was given an alpha-carotene supplement, and the third group was given a placebo. The mice taking the alpha-carotene had a 70 percent reduction in the number of tumors versus those taking the beta-carotene or no supplement at all. From these studies, researchers suspect that alpha-carotene may be a better protector against certain forms of cancer than beta-carotene.

PERSONAL ADVICE

I recommend taking a caretenoid complex along with dark green leafy vegetables and yellow and orange vegetables and fruits. It comes in liquid, tablet, or capsule form. Use as directed.

Alpha-hydroxy Acids

FACTS

Alpha-hydroxy acids (AHAs) are naturally occurring compounds found in foods such as sour milk (lactic acid), grapes (tartaric acid), sugar cane (glycolic acid), apples (malic acid), and citrus fruit (citric acid). For more than a decade, dermatologists have used high concentrations of AHAs (up to 50 percent) for scar removal and facial peels. Today, weaker versions of AHAs are sold in numerous over-the-counter skin care products designed to moisturize and improve the skin. Although they may not be the fountain of youth, for many people, AHAs products can produce noticeable changes in the appearance and quality of their skin.

THE RIGHT AMOUNT

Products range from 2 to 10 percent concentration of AHAs. Most dermatologists consider 5 percent or under to be safe for most people. However, some people may find AHAs irritating at any level, and some may be able to tolerate a higher level. Your best bet is to start out with the weaker products and work your way up. Those with very sensitive skin should stick with the weaker products.

POSSIBLE BENEFITS

Skin Rejuvenator • AHAs have been found to loosen the "cement" binding cells on the skin, permitting the top layer of dead cells to shed more evenly and rapidly, thus revealing smoother, fresher-looking skin underneath. Many studies confirm that AHAs are an effective treatment against extremely dry, flaky skin. They have also been used to treat conditions such as psoriasis. In addition, studies show that these skin products may help erase fine lines and age spots and improve the tone and texture of the skin.

There is some controversy in the medical community over the effectiveness of over-the-counter AHA preparations. The more potent products used by dermatologists are more effective; however, they are also more costly and can cause more skin irritation. Many people, however, find that the milder products are surprisingly effective at a fraction of the cost.

L-Arginine

FACTS

L-Arginine is a nonessential amino acid: since the body produces it on its own, we do not need to get it in food. However, recent studies suggest that L-Arginine may play an important role in maintaining health.

L-Arginine can stimulate the growth and release of growth hormone, which is produced by the pituitary gland. As we age, the level of growth hormone steadily decreases. Some experts believe the decline in L-Arginine production may be responsible for many of the degenerative processes associated with aging.

Good food sources of L-Arginine include nuts, sunflower and sesame seeds, chocolate, popcorn, raisins, and brown rice.

THE RIGHT AMOUNT

L-Arginine is available as tablets and powder. Take 2000 milligrams daily at bedtime, about 2 hours after eating. L-Arginine is often taken in combination with two other amino acids: 2000 milligrams ornithine and 1000 milligrams lysine.

Caution: Do not give L-Arginine to children or to adults with schizophrenia. L-Arginine is reputed to promote herpes,

therefore, people with herpes should not use L-Arginine. Very high dosages can cause deformities of the bones and enlarged joints.

POSSIBLE BENEFITS

Wound Healing • Many studies have demonstrated that L-Arginine supplements can promote wound healing of burns and wounds after trauma such as surgery or injury. If you have been injured recently have undergone surgery, talk to your physician or healer about taking an L-Arginine supplement.

Cancer Fighter • Several studies have confirmed L-Arginine's ability to inhibit the growth of tumors in animals. Studies involving human blood cells show that L-Arginine increased the production of natural killer cells (important immune cells) and other compounds that can thwart the growth of tumors.

Male Infertility • Male seminal fluid contains as much as 50 percent L-Arginine. Several studies have linked a low sperm count to low levels of this important amino acid.

Ascorbic Acid (Vitamin C)

FACTS

If you want to live longer, take your ascorbic acid, or vitamin C. Recent studies suggest that vitamin C supplements (in addition to a diet rich in vitamin C foods) may prevent premature death from heart disease and may even be a more important factor in preventing fatal heart attacks than maintaining a low cholesterol level or eating a low-fat diet.

Vitamin C is also a potent antioxidant and works with other antioxidants in the body to help prevent damage from free radicals that may lead to various forms of cancer.

Vitamin C, a water-soluble vitamin, is necessary for the formation of *collagen*, the substance that binds together the cells of connective tissue. Collagen is also essential for the production of new cells and tissues.

Vitamin C is reputed to be good for colds. In fact, several studies show that although vitamin C can't prevent the common cold, it can lessen a cold's severity by decreasing the histamine level in your bloodstream by up to 40 percent. Histamine causes the runny nose and watery eyes associated with colds and allergies.

Good natural sources of vitamin C include mangoes, kiwi fruit, grapefruit, broccoli, cantaloupe, strawberries, sweet red peppers, sweet potatoes, snow peas, and orange juice.

THE RIGHT AMOUNT

The recommended daily allowance (RDA) for vitamin C is 60 milligrams, for smokers, 100 milligrams. (About half of the U.S. population does not get even 60 milligrams of this vitamin daily.) Studies suggest that the RDA is much too low. I recommend 1000 milligrams daily of calcium ascorbate (the gentlest form of vitamin C for your stomach). Although many people can tolerate up to 10,000 milligrams of vitamin C daily, in some people, excess vitamin C can cause dry nose, diarrhea, excess urination, and skin rashes.

POSSIBLE BENEFITS

Heart Disease • Researchers at the University of California looked at the vitamin C intakes and death rates of more than 11,000 men and women. The study showed a dramatic decline in death from heart disease among men with the highest vitamin C intake, especially among those who took a vitamin C supplement. Merely obtaining the RDA for vitamin C through food did not seem to offer any protection against heart disease. The results were similar among women but less dramatic.

There are several reasons why vitamin C may protect against heart disease. Other studies have shown that vitamin C is particularly effective in intercepting oxidants before they can attack blood lipids. Many researchers believe that when low-density lipoproteins, or "bad" cholesterol, are oxidized, it promotes the formation of plaque, which can cause atherosclerotic lesions in arteries.

Raises Blood Glutathione • Glutathione is one of the most important antioxidants produced in the body. It protects cells from damage inflicted by hydroperoxides (free radicals), a natural by-product of metabolism. Low levels of serum glutathione have been associated with cell damage, depressed immunity, and premature aging. A recent study conducted at Arizona State University showed how glutathione levels fluctuate in humans based on vitamin C intake. People on vitamin C–deprived diets had low levels of glutathione; however, when given a supplement of 500 milligrams of vitamin C, blood glutathione levels bounced back to normal.

Cancer Fighter • Many studies have investigated the association of dietary vitamin C and various forms of cancer. We know from these studies that dietary intake of vitamin C (through food, notably fruits and vegetables) appears to offer some protection against cancers of the lung, cervix, pancreas, mouth, throat, esophagus, colon, and stomach. (In particular, vitamin C may protect against cancers of the stomach because it blocks the formation of nitrosamines in the stomach, which are potential carcinogens.)

There is also some evidence that vitamin C may help to protect against breast cancer, especially in postmenopausal women.

Prevents Cataracts • Cataracts, an opaque covering that can form on the lens of the eye, are particularly common among people over fifty. Researchers at the Laboratory for Nutrition and Vision Research at the U.S. Department of Agriculture's Human Nutrition Center at Tufts University suggest that cataracts may be caused by cellular damage due to oxidation. For example, when vitamin C was added to the diet of guinea pigs, their eyes showed less oxidative damage after exposure to ultraviolet light than in pigs not given vitamin C. In human studies, adults taking antioxidant supplements (including C) were less likely to develop cataracts than those not taking vitamins.

PERSONAL ADVICE

Here's one supplement that everyone should be taking!

Ashwaganda

FACTS

The root of the ashwaganda plant is an important healing herb that is commonly used in Ayurveda, the traditional herbal medicine of India. Ashwaganda is a small shrub that is part of the nightshade family, which includes potatoes, tomatoes, and eggplant.

Although many Western natural healers advise arthritics to avoid eating nightshade plants, in Ayurveda, ashwaganda has long been prescribed to treat arthritis. Recent studies show that ashwaganda may indeed be effective against arthritis and may also be a potent weapon against cancer. In recent years, Ayurveda has become very popular in the West because of its emphasis on the prevention of disease.

THE RIGHT AMOUNT

Ashwaganda teas and other herbal products are available at natural food stores. Ashwaganda is included in many herbal formulas for arthritis. Drink 1 to 2 cups of tea daily, or follow the directions on the package.

Caution: Ashwaganda contains some compounds that may be harmful at very high amounts. Do not exceed the recommended dose.

POSSIBLE BENEFITS

Arthritis • Several Indian studies have confirmed that ashwaganda has anti-inflammatory activity and can help reduce some of the stiffness and swelling associated with arthritis in both animals and humans. In one recent study performed at the University of Poona in Pune, India, forty-two patients with osteoarthritis were given an herbal formula that included ashwaganda and zinc complex. For 3 months, the patients took the herbal formula. Then, after a 2-week period to allow the herbs to wear off, the patients were given a placebo for 3 months. The results: while on the herbal formula, the patients experienced a significant drop in severity of pain and stiffness.

Cancer Fighter • Several animal studies have shown that extract of ashwaganda root can inhibit the growth of tumors in laboratory mice.

Aspirin

FACTS

In 1958 when I started pharmacy school, anyone who would have suggested that aspirin—the wonder drug of the nineteenth century—would be touted as a "hot" anti-aging drug at the dawn of the twenty-first, would have been laughed out of the classroom. However, good old aspirin, chemically known as acetylsalicylic acid, holds great promise for the future as a protector against both cancer and heart disease.

Aspirin is actually a synthetic version of salicum, a natural derivative of the bark of the white willow tree, a longtime herbal remedy for headaches, fever, and arthritis. Until recently, aspirin has been used as an analgesic to treat daily aches and pains. However, recent studies suggest that this drug may be underutilized.

THE RIGHT AMOUNT

To help prevent certain forms of cancer and heart disease, I recommend one baby aspirin (about 81 milligrams) taken every
day. Your physician may suggest a higher dose if you are at risk
of developing heart disease or certain forms of cancer.

**Caution: Do not take aspirin on a regular basis without
first checking with your physician. People with bleeding disorders or who are taking blood thinners (e.g., coumadin and
heparin) should steer clear of aspirin unless advised differently by their physicians. Aspirin can be very irritating to the
stomach and can cause bleeding and ulcers in some people.
People on aspirin should be closely monitored by their physicians for gastrointestinal bleeding, or other problems. If untreated, bleeding ulcers can cause severe problems, including
death.**

POSSIBLE BENEFITS

Heart Disease and Stroke • Will an aspirin a day keep the
cardiologist away? There's strong evidence that it just might.
Aspirin is a blood thinner, that is, it prevents the clumping together of blood platelets, tiny circulating disks that play a key
role in the formation of blood clots. A majority of heart attacks
and strokes are caused by blood clots forming in arteries that
were already narrowed due to atherosclerotic lesions (deposits
of lipids and other cells). By preventing the formation of blood
clots, aspirin may play a significant role in preventing heart attacks and strokes. Consider the results of several recent studies.

- A study of 22,000 healthy male doctors given 325 milligrams of aspirin daily for 5 years (the amount in one
adult aspirin) had 44 percent fewer heart attacks than
those who didn't take the aspirin.
- A study of 87,678 female nurses over 8 years found a 30
percent reduction in risk of first heart attack among
women who took 1 to 6 aspirins per week. In this study,
the aspirin was not prescribed; rather these women took

aspirin on their own to treat headaches or musculoskeletal pain.

- In yet another study of over one thousand recovering heart patients, at the Multicenter Study of Myocardial Ischemia in New Orleans, those who were not taking aspirin were three times more likely to have a fatal heart attack than those who were on the drug.

Cancer Fighter   •   Aspirin is an anti-inflammatory. It blocks the formation of *prostaglandins*, hormonelike substances in the body that can trigger an inflammatory response. By quelling inflammation, aspirin can help to relieve the pain of arthritis and bring down a fever. Prostaglandins are also believed to promote the growth of cancerous tumors; therefore, by nipping prostaglandins in the bud, aspirin may indirectly be a potent cancer fighter.

Based on a study of more than 635,000 people performed by the American Cancer Society, those who took aspirin were at significantly lower risk of dying from digestive tract cancers (esophagus, stomach, rectum, and colon). In fact, men and women who took aspirin at least sixteen times a month were 40 percent less likely to die from these cancers than those who did not. The risk was lowest among men and women who used aspirin regularly for 10 years or more.

Astragalus

FACTS

As we age, our immune system becomes weakened, leaving us more vulnerable to infection and disease. A handful of vitamins and herbs may help to keep the immune system functioning at optimal levels, and astragalus may be one of them. For centuries, Oriental healers have used this herb to treat a wide variety of ailments, ranging from diabetes to high blood pressure,

and have also prescribed it as an immune booster that strengthens the Wei Ch'i, or defensive energy of the body. Western scientists are now beginning to acknowledge that this herb may
indeed have a positive effect on immunity.

Astragalus, which is native to China and Japan, is being
studied in the United States as a possible treatment for AIDS, a
disease characterized by the breakdown of the immune system.

THE RIGHT AMOUNT

Astragalus is available in capsule form at natural food stores.
Take 1 to 3 (400 milligrams) capsules daily.

POSSIBLE BENEFITS

Immune Booster   •   Research by Dr. G. Mavligit of the University of Texas Medical Center in Houston found that a purified extract of astragalus stimulates T cells (one of the key white
cells of the immune system) in healthy animals and helps to
normalize the immune systems of cancer patients with impaired
immunity due to chemotherapy. Other studies have shown that
astragalus can stimulate the production of interferon, a protein
produced in cells that fights against viral invasion. In fact, according to one Chinese study, patients given astragalus root developed less colds than patients not given the root; and when
they did get a cold, they had it for a significantly shorter amount
of time than untreated patients.

Heart Disease   •   In China, astralagus has been used to treat
cardiovascular disease. Animal studies show that this herb can
lower blood pressure and may help to prevent heart attacks by
improving the flow of blood to the heart.

Beta-carotene

FACTS

Beta-carotene, one of six hundred or so naturally occurring plant compounds in the carotene family, is also known as provitamin A. Some of the beta-carotene we eat is converted to vitamin A as the body needs it. Although beta-carotene is an antioxidant, when it is converted to vitamin A, it loses much of its antioxidant properties.

Of all the phytochemicals, beta-carotene is one of the most widely studied. Numerous studies show that people who eat diets rich in beta-carotene have lower levels of cancer and coronary artery disease than those who don't.

Good food sources of beta-carotene include apricots, sweet potatoes, broccoli, cantaloupe, pumpkin, carrots, mangoes, peaches, and spinach.

THE RIGHT AMOUNT

The recommended daily allowance for vitamin A is 5000 international units or 1000 retinol equivalent. Three milligrams of beta-carotene is equal to 5000 international units of vitamin A. Although vitamin A can be toxic at doses higher than 25,000 international units daily, beta-carotene is not believed to be toxic even at high doses. In fact, many studies used dosages as high as 50 milligrams of beta-carotene without any problem.

Most scientists agree that we need at least 6 milligrams (10,000 international units) of beta-carotene daily; many recommend as much as 14 milligrams (23,333 international units) daily. Most Americans ingest about 2 milligrams (3,333 international units).

Beta-carotene supplements are sold separately. In addition, beta-carotene is included in most antioxidant formulas as well as most multivitamins.

Beta-carotene comes in two forms that vary slightly in molecular structure: all-*trans*- and 9-*cis*-beta-carotene. The 9-*cis* form may be better absorbed by the body.

POSSIBLE BENEFITS

Cancer Fighter • A study presented at the 1994 American Cancer Society Science Writer's Seminar showed that beta-carotene can reverse precancerous sores in the mouth, suggesting that it could play a role in preventing oral cancers. People with oral lesions were given 60 milligrams (100,000 international units) of beta-carotene daily. After 6 months, most of the patients experienced a 50 percent reduction or more in the number of mouth lesions, thus reducing their risk of developing oral cancers.

Medical journals worldwide are filled with studies linking low beta-carotene intake and/or low blood levels of beta-carotene to an increased risk of many different forms of cancer, including cancers of the breast, cervix, lung, stomach, colon and rectum, bladder, mouth, and esophagus. For example, in a recent study, researchers in Buffalo, New York, found that women with breast cancer had lower concentrations of plasma beta-carotene than those who were cancer free. A major study in Latin American countries performed by the National Cancer Institute suggested that a high beta-carotene intake was associated with a 32 percent reduction in cervical cancer.

Heart Disease • Recently, many researchers have begun to believe that atherosclerosis (the clogging of arteries with plaque) may be caused by the oxidation of low-density lipoprotein or "bad" cholesterol. Several studies have shown that beta-carotene can significantly block the oxidation of low-density lipoprotein cholesterol, at least in test tubes. Population studies confirm that people with a high intake of beta-carotene have a lower rate of heart disease than those who don't. For example, ongoing research in the Nurses' Health Study show that by eating even one serving of fruits or vegetables daily, you can reduce your risk of heart attack and stroke. Women in the study who took between 15 and 20 milligrams (25,000 to 33,333 international units) of beta-carotene daily had a 22 percent reduced risk of heart attack and a 40 percent reduced risk of stroke.

Immune Protector • Ultraviolet A (UVA) light from the sun not only promotes wrinkles and skin cancer, but may have harmful effects on the immune system. Researchers at Cornell University and Hoffman-LaRouche tested beta-carotene's ability to protect the immune system from UVA damage. In the study, twenty-four healthy men were put on a low-carotene diet for 28 days. Part of the group took a 30-milligram supplement (50,000 international units) of beta-carotene; the others took a placebo. The whole group was exposed to UVA light several times over the next 2 weeks. Blood tests were then taken to measure the amount of beta-carotene and the ability of the blood to respond to various disease-causing antigens. The results: those on the beta-carotene showed a stronger immune response than those on the placebo.

Another study involved twenty-one patients who tested positive for HIV but did not show any signs of AIDS. These patients were given either 180 milligrams (300,000 international units) of beta-carotene daily or a placebo. Of the seventeen patients who actually completed the 4-week study, the beta-carotene group showed significant increases in several blood factors that help to fight infection. This is not to suggest that beta-carotene is a cure for AIDS; however, it does appear to strengthen the body's immune system.

Cataracts • Several studies have shown that antioxidants in general, and beta-carotene in particular, can protect against the formation of cataracts. According to the Nurses' Health Study, women who eat a diet rich in beta-carotene have a 39 percent lower risk of cataracts than those with a low beta-carotene intake.

PERSONAL ADVICE

Eat a diet rich in dark green leafy vegetables and yellow and orange fruits and vegetables to get the broad-spectrum benefits of beta-carotene.

Bilberry

FACTS

The eyes are one of the most important—and vulnerable—organs, particularly as we age. Reading glasses have become one of the hallmarks of middle age. Later in life, cataracts (growths that cloud the lens of one or both eyes) and macular degeneration (which causes a blur or blind spot in the field of vision) are common occurrences that may be treated surgically, although not always successfully. At any age, exposure to TV and computer screens can lead to eye strain. Bilberry, a common herb, is one of the few known substances that may help preserve precious vision.

Bilberry fruit is grown in Europe and Asia and is similar to the North American blueberry. As with most other herbs, although U.S. scientists have ignored it, serious research on bilberry has been done in Europe, where it is widely used to treat and prevent a number of different disorders.

Bilberry contains biologically active compounds called *anthocyanides*, which may have many positive effects on the body.

THE RIGHT AMOUNT

Bilberry is available in capsule form. Take 1 capsule up to three times daily.

POSSIBLE BENEFITS

Eyes • For centuries, herbal healers have used bilberry to treat eye problems. During World War II, Royal Air Force pilots who munched on sandwiches made of bilberry jam before flying their night missions claimed that the jam improved their night vision. Later, studies confirmed that bilberry does indeed enhance eyesight. In 1964, French researchers found that bilberry improved the adaptation to dark after exposure to bright light. However, the improvement was short-lived; within 24 hours after taking the bilberry, the beneficial effects of this herb had worn off. Later, animal studies revealed that bilberry anthocyanosides work by accelerating the regeneration of retinol purple (visual purple), a substance that is required for good eyesight, especially at night.

Strengthens Capillaries • Anthrocyanosides have been used as a treatment for capillary fragility (capillaries are extremely narrow blood vessels), a condition that may increase the risk of infection, traumatic injury, and vascular disease. In addition, studies show that bilberry may be a useful tool in preventing vascular disease, which can cause serious circulatory problems in diabetics.

Bioflavonoids

FACTS

Bioflavonoids are a group of about five hundred compounds that provide color to citrus fruits and vegetables. Once regarded as little more than food dye, many of these compounds are now being investigated by the National Cancer Institute for their potential disease preventive properties.

Some bioflavonoids are potent antioxidants. Bioflavonoids are believed to work in conjunction with vitamin C—each may enhance the function of the other. They also work with vitamin C to keep connective tissues healthy. Bioflavonoids are sometimes referred to as *vitamin P,* short for capillary permeability factor, because they improve the strength of small blood vessels or capillaries. When the capillary walls are weakened, materials from the blood can penetrate the tissues, which can result in easy bruising or hemorrhaging.

One bioflavonoid, rutin, has been used successfully to treat bleeding gums. Bioflavonoids are used by natural healers to treat allergies and asthma. Synthetic versions of these compounds are used in prescription medications for asthma.

The best food sources of bioflavonoids include the white skin and segment part of citrus fruits, apricots, buckwheat, red and yellow onions, blackberries, cherries, rose hip tea, and apples.

THE RIGHT AMOUNT

There is no recommended daily allowance for bioflavonoids. These compounds are not considered a true vitamin, because no deficiency state has been established. Bioflavonoids are usually available in supplements with vitamin C (the usual combination is 500 milligrams vitamin C to 100 milligrams bioflavonoids). Various bioflavonoids are also sold separately as supplements.

POSSIBLE BENEFITS

Heart Disease • Bioflavonoids appear to offer protection against heart disease. Researchers in Holland evaluated the diets of 805 men aged sixty-five to eighty-four. The group who consumed the highest amounts of bioflavonoids had the lowest rate of heart disease. Researchers speculated that the antioxidant action of bioflavonoids may prevent the oxidizing of low-density lipoprotein cholesterol, which can cause atherosclerosis.

Cancer Fighter • Recent studies show that some bioflavonoids may inhibit the action of carcinogens, thus blocking the initiation of cancerous changes in the cells. In addition, the antioxidant properties of bioflavonoids may also help to prevent cancers caused by oxidative damage. (For example, quercetin, which is found in red and yellow onions, has been shown to inhibit the activity of several carcinogens and tumor promoters.)

Antiviral • Some bioflavonoids have been shown to have antiviral activity, especially in combination with vitamin C. For instance, in one study, a combination of 100 milligrams of vitamin C and 100 milligrams of bioflavonoids dramatically accelerated the healing of cold sores caused by the herpes virus. In test tube studies, quercetin and vitamin C were effective against the coxsackie virus and the common cold.

PERSONAL ADVICE

Bioflavonoids in combination with vitamin D may help to relieve hot flashes associated with menopause. Take 1000 milligrams of bioflavonoids and 400 to 800 international units of vitamin D daily.

Boron

FACTS

Until recently, boron wasn't considered to be of particular importance. There's no recommended daily allowance for boron—like other trace minerals, it is needed by the body in minuscule amounts. However, boron may prove the adage "Good things come in small packages." Although the body only needs a tiny quantity of this mineral, boron may play a big role in helping to prevent osteoporosis and may even help your brain to work better.

Boron is found in most fruits and vegetables; however, dried fruits (e.g., prunes and apricots) are the best source.

THE RIGHT AMOUNT

Take 3 milligrams daily. (Do not exceed 10 milligrams daily.) I recommend boron supplements in the form of sodium borate. Boron works best if taken in a good vitamin and mineral supplement including calcium, magnesium, manganese, and riboflavin.

POSSIBLE BENEFITS

Strong Bones   •   Between 15 and 20 million Americans have osteoporosis, characterized by the thinning or wearing away of bones, which make them more vulnerable to breaks and fractures. Complications from osteoporosis are a leading cause of death among the elderly, especially among women. Recent studies suggest that boron may play an important role in helping the body to retain bone mass. Under the direction of Forrest H. Nielson, Ph.D., supervisory nutritionist, U.S. Department of Agriculture, Agricultural Research Services, researchers tested the effect of boron depletion on twelve postmenopausal women. For 119 days, women were given 2000-calorie diets very low in boron (0.25 milligram). The women were later given the same diet supplemented with 3 milligrams of boron for 48 days. Researchers found that the boron supplement reduced the loss of calcium and magnesium in the urine, both of which are minerals that are needed to help build strong bones. In addition, the boron supplement also dramatically elevated levels of serum estrogen and ionized calcium. This is important because women who develop osteoporosis tend to have low serum estrogen levels and low levels of ionized calcium.

A subsequent study of boron depletion in men and women yielded similar results. In both sexes, boron appears to help the body maintain the essential minerals necessary to prevent bone loss.

Brain Function   •   In a U.S. Department of Agriculture study of boron depletion in men and women over forty-five, subjects on a low-boron diet displayed impaired mental functioning when asked to perform simple tasks such as counting and tapping. Electroencephalograms (a test that measures the electrical activity of the brain) showed that low dietary boron, in the researcher's own words, "depressed mental alertness."

Bromelain

FACTS

Bromelain is an enzyme found in raw pineapple. For several decades, natural food enthusiasts have used bromelain to treat many different ailments, ranging from indigestion to arthritis. Bromelain is beginning to enjoy widespread acceptance among older baby boomers who prefer nature's pharmacy over the synthetic brews found in the conventional pharmacy.

THE RIGHT AMOUNT

Fresh, raw pineapple is a good source of bromelain, although supplements offer a more concentrated form of this enzyme. Bromelain is included in many digestive aid formulas sold at natural food stores. In addition, bromelain tablets are available. Take 1 to 3 daily.

POSSIBLE BENEFITS

Digestive Aid • Bromelain helps to break down protein. As we age, a decrease in hydrochloric acid production can prevent the proper digestion and absorption of protein. A daily bromelain supplement may help to compensate for the loss of HCl.

Anti-inflammatory • Bromelain has anti-inflammatory properties that may help to reduce the discomfort caused by rheumatoid arthritis. There haven't been many clinical studies to confirm this; however, there is a good deal of anecdotal evidence. Due to its anti-inflammatory properties, bromelain is also used by athletes to prevent the soreness that accompanies a strenuous workout. It is also believed to facilitate the healing of sports injuries.

Anti-allergic • Bromelain can also help to alleviate allergic symptoms by mediating the inflammatory response that triggers an allergic attack.

Burdock

FACTS

Called *lappa* in Europe and *gobo* in Japan, the burdock root enjoys worldwide recognition as a mild, nourishing herb that may help to keep the body working well from childhood through old age.

For thousands of years burdock root and leaves have been used to treat rheumatism, gout, and skin disorders, such as psoriasis. The herb has also been used by traditional healers as a cancer treatment (along with other herbs) and is considered to be an excellent digestive aid and liver tonic.

Well-known herbalist Christopher Hobbs includes burdock in his list of *adaptogens,* which he defines as important herbs that can be taken daily without any side effects and help "restore to balance all bodily systems." Herbalist Rosemary Gladstar, author of *Herbal Healing for Women,* prescribes burdock for women in all stages of life.

The Japanese, who have the longest life span of any nationality in the world, frequently eat burdock root. Fresh burdock root is available at many greengrocers, Asian markets, and natural food stores in the United States.

THE RIGHT AMOUNT

Burdock root is available as capsules. Take 1 to 3 daily.

POSSIBLE BENEFITS

Cancer Fighter • Burdock root extracts have been shown to inhibit tumor growth in animal studies.

Liver • Burdock leaves and root are believed to stimulate the production of bile by the liver. Bile is essential for the breakdown of fats.

Fights Infection • Studies show that compounds in burdock have antibacterial and antifungal properties.

PERSONAL ADVICE

According to folklore, a lotion made from the leaves of this root should be massaged into the scalp to prevent hair from falling out.

Butcher's Broom

FACTS

Butcher's broom is one of the most popular anti-aging herbs in Europe, and I predict as word gets out about this herb's healing properties, it will have an equally bright future in the United States.

Butcher's broom contains compounds called *ruscogins*, which are similar in structure to steroids. French studies have shown that butcher's broom is a vasoconstrictor; it strengthens veins and reduces capillary fragility (capillaries are tiny blood vessels).

THE RIGHT AMOUNT

Butcher's broom is available in capsule form. Take 400 milligrams daily. Suppositories and ointments are available to treat hemorrhoidal flareups. Use as directed.

POSSIBLE BENEFITS

Varicose Veins • Blood flows to the heart via a network of arteries and away from the heart via a network of veins. Unlike arteries, which are thick and strong, veins are weaker and less elastic and, therefore, are prone to develop certain problems. When veins become swollen and enlarged, they are called *varicosities*. Varicose veins usually occur in the legs, where blood tends to pool due to poor circulation. Most women over forty develop varicose veins in the legs.

Hemorrhoids—swollen anal veins—are a common ailment

of middle age. Obesity and chronic constipation are risk factors for developing hemorrhoids.

Many European studies show that when used over an extended period of time, butcher's broom can greatly relieve the pain and swelling associated with varicose veins and hemorrhoids. In fact, in Europe, this herb is commonly used for these problems.

Caliciferol (Vitamin D)

FACTS

Calcitrol, or vitamin D, is known as the sunshine vitamin because the ultraviolet B rays of the sun trigger oils of the skin to produce this vitamin. Calcitrol can also be obtained through food. Vitamin D works with calcium and phosphorus to produce strong bones.

The risk of vitamin D deficiency increases with age. Many sunscreens filter out the rays that produce vitamin D. In addition, as we age, our bodies are less able to convert vitamin D into the active hormone that is needed for dietary calcium to become incorporated into bones. If you don't eat a diet rich in vitamin D and if you avoid exposure to the sun (which is wise considering the high rate of skin cancer), you may not be getting enough of this vitamin.

Good food sources of vitamin D are fortified low-fat or no-fat dairy products and fatty fish such as sardines, mackerel, salmon, and tuna.

THE RIGHT AMOUNT

The recommended daily allowance for adults is 400 international units. A recent study suggested that women need 500 international units of vitamin D during the winter to prevent bone loss. Talk to your doctor or natural healer about taking a vitamin D supplement; excessively high doses can be toxic.

POSSIBLE BENEFITS

Osteoporosis • Decreased activity and less exposure to sun can result in wintertime bone loss. According to one study conducted at Tufts University, a vitamin D supplement may help to prevent this loss. In the study, 249 healthy postmenopausal women with a dietary intake of about 100 international units of vitamin D daily were selected to receive a calcium supplement of 800 milligrams per deciliter daily. One-half of the group was given an additional supplement of 400 international units of vitamin D daily. The rest were given a placebo. Researchers then measured the patients' spinal bone mineral density in the summer months and in the winter months. As expected, women in both groups showed an increase in spinal bone mineral density in the summer. However, the women taking the vitamin D supplement showed significantly less bone loss during the winter than those taking the placebo. Based on this study, it would seem wise to take at least 400 international units of vitamin D daily in addition to eating a calcium-rich diet.

Calcium

FACTS

For a lifetime of strong bones, normal blood pressure, and even some protection against cancer, calcium is just what the doctor ordered. Unfortunately, few Americans are filling their prescriptions.

According to a recent U.S. Department of Agriculture survey, most Americans are falling seriously short of this mineral, and the results can be devastating in later life.

Calcium is used for building strong teeth and bones and in maintaining bone strength. It is also important for maintenance of cell membranes, blood clotting, and muscle absorption.

Good sources of calcium are low-fat and nonfat dairy products, kale, broccoli, canned salmon or sardines with bones, and calcium-fortified fruit juice.

THE RIGHT AMOUNT

The recommended daily allowance for adults up to twenty-five is 1200 milligrams, and from twenty-five to fifty, 800 milligrams. Most women and younger men consume less than half the calcium that they need. Postmenopausal women should get 1500 milligrams of calcium daily, but few do.

It may be difficult to obtain all the calcium you need through diet alone. However, recently, several brands of calcium supplements, notably those made from bone meal, dolomite, or oyster shells, tested high in lead. Therefore, I recommend using calcium citrate, which is both safe and effective. Vitamin D helps facilitate calcium absorption.

POSSIBLE BENEFITS

Strong Bones • Twenty-five million Americans—80 percent of them women—have osteoporosis, a condition characterized by low bone mass and increased susceptibility to fractures, primarily in the hip, spine, and wrist. In the United States, osteoporosis is responsible for about 1.3 million fractures per year. Postmenopausal women are particularly vulnerable to this problem; in fact, one-third of all women in their eighties will experience a hip fracture. Complications from osteoporosis are a leading cause of death among elderly women. Recent studies suggest that calcium may play a leading role in helping to reduce bone loss that can lead to osteoporosis.

In a recent French study, more than sixteen hundred postmenopausal women were given 1200 milligrams of calcium and 800 international units of vitamin D daily for 18 months. Another group was given a placebo. The results: a 43 percent reduction in hip fractures among the vitamin-supplemented group. In addition, in the group on calcium and vitamin D, bone density rose 2.7 percent on the hip, whereas density dropped 4.6 percent in the untreated group.

Calcium alone may not be enough to prevent osteoporosis: other studies show that exercise may also play a preventive role as well as postmenopausal estrogen replacement therapy. In fact, for some women, a combination of all three may be their strongest defense against this bone-breaking disease.

Lowers Blood Pressure • High blood pressure, pressure over 140/90, is associated with an increased risk of heart disease and stroke. (The top number, *systolic pressure*, is generated when the heart contracts and pushes blood through the artery. The bottom number, the *diastolic pressure*, is the pressure in the arteries when the heart muscle relaxes between beats.) Several studies have established that calcium supplements can lower blood pressure. A 13-year California study of 6634 men and women showed that people who consumed 1000 milligrams of calcium daily reduced their risk of developing hypertension by 20 percent. Another study of children (the Framingham Children's Study) revealed that the children who ate the most calcium-rich foods had the lowest blood pressures. As we age, blood pressure tends to rise; therefore, adding calcium to your diet may help to prevent developing serious hypertension.

Cancer Protection • Several studies have linked low intake of calcium and vitamin D with an increased risk of colon cancer. For example, a 19-year study of more than 1500 men in Chicago found that an intake of more than 375 milligrams of calcium daily (roughly the amount in one glass of milk) was associated with a 50 percent reduction in the rate of colon cancer as compared to an intake of over 1200 milligrams, which was associated with a 75 percent decrease in colon cancer. Researchers suspect that calcium may bind with fatty acids, thus preventing them from irritating the colon walls. Low intakes of calcium may also increase the rate of excretion of vitamin D, which also appears to play a role in helping to prevent colon cancer. Think of it this way: 2 cups of nonfat milk or calcium-fortified orange juice and two servings of low-fat yogurt may be all that it takes to prevent this potentially lethal cancer.

Capsaicin

FACT

Capsaicin (also known as cayenne), a compound derived from hot chili peppers, gives new meaning to the phrase "Hot 100." Capsaicin is the substance that gives chilies their unique bite. Hot chilies have been used in cooking for thousands of years. Herbal healers have prescribed them for various ailments ranging from asthma to arthritis to even indigestion. (Contrary to popular belief, hot foods do not cause stomach distress in a healthy stomach, although they may irritate ulcers. In fact, chilies actually stimulate the production of saliva and gastric acids, which *aid* digestion.) In recent years, capsaicin has gained the respect of traditional medical practitioners and, ironically, is now considered one of the most important "new" compounds in medicine. Capsaicin has many different affects on the body, and some of them may indeed help to extend life. However, even if capsaicin does not promote longevity, I believe that it can at the very least improve the quality of life for older adults, especially for those in chronic pain.

THE RIGHT AMOUNT

Capsaicin (cayenne) is available in many different forms including capsules, tea, and ointment. Take 1 to 3 capsules daily, or drink 1 cup of tea daily. Capsaicin ointment may be used on the skin for relief of shingles and arthritic pain. Some people may find the ointment irritating, so check with your doctor before using it.

POSSIBLE BENEFITS

Heart Disease • In animal studies, capsaicin has had a favorable effect on blood lipid levels, which can help reduce the risk of heart disease and stroke. According to a 1987 study published in *The Journal of Bioscience*, rats fed a diet high in capsaicin experienced a significant reduction in blood triglycerides and low-density lipoproteins, or "bad" cholesterol. (Triglycerides over 190 milligrams per deciliter for women and over 400 milligrams per deciliter for men are believed to increase the risk of heart attack.)

Pain Relief • When you rub capsaicin cream on your skin, you immediately feel a hot, burning sensation that eventually tapers off. Recently, scientists have learned that capsaicin stimulates certain nerve cells to release a chemical called *substance P*, which sends pain signals throughout the nervous system. Capsaicin quickly depletes the cells of substance P, thus temporarily blocking their ability to transmit any more pain impulses. Capsaicin skin cream is now used topically to treat various ailments, including shingles, a particularly painful rash caused by the reactivation of the chicken pox virus that often strikes older adults. Shingles usually disappears within 3 or 4 weeks; however, in older adults or in people with weakened immune systems, it can linger on in the form of postherpetic neuralgia, a very painful and distressing ailment. A potent form of capsaicin cream (marketed as Zostrix) is one of the few treatments that has offered any relief to the victims of postherpetic neuralgia. In addition, Zostrix has been used quite effectively to treat diabetic neuropathy, a condition characterized by severe foot and ankle pain. Several over-the-counter creams containing capsaicin are also used to treat the pain and stiffness of arthritis. (If you use a cream containing capsaicin, be careful to avoid getting it in your eyes.)

Mood Enhancer • When you bite into a hot chili pepper, you feel a rush of heat that can quite literally bring tears to your eyes. The body responds to this "pain" by releasing *endorphins*, chemicals in the brain that have a pain-relieving effect similar to morphine. Capsaicin may be nature's way of helping you to beat the blues.

PERSONAL ADVICE

Cayenne tea can have a mild, stimulating effect. When you're feeling down, have a cup for a quick pick-me-up.

L-Carnitine

FACTS

If you're at risk of developing coronary artery disease (the number one killer in the United States of both men and women), here's a potential life extender that you should know about. L-Carnitine is a nonprotein amino acid that is found in heart and skeletal muscle. Its primary job is to carry activated fatty acids across the mitochondria—the so-called powerhouse of the cell—providing heart and skeletal cells with energy.

L-Carnitine is widely used in Japan as a treatment for heart disease and is growing in popularity in the United States. Enthusiasts claim that L-Carnitine can protect against heart disease and can improve physical stamina and endurance during exercise.

Severe L-Carnitine deficiency is fairly rare and is associated with muscle weakness and cramps after exercise. People with kidney disease, severe infection, liver disease, and other medical problems may develop L-Carnitine deficiency. Some researchers believe that subtle forms of L-Carnitine deficiency, which may go unnoticed, may increase the risk of having a heart attack.

Red meat—beef and lamb—and dairy products are the best natural sources of L-Carnitine. Unfortunately, these foods are also high in saturated fat, which can promote heart disease. Therefore, an L-Carnitine supplement may be preferable to loading up on meat.

THE RIGHT AMOUNT

There is no recommended daily allowance for L-Carnitine. The average American consumes between 100 and 300 milligrams of this amino acid daily. L-Carnitine is available in capsule form at natural food stores. Take two 500-milligram capsules daily. In rare cases, people taking over 1 gram of carnitine per day may develop a fishy odor, which is caused by the breakdown of carnitine by intestinal bacteria. The odor usually disappears when the dose is cut back; however, if it is troublesome, you may want to discontinue use.

Caution: There are two kinds of carnitine: L-carnitine and D-carnitine. Some studies suggest that D-carnitine may be toxic, therefore, stick to products containing only L-carnitine. If you have a heart condition, do not take this or any other supplement without first consulting with your physician. In high doses (over 3 grams per day), L-carnitine may cause cramps or diarrhea.

POSSIBLE BENEFITS

Heart Disease • Ischemia is the reduction in the oxygen supply to the heart usually caused by the narrowing of a coronary artery, often due to atherosclerotic deposits or an arterial spasm. Several studies show that ischemia can result in a reduction in carnitine in heart muscle. L-Carnitine supplements appear to raise carnitine levels in heart patients and increase their endurance. In one study involving eighteen patients with coronary artery disease, exercise sessions were performed 2 weeks apart. Prior to exercise, one group of patients received carnitine, and the other received a placebo. Those on carnitine maintained lower blood pressure and were able to exercise longer and harder prior to experiencing angina or chest pain (a sign of ischemia). Other studies of heart patients have yielded similar results. We don't know for sure whether L-Carnitine supplements can actually prevent ischemia, but these studies suggest that it might.

In another study, twenty-six patients with high blood lipid levels were treated with 3 grams of oral L-Carnitine per day. The result: a dramatic decline in total serum cholesterol and serum triglyceride. (Cholesterol levels over 200 milligrams per deciliter may increase your risk of having a heart attack. Triglyceride levels over 400 for men, and 190 for women are believed to increase the risk of heart disease.) In other studies, L-Carnitine has been shown to raise high-density lipoproteins, or "good" cholesterol.

Improves Workout • I have heard anecdotal evidence that L-Carnitine can improve stamina and strength during a workout; however, there is no scientific evidence.

Alzheimer's Disease • The brain tissue of mammals is a rich source of carnitine. Some studies suggest that L-Carnitine may be effective in slowing down the progression of Alzheimer's disease. Several European studies have reported that a daily supplement of L-Carnitine (about 2 grams daily) can slow the mental deterioration typical of this disease. (Dietary intakes of L-Carnitine average 100 to 300 milligrams daily in the United States.) However, U.S. researchers did not report good results from a major trial testing L-Carnitine on Alzheimer's patients.

Centella (Gotu Kola)

FACTS

Although most people can maintain good health throughout their lifetime, there are times when an accident or illness may result in prolonged bed rest or reduced activity. Centella (also called gotu kola) can help you get back on your feet faster by preventing dangerous complications that can result during an extended period of inactivity.

THE RIGHT AMOUNT

Centella is available as capsules or extract. Take 1 capsule up to three times daily. Mix 5 to 10 drops of extract in a cup of liquid. Take up to three times daily.

Caution: Do not use this herb during pregnancy. People with an overactive thyroid should avoid this herb.

POSSIBLE BENEFITS

Circulatory Disorders • Patients confined to bed can develop venous insufficiency, a condition that seriously impairs the flow of blood throughout the body, especially in the feet and legs. In some cases, the veins may become inflamed, resulting in phlebitis, a painful and potentially serious condition. Compounds in centella have been shown to strengthen and tone veins and capillaries and may help prevent circulatory problems. In addition, studies show that centella has been used successfully to treat patients suffering from problems related to venous insufficiency.

Wound Healing • Used externally or taken internally, centella can accelerate the healing of wounds, skin ulcers, and other sores.

PERSONAL ADVICE

According to herbalist Christopher Hobbs, legend has it that if you eat a leaf of centella each day, your life span will be extended one thousand years.

Choline

FACTS

Thousands of years ago, Chinese healers recommended foods such as eggs and meat for mental alertness and foods such as fruits and grains for a more relaxed state. Until recently, modern psychiatry dismissed such notions as pure hokum, but we now know that the chemicals in foods can indeed have a profound effect on our thought processes and mental well-being.

For example, egg yolks contain a compound called *phosphatidylcholine*, which is a major source of choline in the body.

Recent studies suggest that choline may prove to be a memory tonic.

The brain consists of millions of tiny neurons or cells that are connected by long tendrils called *axons*. The cells "talk" to each other via chemicals called *neurotransmitters*. The brain uses choline to make acetylcholine, a neurotransmitter that plays a role in memory function.

Other good food sources of choline include soybeans, cabbage, peanuts, and cauliflower.

THE RIGHT AMOUNT

Choline is available in tablet and liquid form at natural food stores. Take 1000 milligrams daily.

POSSIBLE BENEFITS

Memory Booster   •   Some researchers believe that as we age, we begin to produce less acetylcholine or the acetylcholine that is produced is less efficient, which is why many older people become forgetful. There is some evidence that choline deficiency may result in memory loss. Alzheimer's patients have lower levels of choline than normal. However, attempts to reverse the condition with choline supplements have so far been ineffective. Some researchers believe, however, that choline supplementation may slow down memory loss.

In another study, a drug that interferes with acetylcholine was given to college students. The students began to show signs of forgetfulness similar to those seen among the elderly. In fact, many common drugs, including antihistamines, antidepressants, and antispasmodics, may block acetylcholine and can cause short-term memory loss. Older people in particular are especially vulnerable to drug-induced memory loss and are quick to assume that lapses in memory are a natural part of the aging process. Very often, memory is restored when the drugs are stopped.

Chromium

FACTS

When you were a kid, nobody ever told you, "Take your chromium or no dessert!" Now that you're *not* a kid anymore, I'd like to remind you, "Take your chromium." As we age, we need this mineral more than ever.

Chromium is a trace mineral that works with insulin to help the body utilize sugar and metabolize fat. Recent studies suggest that chromium protects against heart disease and diabetes and may even help to firm up flabby muscles. What's even more exciting is the fact that a preliminary study hints that chromium may improve longevity.

Chromium is found in broccoli, whole wheat English muffins, brewer's yeast, meat, cheese, and shellfish.

THE RIGHT AMOUNT

There is no recommended daily allowance for chromium. In 1980, the National Research Council, National Academy of Sciences, recommended 50 to 200 micrograms of chromium daily. Richard Anderson, Ph.D., of the U.S. Department of Agriculture's Human Nutrition Research Center—a leading authority in chromium—says that people need at least 50 micrograms daily of chromium. However, he concedes that most Americans fall short of this amount. Studies show that serum chromium levels decrease with age, which means that adults over fifty are often short on chromium.

I recommend taking a minimum of 200 micrograms of chromium daily.

POSSIBLE BENEFITS

Improves Glucose Tolerance • Insulin helps the body to metabolize or break down glucose, or blood sugar, in a form that can be utilized by cells for energy. Animal studies show that chromium helps regulate the release of insulin by acting on insulin-producing cells or beta cells. Beta cells in the pancreas manufacture and store insulin until a rising blood sugar level signals to them to release it. In a U.S. Department of Agriculture study, one group of laboratory rats was fed a chromium-rich diet; the other was fed a chromium-deficient diet. Each group of rats was given a glucose solution to stimulate insulin. The rats fed the chromium-deficient diet secreted up to 50 percent less insulin during the test than the rats given the chromium-sufficient diet. Based on this study, it appears as if chromium directly stimulates the production of insulin as the body needs it.

Human studies show that chromium supplements can normalize blood sugar levels in half the people with high blood sugar.

As people age, there is a tendency to develop type II diabetes mellitus, a condition characterized by high blood glucose levels often caused by the body's failure to produce enough insulin. Researchers are hopeful that chromium may help to perk up insulin production in older adults, thus reducing the risk of developing this form of diabetes.

Lowers Blood Lipids   •   Several studies have shown that chromium can cut serum cholesterol levels and triglycerides, another form of blood lipid that may help to promote heart disease. In a study published in *The Western Journal of Medicine*, twenty-eight volunteers with elevated cholesterol (220 to 320 milligrams per deciliter) were given either 200 micrograms of chromium picolinate supplement or a placebo. After a 6-week period, those on the chromium showed an average 7 percent drop in cholesterol, thus reducing their risk of heart disease by 14 percent. Low-density lipoprotein, or "bad" cholesterol, levels dipped by more than 10 percent.

Muscle Builder   •   Chromium picolinate supplements are being promoted as a new and safe way to build muscle. Several studies have shown that supplements of chromium picolinate can increase muscle mass. However, it only works for people who exercise regularly. Therefore, if you want to firm up the flab, take a chromium supplement along with a sensible exercise regime. Sorry, couch potatoes, simply popping a chromium pill without exercise is not effective. (As we went to press, a recent study suggested that this popular form of chromium, chromium picolinate, may cause chromosomal damage on animal cells in high doses. We do not know whether this is significant for humans or not.)

Longevity • I've saved the best for last. A researcher at Bemidji State University in Minnesota fed chromium picolinate and two other chromium supplements to a small group of laboratory rats. The results: the rats on the chromium picolinate lived an average of 1 year longer than the rats on the other form of chromium. The chromium picolinate increased the average life span of the rats by one-third. Although we don't know whether chromium will help humans live longer, we do know that chromium can help prevent heart disease and diabetes, which can cut life short.

Cinnamon

FACTS

Cinnamon has been a highly prized spice since ancient times and is used in many different cuisines. However, modern scientists are finding some new uses for this venerable spice. Recently, researchers have discovered that cinnamon (and a handful of other spices) may help control blood sugar levels by increasing the efficiency of insulin.

THE RIGHT AMOUNT

Use this spice freely on cereal, fruit, yogurt, and even toast. I make it a point to eat about 1 teaspoon of cinnamon daily.

POSSIBLE BENEFITS

Diabetes • About one in four Americans have a genetic tendency to develop *diabetes,* a condition characterized by the inability of the body to metabolize and use foods properly. As a result, diabetics develop excessive amounts of blood sugar that is not utilized and is secreted into urine. In many cases, the diabetic does not produce enough *insulin,* the hormone that helps to regulate blood sugar. Insulin is produced by beta cells in the pancreas, and over time, these beta cells can wear out. If untreated, diabetes can lead to severe complications including heart disease. Most cases of diabetes occur later in life; in fact, a sixty-five-year-old is sixty times more likely to develop diabetes than someone under twenty. Even if you have a tendency to develop diabetes, it is not inevitable that you will. Some physicians believe that the condition can be delayed or even avoided through proper diet. People who are overweight, especially women, are at much higher risk of developing diabetes than normal-weight people. A high-fat, high-calorie diet may overwhelm the beta cells, hastening the onset of diabetes. However, some foods and spices appear to help keep blood sugar levels under control. In recent test tube studies, cinnamon appeared to significantly increase the ability of insulin to metabolize glucose.

Citrus

FACTS

Will eating citrus fruit make you live longer? The National Cancer Institute (NCI) is banking on it. The NCI is spending millions of dollars to study compounds found in oranges, grapefruit, lemons, and limes for their potential cancer-fighting properties.

Citrus fruits contain a virtual drug store of phytochemicals that may help to ward off disease. However, they are best known for being an excellent source of vitamin C, a potent antioxidant and enemy of the common cold. In addition, citrus fruits offer other important minerals including potassium, which controls blood pressure, and a fair amount of fiber, which is good for most everything.

THE RIGHT AMOUNT

Make one of your "five a day" a citrus fruit.

POSSIBLE BENEFITS

Cancer Fighter • The NCI is investigating *limonene*, a citrus oil that has been shown to shrink mammary tumors in rats and, even better, prevented the growth of new tumors. Given the fact that breast cancer is a virtual epidemic in the United States, limonene may prove to be of great importance.

Citrus also contains compounds called *bioflavonoids* (also known as vitamin P), which provide the yellow and orange color of these fruits and maybe much, much more. Some bioflavonoids are antioxidants that help prevent damage to cells inflicted by free radicals. Others help to prevent the spread of malignant cells throughout the body. Researchers hope that one day a form of bioflavonoids may be used to treat various forms of cancer.

In addition, citrus contains *terpenes*, compounds that help produce enzymes that deactivate carcinogens (and also limit the production of cholesterol), which may also prove to be a useful tool in the fight against cancer.

Heart Disease • Most heart attacks and strokes are caused by tiny blood clots that form in arteries that are already narrowed by atherosclerotic lesions. Citrus contains *coumarins*, natural blood thinners that may help prevent the formation of dangerous clots.

Pectin, a compound found in the pulpy membranes that separate individual sections in grapefruits and oranges, can lower blood cholesterol levels, thus reducing the risk of heart attack and stroke. Grapefruit pectin is the most effective. In a recent study at the University of Florida College of Medicine, people with high cholesterol levels were given grapefruit pectin (in a powdered form) daily. Within 16 weeks, the group's cholesterol dropped on average 7.6 percent; low-density lipoproteins, or "bad" cholesterol, were cut by 10 percent. Although the powdered form of grapefruit may be more potent than the natural pectin, researchers believe that whole grapefruit can also lower cholesterol, although perhaps not as much. However, since most people only eat the grapefruit sections and not the membrane containing the pectin, they miss out on the cholesterol-lowering benefit.

Club Moss

FACTS

For centuries, Chinese healers have routinely prescribed a tea brewed from an oriental club moss (*Huperzia serrata*) to reverse memory loss in older people. Western scientists, who tended to dismiss all folk medicine, have tried to no avail to concoct their own drug to reinvigorate people's memories. In 1986, skepticism gave way to hope when researchers at the Shanghai Institute of Materia Medica reported that they had isolated natural compounds in club moss called *huperzine A* and *huperzine B,* which, according to animal tests, helped to improve learning, memory retrieval, and memory retention. (Huperzine A appeared to be the more effective.)

What Western scientists found most intriguing about huperzine was that it raised acetylcholine levels by inhibiting acetylcholinesterase, an enzyme that breaks down acetylcholine. Acetylcholine is a chemical found in the brain that is directly involved in memory and awareness. People with Alzheimer's disease, a life-threatening disorder characterized by severe memory loss and dementia, have lower than normal levels of acetylcholine. Because there is no treatment or cure for

Alzheimer's, any compound that can raise acetylcholine levels is considered a potential weapon against this debilitating disease. Researchers at the Mayo Clinic in Jacksonville, Florida, have been studying huperzine as a potential drug for Alzheimer's. They have recently licensed the use of huperzine A to a pharmaceutical company that is seeking the Food and Drug Administration's permission to test the drug on humans.

THE RIGHT AMOUNT

Drink 1 or 2 cups of brewed club moss tea daily. There are several different types of club moss; be sure that the tea is *Huperzia serrata* and not some other species of club moss. (The species of club moss native to the United States has not yet been studied, so there is no way of knowing whether it would be effective.) Depending on where you live, getting true club moss may be a bit of a challenge; however, it should be available at major herb stores around the country. If you live in an area with a large Chinese population, check out some of the local herb shops.

POSSIBLE BENEFITS

Memory Enhancer • Several animal studies confirm huperzine A's positive effect on memory. In one study, laboratory mice were taught how to run through an electric grid without getting a shock. After the training, the mice were given either an electric shock or a drug to induce amnesia. One group of mice was given huperzine immediately after the amnesia treatment, the other group was not. Twenty-four hours later, the mice were placed back on the electric grid to see how much they retained from their earlier training. The mice given huperzine performed significantly better than the untreated mice. Will huperzine work as well on humans? There are some promising signs that it will. For example, Chinese studies have shown that huperzine can help to improve memory function in stroke victims. More studies are needed before we know for sure whether huperzine will offer relief from Alzheimer's disease and whether it really is a potent memory tonic. However, in the meantime, it can't hurt to include a cup or two of club moss tea in your daily diet.

Cobalamin (Vitamin B_{12})

FACTS

Cobalamin, also known as vitamin B_{12}, plays many important roles in the body. It aids in the production of red blood cells, is essential for the normal functioning of the nervous system, and also helps to metabolize protein and fat. Most recently, B_{12} has been touted as the "brain vitamin," because a lack of this important vitamin can severely hamper mental agility in people of all ages. B_{12} deficiency is quite common among the elderly population. In fact, as many as 10 percent of people over sixty may have low blood levels of this vitamin, and the results can be devastating.

B_{12} is found in meat, fish, eggs, and dairy products.

THE RIGHT AMOUNT

The recommended daily allowance for B_{12} is 2 micrograms for men and women. B_{12} is available as capsules, tablets, a nasal gel, and a sublingual form that dissolves under the tongue.

POSSIBLE BENEFITS

Brain Booster • According to a recent study performed at the University Hospital of Maastricht in the Netherlands, otherwise healthy people with low blood levels of B_{12} did not perform as well on mental tests as people with higher blood levels of this vitamin, regardless of age.

Neurologic Symptoms in Older Adults • Vitamin B_{12} deficiency can cause severe neurologic and psychological symptoms in older people, ranging from numbness or tingling in the arms or legs (peripheral neuropathy) to balance problems, to confusion and even dementia. If caught in time, many but not all of these problems can be reversed with B$_{12}$ supplements. Unfortunately, many people are likely to dismiss confusion or erratic behavior in the elderly as part of the natural aging process and may not look for other causes. However, several studies show that B$_{12}$ deficiency is extremely widespread among people over sixty. In fact, according to a recent study of one hundred people between ages sixty-five and ninety-three performed at New York Medical College, more than twenty-one had *low* B$_{12}$ levels (of which two had peripheral neuropathy) and sixteen had *very low* levels (of which three had peripheral neuropathy and one suffered from mental deterioration).

Why is B$_{12}$ deficiency so common among older adults? As people age, they are prone to develop a condition called *atrophic gastritis*, characterized by less gastric acid and an increased amount of bacteria in the upper small intestine and stomach. The combination of a low level of gastric acid and the presence of bacteria is believed to hamper the ability of the body to utilize the B$_{12}$ in food. Antibiotics may be prescribed to reduce the level of bacteria, which may help increase the level of B$_{12}$ derived from food. However, B$_{12}$ supplements may be better absorbed than B$_{12}$ bound to food.

If an older person shows signs of neurologic or psychological disturbances and other physical causes have been ruled out, he or she should be checked for B$_{12}$ deficiency. In fact, some researchers now believe that every adult over sixty-five should be checked for B$_{12}$ deficiency since the long-term consequences can be devastating.

PERSONAL ADVICE

I personally recommend the nasal gel or sublingual form, which bypasses the stomach and is directly absorbed into the bloodstream.

Coenzyme Q_{10}

FACTS

An *enzyme* is a protein found in living cells that brings about chemical changes. A coenzyme works with an enzyme to produce a particular reaction. Coenzyme Q_{10} is found in every cell in the body and is essential in facilitating the process that provides cells with energy. As we age, levels of cozenzyme Q_{10} begin to fall. However, exercise can raise levels of coenzyme Q_{10}.

Coenzyme Q_{10} can be synthesized by the body or obtained from food. Deficiency states can occur, particularly among the elderly.

Since 1974, coenzyme Q_{10} has been used successfully to treat heart disease in Japan—6 million Japanese take it annually. Recent studies suggest that coenzyme Q_{10} may play a vital role in thwarting the aging process. It can also increase your energy level, especially in people who do not exercise.

THE RIGHT AMOUNT

Coenzyme Q_{10} is available as capsules. Take 30 milligrams daily.

POSSIBLE BENEFITS

Heart Disease • Several studies have shown that coenzyme Q_{10} can increase stamina and reduce angina in heart patients. In one Japanese study, researchers selected ten men and two women with chronic unstable angina (chest pain) between the ages of forty-five and sixty-six. The 12-week study was divided into three phases. In phase 1, patients were given a placebo. In phase 2, half the patients were given a placebo, and the others were given 150 milligrams of coenzyme Q_{10} daily (50 milligrams three times a day). In phase 3, the group on the placebo was given coenzyme Q_{10}, and the group that had been given coenzyme Q_{10} was now given a placebo. During each phase, exercise tests were performed by patients on a treadmill. Patients on the coenzyme Q_{10} had fewer attacks of angina and were able to exercise longer than those not on the medication. In addition, those on the coenzyme Q_{10} required fewer nitroglycerin tablets to relieve the pain of angina than those on the placebo.

In Japan, coenzyme Q_{10} is used to treat congestive heart failure. It works by increasing the strength of the heart muscle.

Studies have shown that coenzyme Q_{10} may lower blood pressure.

Antioxidant • Animal studies have shown that coenzyme Q_{10} inhibits *lipid peroxidation,* a process that promotes the formation of *free radicals,* unstable oxygen molecules that can cause damage and malignant changes in cells. Free radicals may contribute to heart disease, premature aging, and even cancer. Antioxidants such as coenzyme Q_{10} may prevent cells from being damaged by free radicals.

PERSONAL ADVICE

Coenzyme Q_{10} is very effective in preventing toxicity from a large number of drugs used to treat cancer, high blood pressure, and other diseases.

Cranberry

FACTS

Urinary tract infections (UTIs), characterized by painful urination, blood or pus in the urine, fever, low back pain, or cramps, are more common among older men and women. In men, enlargement of the prostate gland, a common condition affecting nearly half of all men over fifty, can promote UTIs. Postmenopausal women in particular suffer more UTIs than younger women due to vaginal dryness caused by lower estrogen levels.

Once an infection has taken hold, it must be properly treated with medication, and sometimes, several drugs must be used before the infection is gone. However, studies have shown that cranberry juice can help prevent these annoying and painful infections from occurring in the first place.

THE RIGHT AMOUNT

Drink 1 to 2 glasses of cranberry juice daily. Cranberry concentrate is available in capsule form at natural food stores. Take 2 to 6 capsules daily.

POSSIBLE BENEFITS

Prevent UTIs • UTIs are caused by *Escherichia coli* bacterium, which tends to adhere to the walls of the urinary tract. Recently, researchers at Alliance City Hospital in Ohio discovered that cranberry juice prevented *Escherichia coli* from sticking to the endothelial cells of the urinary tract; thus, the potentially dangerous bacterium was flushed out in the urine.

Cruciferous Vegetables

FACTS

Population studies of dietary habits—so-called epidemiological studies—have shown that people who eat a diet high in cruciferous vegetables (e.g., cabbage, broccoli, brussels sprouts, kale, and cauliflower) have lower rates of cancer than people who don't. Because of its possible role in fighting cancer, researchers at the National Cancer Institute have begun investigating the cruciferous family to isolate its potential cancer-fighting properties.

THE RIGHT AMOUNT

I recommend at least two servings (1 cup) of these vegetables daily.

POSSIBLE BENEFITS

Cancer Fighter • Researchers at the Institute for Hormone Research in New York have found that *indoles*, a group of phytochemicals in cruciferous vegetables, may be a powerful weapon against cancer. Indoles appear to alter the biological pathway that converts certain estrogens into more potent forms that can trigger the growth of tumors in estrogen-sensitive sites, such as the breast. Women with breast cancer tend to have higher blood estrogen levels than normal, and any substance that controls the amount of estrogen circulating in the bloodstream may have a protective effect against certain forms of breast cancer.

Researchers at Johns Hopkins School of Medicine in Baltimore recently found what may be an even more vigorous cancer fighter in cruciferous vegetables: *sulforaphane*. Sulforaphane stimulates the action of protective enzymes that help the body fight against tumor growth. (See Sulforaphane, p. 150.) In fact, one researcher said that sulforaphane may be one of the most potent protective agents against cancer discovered to date!

Antioxidant Boost • Cruciferous vegetables are excellent sources of beta-carotene, vitamin C, selenium, and vitamin E. Antioxidants may help to prevent the cellular damage caused by free radicals, which may be responsible for many different forms of cancer and heart disease.

Fiber Boost • Cruciferous vegetables are an excellent source of fiber, which helps to prevent constipation and digestive diseases, such as diverticulosis, but also may help to prevent cancer of the colon, breast, lung, and cervix.

Dandelion

FACTS

To most suburbanites, dandelions are just troublesome weeds. But to practitioners of herbal medicine, they are a veritable gold mine. Herbalists have long used dandelions to treat liver ailments and digestive disorders. Like so many other herbs these days, dandelions are being rediscovered by men and women who are determined to maintain a lifetime of good health.

Dandelion is an excellent source of beta-carotene and lutein, two members of the carotenoid family that may protect against certain forms of cancer.

THE RIGHT AMOUNT

Dandelions can be eaten fresh in salads. Dandelion tea and capsules are available at natural food stores. Drink 1 cup of tea daily or take 1 to 3 capsules daily. Dandelion is included in many herbal formulas designed to promote good digestion and improve liver function.

POSSIBLE BENEFITS

Liver • The liver weighs a mere 3 to 4 pounds, but it is worth its weight in gold several times over. The liver performs many vital jobs in the body including the detoxification of poisons and impurities that may enter the bloodstream; the production of sex hormones, proteins, and enzymes; and the breakdown of fat. Animal studies show that dandelion extract can stimulate the production of bile by the liver, which is essential for the metabolism of fat. Herbalists believe that dandelion is an overall tonic for the liver, generally improving the liver's ability to function.

Digestive Aid • Dandelion, like other "bitters," can help treat digestive problems, such as gas and bloating. This herb can also help to prevent constipation.

Menopause • Dandelion, which is rich in plant estrogens, is often prescribed to relieve some of the discomfort of menopause caused by a sharp dip in estrogen levels. Dandelion has a mild diuretic effect, which can help eliminate menopausal water retention. However, unlike other diuretics, it is rich in potassium and does not sap the body of this vital mineral.

Dong Quai

FACTS

Known in the West as dong quai and in the Far East as tang keui, this member of the angelica family is a highly esteemed anti-aging herb. According to Ron Teeguarden, author of *Chinese Tonic Herbs,* dong quai is the "ultimate woman's tonic herb." It is widely used throughout Asia to help ease the symptoms of menopause.

In younger women, dong quai is used to regulate menstrual disorders.

THE RIGHT AMOUNT

Dong quai is available in tablet or capsule form and is included in many "change of life" supplements sold at natural food stores. Take 2 tablets or capsules twice daily.

POSSIBLE BENEFITS

Menopause • Chinese healers consider dong quai to be a hormone regulator that maintains hormones within normal levels. Dong quai contains hormonelike compounds that may relieve hot flashes, vaginal dryness, and other symptoms of menopause. It is also rich in vitamin E, which may also explain why women may find it useful for menopause. Dong quai has a mild sedative effect, which can help relieve stress.

Heart Disease • Studies show that this herb can lower blood pressure in both men and women and slow down the pulse rate.

Anemia • Chinese women use dong quai as a "blood builder." Dong quai is a rich source of iron and may help to prevent iron deficiency anemia.

Diabetes • Dong quai has been shown to regulate blood sugar, thus helping to prevent high concentrations of glucose or blood sugar that can lead to diabetes.

PERSONAL ADVICE

Next time you're eating at a Cantonese Chinese restaurant, try ordering the dong quai duck.

Echinacea

FACTS

Echinacea is living proof that the more things change, the more they stay the same. Native Americans first used this beautiful purple cornflower as a remedy for toothaches, sore throats, and even snake bites. European settlers brought echinacea back to Europe, where it quickly became a popular herbal remedy. Around the turn of the century, scientists who had studied the effect of echinacea on blood cultures recognized that this herb could boost the immune system by stimulating the production of white blood cells. Physicians as well as herbalists used echinacea to treat infection and cancer. Once antibiotics were discovered, interest in herbs such as echinacea waned. However, as interest in preventive medicine increased in the 1980s, researchers began to look for ways to keep people healthy. Anything that could bolster the immune system attracted great attention, and interest in echinacea was revived. Today, as we approach the twenty-first century, echinacea is now being touted as a hot "new" immunostimulant.

THE RIGHT AMOUNT

Echinacea is available in capsule and extract forms at most natural food stores and herb shops. (Some preparations are made from the roots of the *Echinacea angustifolia* plant; others are made from the roots or leaves of *Echinacea purpurea*.) Either form of echinacea may be included in herbal preparations designed to boost the immune system.

I find that the capsules are the easiest. Take 1 capsule three times daily. If you prefer to use extract, mix 15 to 30 drops in liquid every 3 hours up to three times daily. Many of the active compounds in echinacea can be destroyed during processing. Freeze-drying is the most effective way to preserve this herb's healing properties.

POSSIBLE BENEFITS

Antiviral • Several studies have shown that echinacea prevents the formation of an enzyme called *hyaluronidase*, which destroys a natural barrier between healthy tissue and unwanted pathogenic organisms. Thus, echinacea helps cells maintain their natural line of defense against bacteria and viruses.

Several studies have shown that echinacea may be an effective treatment against colds, ear infections, and flu. A recent German study of 180 patients between the ages of eighteen and sixty showed that echinacea extract (four droppers daily) were significant in relieving the symptoms and duration of flulike infections. (There's no reason to believe that capsules would not work as well.) Other European studies have shown that echinacea is useful in the treatment of ear infections in children.

In 1978, a study of echinacea in *Planta Medica* showed that a root extract destroyed both herpes and influenza virus.

Cancer Fighter • Several animal studies show that echinacea can inhibit the growth of certain types of tumors, probably by stimulating the production of key lymphocytes, which in turn accelerate the body's own defenses. Echinacea has also been used to restore normal immune function in patients receiving chemotherapy.

Antifungal   •   At least one study has shown that echinacea (taken orally and applied vaginally in cream form) may be an effective treatment against yeast infection (*Candida albicans*), a particularly persistent infection. Even better, this treatment appears to help prevent the infection from recurring.

Ellagic Acid

FACTS

Ellagic acid, a polyphenolic compound found in fruit, is attracting a great deal of attention among cancer researchers because it appears to be a potent cancer fighter.

Strawberries, grapes, and cherries are a good source of ellagic acid.

THE RIGHT AMOUNT

There is no recommended daily allowance for ellagic acid. As of yet, there is not enough information to recommend a specific amount of ellagic acid; however, I advise people to eat at least one serving daily of a fruit with this substance (one serving = ½ cup of fruit).

As of this writing, ellagic acid is not available in supplement form. Even if it were, I generally advise people to try to get their phytochemicals from food whenever possible.

POSSIBLE BENEFITS

Cancer Fighter   •   Animal studies show that ellagic acid counteracts synthetic and naturally occurring carcinogens, thus preventing healthy cells form turning cancerous. Ellagic acid is also an antioxidant, which may block the destructive effects of free radicals.

Ellagic acid's ability to counteract carcinogens is very promising. For example, in one Japanese study, laboratory rats were fed a diet high in various polyphenol compounds. One group was given ellagic acid exclusively. The rats were later exposed to a potent carcinogen to induce tongue cancer. All of the rats on the various polyphenolic compounds had a reduced incidence of cancer; however, those on the ellagic acid remained entirely cancer free. The researchers speculated that ellagic acid (and other polyphenols) may help to prevent cancer in other tissues, including the skin, lung, liver, and esophagus.

In another study, researchers tested the effect of ellagic acid on a nicotine-derived carcinogen found in cigarette smoke. The study revealed that the ellagic acid (and other polyphenols) blocked the carcinogenic effect of the nicotine compound on animal cells.

More research needs to be done to determine if ellagic acid will work in a similar way on humans. However, until the results are in, eating foods rich in ellagic acid can't hurt, and it just might help.

Fenugreek

FACTS

Fenugreek is an herb that is used as a spice to flavor curry and chutney. Since ancient times, it has been valued for its medicinal properties. Fenugreek is reputed to be an aphrodisiac. It has been used to treat impotence in men and discomfort associated with menopause in women. Modern scientists believe that fenugreek may play a role in helping to prevent or postpone adult-onset diabetes.

THE RIGHT AMOUNT

Fenugreek tea is available at natural food stores. It is also available in capsule form. Drink 1 to 2 cups daily. Take 1 capsule up to three times daily. It is also included in many herbal formulas for women.

Caution: Do not use fenugreek during pregnancy.

POSSIBLE BENEFITS

Menopause • Fenugreek contains steroidal saponins, which are similar to sex hormones produced by the body and, therefore, may play a role in regulating hormone levels. In fact, herbal healers recommend fenugreek for hot flashes and depression associated with menopause.

Diabetes • According to U.S. Department of Agriculture researcher James A. Duke, Ph.D., fenugreek (along with a handful of other herbs and spices) may help slow the onset of adult diabetes. Fenugreek seeds contain at least six different compounds that can help control blood sugar levels, thus preventing a sugar surge that may create problems for many older people who may not produce enough insulin or may be insulin resistant.

Fiber

FACTS

There's one thing that advocates for alternative medicine and mainstream groups like the American Medical Association can agree on: Americans should eat more fiber.

Fiber is a catchall phrase for the nonnutritive food substances found in plants that are not digested or absorbed by the body—so-called roughage. Although there is compelling evidence that a diet high in fiber may help to ward off a number of deadly diseases, the American diet is woefully low in fiber. In fact, the average American consumes about 10 grams of fiber daily, less than half of the 30 grams of fiber recommended by most doctors and medical researchers.

There are two types of fiber: soluble and insoluble.

Soluble fiber, which includes pectin and plant gums, binds with bile in the intestine and is excreted in the feces. Scientists believe that the liver compensates for the loss of bile by producing more bile salts in which cholesterol is a necessary ingredient. By reducing the amount of cholesterol circulating in the blood, soluble fiber helps to lower blood cholesterol levels.

Insoluble fiber contains compounds called *cellulose* and *hemocelluloses*, which absorb water and can improve the functioning of the large bowel. Insoluble fiber softens and bulks waste to help move it more quickly through the colon, thus helping to prevent constipation and reducing exposure to pesticides or naturally occurring carcinogens in food.

Good sources of soluble fiber include apples, oat bran, broccoli, carrots, dried peas and beans, potatoes, strawberries, and other fruits and vegetables.

Good sources of insoluble fiber include celery, leafy green vegetables, whole grains, kidney and pinto beans, apples, and other fruits and vegetables.

THE RIGHT AMOUNT

I recommend 30 to 35 grams of fiber daily. In order to achieve this goal, you must be diligent about consuming daily at least five servings of fruits and vegetables daily (½ cup or one medium size fruit = one serving) and roughly six servings of whole grains (one piece of whole grain bread or ½ cup of whole grain cereal = one serving).

Caution: If you're adding fiber to your diet, go slow! Introduce it gradually. If you gobble up too much fiber too quickly, you may develop gas and cramps. Drinking 6 to 8 glasses of water daily will help relieve gas.

If you have any rectal bleeding or blood in your stool, contact your doctor immediately.

POSSIBLE BENEFITS

Cancer Fighter • In 1970, British physician Dr. Denis Burkitt published a study in which he noted that in countries where the population ate a diet high in fiber, cancer of colon and rectum—a leading cause of death in the United States—was relatively rare. Other studies have confirmed the link between colorectal cancer and fiber. For example, a study at the Harvard School of Public Health recently examined the diets of seven thousand men. Researchers found that men who consumed the highest amount of saturated fat and the lowest amount of fiber were four times more likely to develop colon polyps, often a precursor to cancer.

Fiber may also offer protection against breast cancer, the second leading cause of cancer deaths among women. Studies have shown that women who develop breast cancer typically have higher levels of blood estrogen than women who remain cancer free. A recent study sponsored by the American Health Foundation attempted to see if fiber could lower blood estrogen levels. In the study, women were given 15 to 30 grams daily of wheat, corn, or oat bran. At the end of 2 months, the women on the wheat bran experienced a dramatic drop in blood estrogen levels, but not the women on the other forms of fiber.

Heart Disease • Several studies have shown that soluble fiber can lower blood cholesterol levels, which decreases the risk of coronary artery disease and stroke. For example, psyllium, derived from the ground-up husks of the psyllium plant, is used as a laxative (Metamucil) and in cereal as a cholesterol-lowering agent. In fact, according to one study performed at the University of Kentucky Medical Service, a diet rich in psyllium flake cereal can reduce blood cholesterol levels by 12 percent. Based on this study, psyllium appears to be especially effective in lowering low-density lipoproteins, or "bad" cholesterol. (Psyllium can cause an allergic reaction in some people.)

Oat bran is another popular cholesterol buster. Studies show that by eating roughly three packets of instant oatmeal daily, you can cut your total cholesterol level by about six points, thus reducing your risk of heart attack.

Dried beans are also a potent cholesterol cutter. A recent study showed that by eating 4 ounces of cooked beans daily, people with cholesterol levels of over 200 milligrams per deciliter can reduce total cholesterol by as much as 20 percent.

Gastrointestinal Disorders • Insoluble fiber can help to ward off the kinds of gastrointestinal ailments that plague middle age and beyond. First, fiber can prevent constipation—infrequent bowel movements or hard stool that is difficult to pass. Constipation is not just uncomfortable, but it can promote *hemorrhoids*, varicose veins in the area of the anus and rectum. People with a chronic history of constipation are also more likely to develop diverticular disease (diverticulosis and diverticulitis), which affects more than one-third of all adults over fifty. *Diverticulosis* is characterized by the presence of diverticula, saclike herniations that can form in any part of the gastrointestinal tract, but more often than not in the colon. Symptoms of diverticulosis may vary from no symptoms at all to cramps, constipation, or diarrhea. Diverticulosis can develop into a more serious condition, *diverticulitis,* if the diverticula become inflamed. Diverticulosis is quite common among older people and is usually treated with a high-fiber diet. (Diverticulitis is treated with antibiotics and a low-fiber diet.)

Flax

FACTS

As far back as 8500 years ago, flax was a normal part of a diet that included other wild cereal grasses such as barley. In modern times, flax has been used primarily as a source of linen and linseed oil. Today, however, researchers at the National Cancer Institute are exploring the potential anticancer properties of an edible form of flaxseed. If their expectations are proven correct, flax may once again become a dietary mainstay.

THE RIGHT AMOUNT

Flaxseed oil is available as capsules or liquid at natural food stores. Take 1 to 3 capsules or 1 to 3 tablespoons daily. Ordinary flax can become rancid very quickly. Use only products that include stabilized flax. Vitamin-fortified, stabilized flaxseed baked products are available at some natural food stores and through mail order.

POSSIBLE BENEFITS

Cancer Fighter • Flax contains twenty-seven anticancer compounds including fiber, pectin, tocopherol (vitamin E), and sitosterol. Flax is also an excellent source of lignans, which are converted in the gut into compounds that are similar in structure to natural estrogens produced by the body. Lignans are believed to deactivate potent estrogens that can cause tumors to grow; like other phytoestrogens, they bind to estrogen receptor sites on cells in place of the more potent estrogens. Studies have shown that people who consume diets rich in lignans have lower levels of cancer of the breast and colon.

Folic Acid

FACTS

In recent years, pregnant women have been urged to take 400 micrograms of this B vitamin daily to prevent neural tube defects in their babies. But folic acid is not just for the very young—it's for people of all ages, especially those who want to live to be a ripe old age.

Folic acid helps in the formation of red blood cells and in nucleic acids, RNA and DNA, the genetic material in the cells.

Folic acid is derived from the word *foliage* because it is found in dark green leafy vegetables such as spinach and broccoli. It is also found in dried beans, frozen orange juice, yeast, liver, sunflower seeds, wheat germ, and fortified breakfast cereals.

THE RIGHT AMOUNT

The recommended daily allowance for folic acid is 400 micrograms, roughly the amount in 1½ cups of boiled spinach or ½ cup of peanuts. Women on average get only one-half of the recommended daily allowance. Supplements of 400 micrograms are sometimes supplied in B-complex formulas. One hundred micrograms of folic acid is the usual amount found in supplements.

POSSIBLE BENEFITS

Heart Disease • Folic acid may help to prevent the number one killer of both men and women in the United States—heart disease—by helping to maintain normal levels of homocysteine, an amino acid found in the body. In a recent study performed at Harvard Medical School, men with even a *slightly* elevated level of homocysteine were three times more likely to have a heart attack than men with the lowest levels. Based on the study, when given a folic acid supplement, homocysteine levels dropped back to normal in most men. Researchers at Harvard say that patients who are believed to be at high risk of having a heart attack should have their homocysteine levels checked. Here's my advice: even if you're not at high risk of having a heart attack, it just makes good sense to eat a diet rich in folic acid.

Cancer Fighter • Researchers at Brigham and Women's Hospital in Boston have linked a diet low in folic acid to a change in DNA that may allow cancer-causing genes to be expressed. In their study of 26,000 men and women, those with the lowest intake of folic acid had the highest level of adenomas (precancerous tumors) of the colon or rectum. At Tufts University, researchers are studying whether very high does of folate—about twenty times the current recommended level of 400 micrograms—can help prevent colon cancer in people with precancerous polyps.

Low levels of folic acid have also been linked to cervical cancer. Each year, 6000 women die of cervical cancer in the United States. Cervical dysplasia—cell abnormalities that if left untreated, often lead to cancer—can be caused by an infection with the human papillomavirus. (Cigarette smoking, multiple sex partners, and early age at first intercourse are also believed to increase the risk of cervical cancer.) In a recent study performed at the University of Alabama, 300 women with cervical dysplasia were compared with 170 healthy women. These women were interviewed about their lifestyle and eating habits. As part of the study, blood levels for certain vitamins were also checked. The results: women with the highest levels of folic acid had the lowest levels of cervical dysplasia, even if they were infected with the human papillomavirus. The researchers concluded that folic acid may offer some protection against this potentially lethal virus.

Fo-ti

FACTS

According to Chinese legend, this herb (known as *ho shou wu* in China) can help prevent hair from turning gray. Fo-ti is a favorite longevity herb among Chinese herbalists. Although there is little evidence to prove that fo-ti can help maintain hair color, recent studies show that this herb may offer real protection against heart disease.

THE RIGHT AMOUNT

Fo-ti is available as capsules at natural food stores. Take 1 capsule up to three times daily.

POSSIBLE BENEFITS

Heart Disease • Several Chinese studies have shown that fo-ti can lower blood cholesterol levels, thus helping to protect against heart attack. In addition, this herb contains flavonoid-like compounds that strengthen and dilate blood vessels, improving the flow of blood to the heart.

PERSONAL ADVICE

The Chinese have a mystical reverence for fo-ti. According to Chinese folklore, the older the root, the more powerful its rejuvenating properties!

Gamma-linolenic Acid

FACTS

Gamma-linolenic acid (GLA) is a fatty acid that is extracted from the seeds of evening primrose or borage plants. For centuries, herbalists have valued both plants for their medicinal properties. Today, GLA is marketed as evening primrose oil and can be found in most natural food stores. GLA is a very popular over-the-counter treatment in Canada and Europe (especially Britain) for a wide range of ailments ranging from premenstrual syndrome to skin rashes. Recent studies suggest that GLA may help prevent cardiovascular disease, provide relief for rheumatoid arthritis, and may even be used one day as a cancer treatment.

THE RIGHT AMOUNT

GLA is available in capsule form. Take 250 milligrams up to three times daily.

POSSIBLE BENEFITS

Reduces Inflammation   •   In a study reported in the November 1, 1993, issue of *Annals of Internal Medicine*, researchers at the University of Pennsylvania's Graduate Hospital in Philadelphia gave capsules containing 1.4 grams of GLA daily to nineteen people with rheumatoid arthritis (RA), an autoimmune disorder characterized by inflamed and painful joints. Eighteen other RA patients received a placebo. After six months, the group on the

GLA showed less pain and less signs of inflammation than the patients taking the placebo. The research team did not find any adverse side effects associated with GLA. More studies need to be done to see if GLA is an effective treatment for RA.

Heart Disease • Several studies have shown that GLA may lower cholesterol levels in some people. In one Canadian study, patients taking 4 grams of evening primrose oil daily experienced a 31.5 percent decline in cholesterol after 3 months. However, other studies have shown that GLA has only a small effect on lowering cholesterol.

In a study conducted at McMaster University in Hamilton, Canada, researchers tested GLA's ability to prevent blood clots. Rabbits were fed various fatty acids, including GLA, for a 4-week period. The researchers found that GLA appears to inhibit platelets (blood cells involved in the formation of blood clots) from adhering to the walls of blood vessels. Thus, GLA may help to prevent blood clots, a major cause of heart attack and stroke.

Cancer Fighter • A recent study performed at Nazam's Institute of Medical Sciences in India has shown that GLA can selectively kill tumor cells. In a clinical trial, six patients with gliomas, a particular type of tumor, were given GLA. All the patients showed mild improvement. This doesn't mean that GLA is a cure for cancer; however, one day GLA may prove to be an effective treatment in conjunction with other therapies against certain types of tumors.

Genistein

FACTS

Genistein is a hot "new" anticancer compound that's actually been around for thousands of years, but until recently, nobody has noticed. Genistein is a recently identified isoflavone found in soy and soy-based products. For decades, scientists have been mystified as to why the incidence of many different forms of cancer in Asia is so much lower than in the United States. (For example, the breast cancer rate in the United States is 22.4 per 100,000; in Japan it's 6 per 100,000.) Recent studies suggest that genistein could be a potent cancer fighter.

Good sources of genistein include whole soy beans, tofu (bean curd), soy flour, soy milk, and rehydrated vegetable protein, which can be used in place of chopped meat in foods such as tacos and chili. (Soy sauce does not contain genistein.)

THE RIGHT AMOUNT

Eat one or two portions of soy foods per day (about 3 ounces).

POSSIBLE BENEFITS

Cancer Fighter • Since 1987, several hundred papers have been published on genistein's role as a possible cancer fighter. In 1993, a German study published in *The Proceedings of the National Academy of Sciences* found that in test tube studies, genistein blocks a process called *angiogenesis*, which is responsible for the growth of new blood vessels. The researchers speculate that genistein may indirectly prevent the growth of tumors by thwarting the formation of new blood vessels that are necessary to nourish them. In other words, genistein literally starves little tumors before they can grow into bigger problems. The researchers go on to note that in animal studies, soy products have inhibited the formation of mammary tumors, and they logically conclude that genistein may be the compound protecting Japanese women from breast cancer.

Autopsies of Japanese men show that prostate cancer is as common among Japanese men as it is among American men, but the cancer seems to grow much more slowly, so slowly in fact, that many die without ever developing clinical disease. Until recently, there was no explanation for this phenomenon. However, researchers now suspect that genistein is actually blocking the growth of these tumors. Finnish researcher Herman Aldercreutz and colleagues compared blood plasma levels of isoflavones in Japanese and Finnish men. The levels of isoflavones were more than 100 times higher among the Japanese men, with genistein occurring in the highest concentration of any other isoflavone. The researchers concluded "a life-long high concentration of isoflavonoids in plasma (Japanese children have as high a urinary excretion as adults) might explain why Japanese men have small latent carcinomas that seldom develop to clinical disease" (*The Lancet*, November 13, 1993).

Researchers Greg Peterson and Stephen Barnes of the University of Alabama tested whether genistein could block the growth of non-estrogen-dependent human breast cancer cells. In this study, they showed that genistein thwarted the growth of breast cancer in vitro and that the presence of an estrogen receptor is not necessary for isoflavones to inhibit tumor growth. This suggests that the protective effect of isoflavones may not be due to their effect on hormones, but rather, the particular ability of genistein to block cell growth.

Genistein holds great promise as a potential cancer protector. However, more studies need to be done to confirm whether this is true.

Heart Disease • Genistein is believed to inhibit the action of enzymes that may promote cell growth and migration. Some researchers speculate that by blocking the action of these enzymes, genistein may also prevent the growth of cells that form plaque deposits in arteries, much the same way that genistein may prevent the growth of tumors.

Ginger

FACTS

Ginger root is one of the most widely used herbs in the world. In China, where it is highly regarded as a "warming herb," it was mentioned in the famous *Shen Nung Herbal*, which dates back to 3000 B.C. Ginger is also a major medicinal herb in Ayurvedic medicine, the Indian system of traditional medicine, which is rapidly gaining popularity in the West. In the United States, the National Cancer Institute has included ginger in its Experimental Food Program, which is exploring the cancer preventive compounds in different foods.

Herbal healers in the West have long prescribed ginger as a treatment for nausea and morning sickness.

THE RIGHT AMOUNT

Fresh ginger is sold at supermarkets and greengrocers. It can be used in cooking or made into a tea. Ginger capsules and teas are available at natural food stores. Take 1 capsule up to three times daily, or drink 1 to 2 cups of ginger tea.

POSSIBLE BENEFITS

Cancer Fighter • Ginger is abundant in a compound called *geraniol*, which may be a potent cancer fighter. In a recent study, Dr. Charles Ellson of the University of Wisconsin, Nutrition Science Department, found that only 0.1 percent of geraniol increased the survival rate of rats with malignant tumors. In addition, studies have shown that geraniol can enhance the effectiveness of other anticancer drugs. More studies are being done to determine if geraniol will have similar effects on people.

Heart Disease • Several studies have shown that ginger can prevent platelet aggregation, that is, it can prevent blood cells from sticking together and forming blood clots. If a clot lodges in an artery leading to the heart or the brain, it can cause a heart attack or stroke. In one Indian study, twenty healthy male volunteers were fed 100 grams of butter daily, which significantly increased their rate of platelet aggregation. However, when ten of the men were given 5 grams of dry ginger divided into two doses with the fatty meal, the ginger appeared to inhibit the degree of platelet aggregation.

Migraine • A Danish study showed that ginger may help prevent migraine headaches, and may relieve some of the symptoms of these headaches such as pain and nausea. Studies show that ginger has anti-inflammatory activity, which could explain why it would work as a pain reliever.

Ginkgo

FACTS

Do you have difficulty remembering the names of people even if you've just been introduced to them? Do you find yourself becoming more forgetful? Becoming forgetful is one of the most negative stereotypes of aging, and the bad news is, there's some truth to it. A recent survey of nearly fifteen thousand adults over age fifty-five revealed that about three-quarters of them had some difficulty remembering things. The good news is, the leaf from an ancient tree may help to perk up your memory. Recent studies suggest that extract from the ginkgo tree leaf may help improve memory, maintain mental sharpness, and provide many other life-extending benefits.

The ginkgo tree, which dates back to before the Ice Age, is one of the hardiest trees known to humankind. Some live as long as four thousand years! Although the ginkgo kernel has been used in Oriental medicine for hundreds of years, it was only in the 1970s that European researchers began investigating the potential medicinal properties of the ginkgo leaf. Today, ginkgo is one of the most commonly prescribed drugs in Europe for a wide range of problems ranging from memory loss to tinnitus (ringing in the ears) to hemorrhoids to headaches.

Although ginkgo products are sold in natural food stores, ginkgo may soon be used as a serious drug in the United States. In 1988, a chemist at Harvard synthesized a ginkgo compound called *ginkgolide B*, which, among other things, is being tested as a potential drug for asthma and to help prevent the rejection of transplanted organs.

THE RIGHT AMOUNT

Ginkgo, which is growing in popularity, is available in most natural food stores and even many drug stores. I recommend a supplement called Ginkgo 24 containing a solution of 24 percent ginkgo biloba in a 50:1 extract. Take 60-milligram capsules or tablets three times daily. The effects of ginkgo are short-lived—the dose lasts for only a few hours. There is no known toxicity.

POSSIBLE BENEFITS

Memory Booster • There are several reasons why older adults may have difficulty remembering. Stress, lack of physical exercise, poor mental stimulation, and even subtle vitamin deficiencies may impair cognitive function. However, there is also a natural slowing down in mental processes due to decreased levels of certain chemicals in the brain. Electrical impulses or messages from the brain are transmitted along nerve cells called *neurons*. Neurons have long tendrils called *axons*, which overlap onto another neuron. Neurons "communicate" with each other via chemicals called *neurotransmitters*, notably dopamine and noradrenaline. As we age, there is a decreased production of neurotransmitters, thus resulting in reduced alertness and memory retention. Animal studies have shown that ginkgo increases the level of dopamine, which improves the body's ability to transmit information. Several human studies have shown that ginkgo can improve mental performance among elderly people who have shown deteriorating mental function. Studies of younger people suggest that high doses of ginkgo can improve short-term mental processes. In his book, *Next Generation Herbal Medicine*, herbalist Daniel Mowrey, Ph.D., suggested that one day, college students may use ginkgo to help them cram for exams.

Improves Circulation • Studies also show that ginkgo improves the blood flow to the brain (and to other vital organs), providing oxygen and nutrients the brain needs to function at peak capacity. As we age, circulation is often impaired by plaque deposits in the arteries delivering blood to the brain and other organs. Ginkgo helps to dilate or relax arteries and veins, thus improving blood flow throughout the body.

Antioxidant • Ginkgo is rich in flavonoids, potent antioxidants that protect the body against free radicals or unstable molecules that can cause damage to healthy cells. Heart disease, cancer, and even arthritis are just some of the diseases that are believed to be caused or worsened by free radical damage.

Prevents Blood Clots • Studies show that ginkgo inhibits blood cells from sticking together, thus preventing the formation of blood clots that can lead to heart attack or stroke. (If a clot lodges in an artery leading to the heart, it can cause a heart attack. If it lodges in an artery leading to the brain, it can cause a stroke.)

PERSONAL ADVICE

Try taking ginkgo capsules for hemorrhoids. Many people swear that is it is one of the most effective agents for helping to control bleeding and itching due to irritated hemorrhoids.

Ginseng

FACTS

Of all the substances listed in the anti-aging hot hundred, ginseng may be the most widely used. For five thousand years, the Chinese have revered this herb as a cure-all for nearly every ailment, from impotence to heart disease, and as an overall antidote to the ravages of aging. In recent years, ginseng has been promoted in the West as a tonic and a rejuvenator, which has generated a great deal of interest in this herb. At last count, there were more than three thousand scientific studies performed on ginseng. Most of these studies were done in the Orient or in the former Soviet Union, where ginseng (a home-grown variety) is routinely given to athletes to improve stamina and performance. Although more research needs to be done, there is strong evidence that ginseng has many positive effects on the body and the mind.

There are three different types of ginseng: panax ginseng is grown in China; American ginseng (*Panax quinquefolius*) is grown in the United States. Siberian ginseng (*Eleutherococcus senticosus*), grown in Siberia, is actually not ginseng at all, but a close relative that has similar affects. All forms of ginseng have similar properties, with some differences. Chinese ginseng is considered the strongest form of ginseng; American ginseng is milder and is highly prized in the Orient.

THE RIGHT AMOUNT

Ginseng comes in many forms including capsules, tea, and powder. I recommend American or Siberian ginseng; some people may find panax ginseng too stimulating, especially at night. For capsules, take 1 up to three times daily. For tea, drink 1 cup daily. If you use powder, mix 5 to 10 grams in liquid daily. Excess use of ginseng can make some people very jittery; do not exceed the recommended dose.

Caution: In rare cases, ginseng, which has a mildly estrogenic effect on the body, can cause vaginal bleeding in post-menopausal women. If this happens, be sure to tell your doctor that you are using ginseng; vaginal bleeding can be mistaken as a symptom of uterine cancer. Do not use ginseng if you have high blood pressure or an irregular heartbeat.

Be sure to buy ginseng products from a reputable company. Ginseng is expensive, and many unscrupulous distributors may try to pass off cheaper products as ginseng.

POSSIBLE BENEFITS

Stimulant • Oriental healers contend that ginseng improves mental performance, especially in older people. Animal studies confirm that ginseng may improve the capacity to learn. For example, rats given ginseng were able to run through a maze faster to find a food reward than were untreated rats. Several human studies found that people taking ginseng made fewer mistakes and may even complete tasks faster than people not taking ginseng. There are several theories as to why ginseng may have a positive effect on learning. Some researchers speculate that ginseng may indirectly stimulate the production of stress hormones that can increase stamina and prevent fatigue. However, ginseng also contains choline, a chemical in the brain that is essential for learning and memory retention, which may also help to perk up mental activity (see Choline, p.52). More studies are needed to determine ginseng's exact effect on mental functioning.

Antioxidant • Ginseng contains antioxidants, substances that prevent cellular damage due to oxidation, exposure to unstable molecules called free radicals. Free radicals are believed to be responsible for promoting mutations in cells that could lead to cancer. In addition, free radicals may play a role in heart disease by promoting the formation of low-density lipoproteins, or "bad" cholesterol.

Cancer Fighter • Researchers at Japan's Kanazawa University found that unpurified saponins, compounds found in ginseng, inhibited the growth of cancer cells and actually converted diseased cells into normal cells.

Lowers Cholesterol • Japanese researchers showed that rats who were fed a high-cholesterol diet showed a drop in cholesterol and a rise in beneficial high-density lipoprotein, or "good" cholesterol, after being fed ginseng.

Antistress • Soviet scientist I. I. Brekhman, Ph.D., first coined the term *adaptogen* to describe ginseng. According to studies performed by Brekhman, ginseng helps the body to better cope with stress by normalizing body functions. For example, if blood sugar levels drop too low or blood pressure rises too high, Brekhman contends that ginseng somehow brings the body back to normal levels. Although the concept of an adaptogen may seem foreign to Westerners who take medication only when they are sick, it is in keeping with traditional Chinese medicine, which uses ginseng and other herbs as a tonic to maintain overall health.

Menopause • Ginseng contains compounds that are similar in action to estrogen, the female sex hormone. Many women use ginseng to help control some of the unpleasant side effects of menopause, such as hot flashes, which may occur when estrogen levels decline. (Interestingly enough, in countries where ginseng is commonly used, such as China and Japan, menopause is not considered a "medical problem," nor do post-menopausal women routinely take estrogen supplements.)

PERSONAL ADVICE

Take ginseng 1 hour before eating. Vitamin C can interfere with the absorption of ginseng, so if you take a C supplement, wait 2 hours before or after taking ginseng to do so.

Glutathione

FACTS

I call glutathione the "triple-threat anti-aging amino acid" because it is synthesized from three amino acids: L-cysteine, L-glutamic acid, and glycine, all of which are found in fruits and vegetables. Glutathione is a potent antioxidant that is synthesized by our own body cells. Studies have shown that glutathione may help protect against cancer, radiation poisoning, and the detrimental effects of cigarette smoke and alcohol abuse. Glutathione is a popular supplement in Japan, the country with the longest life span in the world. Although many mainstream U.S. scientists have dismissed glutathione supplements as worthless, a recent study sponsored by the Human Nutrition Research Center on Aging at Tufts University suggests that glutathione supplements may help keep an aging immune system healthy.

THE RIGHT AMOUNT

Glutathione is present in fruits and vegetables; however, cooking can reduce its potency. I recommend taking 50-milligram capsules one or two times daily.

POSSIBLE BENEFITS

Immune Booster • Simin N. Meydani, Ph.D., a well-known researcher in the field of nutrition who discovered that vitamin E had a positive effect on the immune system of elderly people, investigated whether glutathione would have a similar effect on aging white blood cells in animals and humans. In both animal and human studies, Dr. Meydani found glutathione gave the immune system a much-needed boost. It not only improved the blood cells' ability to produce substances that can help ward off infection, but it also reduced the amount of inflammatory substances produced by the cells. Interestingly enough, glutathione had a greater effect on the sluggish cells of older people than on younger ones. More research needs to be done before we can say that glutathione is a bona fide immune booster, but the preliminary evidence looks good.

Anti-inflammatory • Glutathione has been used as treatment for allergies and arthritis, both conditions that are caused by an inflammatory response in the body.

PERSONAL ADVICE

Here's more evidence that when it comes to aging well, the adage Use it or lose it! takes on new importance. Studies suggest that exercise may increase the level of antioxidants such as glutathione in older people.

Grapeseed Extract

FACTS

Grapeseed extract is touted as a potent anti-aging compound in France, and is fast gaining popularity in the United States.

Grapeseed extract contains a unique type of bioflavonoids called *proanthocyanidins*, which are synergistic with vitamin C, that is, they greatly enhance the activity of vitamin C. In fact, some researchers believe that grapeseed extract helps vitamin C enter cells, thus strengthening the cell membranes and protecting the cells from oxidative damage.

Proanthocyanidins are also found in cranberries, cola nuts, and other fruits and vegetables.

THE RIGHT AMOUNT

Grapeseed extract is sold in capsule form at natural food stores. Take 1–2 (30–100 milligrams) of grapeseed extract daily.

POSSIBLE BENEFITS

Cancer Fighter • Grapeseed extract is a potent antioxidant and free radical scavenger. Free radicals are unstable oxygen molecules that can attack normal cells, destroying them or causing them to mutate. Free radical damage can also lead to the kind of unfettered cell growth associated with cancer. Vitamin C is a potent antioxidant in its own right, but studies suggest that it may be even more effective when combined with proanthocyanidins such as grapeseed extract. In fact, according to researchers at the Department of Pharmacy of Nagasaki University School of Medicine in Japan, test tube studies showed that the bioflavonoids in grapeseed extract had stronger antioxidant activity than vitamin C.

Heart Disease • Several studies have confirmed that antioxidants like grapeseed extract can prevent the oxidation of blood lipids, such as low-density lipoprotein, or "bad" cholesterol, which can promote the formation of plaque or fatty deposits in the arteries.

Anti-inflammatory • Grapeseed extract has been used as an anti-inflammatory to treat common ailments such as arthritis and allergies. Many bioflavonoids inhibit the release of certain enzymes that can promote inflammation. In the case of arthritis, free radical damage may also contribute to joint pain and swelling associated with this condition.

Circulation • Capillaries are tiny blood vessels that can be easily destroyed by free radical damage. In addition, as we age, cells lose collagen, a protein fiber that is important for the growth and repair of cells including capillary cells. Weakened capillaries can lead to easy bruising and a tendency to develop varicose veins. Grapeseed extract helps strengthen capillaries in two ways. By protecting against free radical assault, grapeseed extract may help prevent weakening of capillaries. In addition, since vitamin C is essential for the production of collagen and grapeseed extract enhances the performance of vitamin C, it is indirectly involved in collagen production.

Green Tea

FACTS

If there was an Olympic competition for longevity, the Japanese would be the world champions. The Japanese have a longer life span than any other nationality, even though they are heavy smokers. What's their secret? Some researchers in the United States and Japan are looking for the answer in a cup of tea—no, they're not reading tea leaves, they're reading some impressive studies that suggest that phytochemicals found in green tea may help fight against cancer and heart disease.

Green tea, derived from the tea plant, is a rich source of potentially beneficial compounds called *catechins*. As tea undergoes processing, it loses some of its precious catechins to oxidation. Green tea is very lightly processed, thus retaining more of its catechins than the heavily processed dry black tea that is sold in the United States.

THE RIGHT AMOUNT

Sip 1 or 2 cups of green tea daily. Real green tea is found in natural food stores or Asian markets. Green tea extract tablets are also available. Take 1–2 tablets daily.

POSSIBLE BENEFITS

Cancer Fighter • Researchers at the American Health Foundation in New York exposed mice to nitrosamines, a potent cancer-causing agent in cigarette smoke. One group of exposed mice was given green tea, the other was not. The results: there were 45 percent fewer cases of lung cancer among the teetotaling mice. In other studies of lab mice, green tea helped to slow the rate of tumor growth in mice exposed to ultraviolet radiation.

Does this mean that green tea will work as well in humans? There's some evidence that it might. The cancer rate in central Japan is lower than anywhere else in Japan; coincidentally, it is the place where green tea is produced and where the people drink more of the stuff than anywhere else in the country. More studies remain to be done before we'll know for sure whether or not green tea is a bona fide cancer protector; however, drinking a cup or two of tea a day can't hurt and just may help.

Cholesterol Buster • Animal studies show that green tea catechins can reduce cholesterol levels in laboratory rats fed a diet high in saturated fat and cholesterol. Human studies have shown that people who eat a high-cholesterol diet (averaging three egg yolks in one meal) can maintain normal cholesterol levels by sipping green tea with their meals. I'm not suggesting that green tea will work this well for everyone or that you can eat a high-fat diet as long as you wash it down with green tea. However, adding green tea to an already sensible diet may be a good way to keep cholesterol levels in check.

PERSONAL ADVICE

Coffee drinkers take note: on average, brewed tea contains one-half the caffeine found in coffee and is probably twice as good for you.

Hawthorn

FACTS

Heart disease is the number one killer of both men and women in the United States, which is why I believe this "heart healthy" herb will become very hot as the baby boom generation reaches middle age and beyond.

Since the 1700s, European herbalists have used preparations made from the hawthorn plant as a tonic for the heart. Today, this herb is widely used throughout Europe, notably in France, England, Russia, and Germany, and is gaining in popularity in the United States.

THE RIGHT AMOUNT

Hawthorn is available in capsule form or as a tea at natural food stores. Take 1 capsule up to three times daily. (Preparations sold in the United States are made from the hawthorn berry.) Drink 1 to 3 cups of tea daily.

Caution: If you are on any medication for your heart, do not discontinue or alter your dose without talking with your physician or healer.

POSSIBLE BENEFITS

Heart Disease • Hawthorn is a well-researched herb, especially in Europe. Animal and human studies show that hawthorn has many positive effects on the cardiovascular system. Hawthorn is rich in bioflavonoids, compounds that strengthen capillaries, thus improving the flow of blood throughout the body. Studies on humans and dogs have shown that hawthorn can reduce blood pressure during exertion; animal studies also show that this herb can increase the contractility of the heart muscle, strengthening the heart's ability to pump blood. In fact, in Europe, hawthorn may be prescribed along with the drug digitalis to regulate the heartbeat; the addition of hawthorn reduces the required dose of digitalis. Other studies have shown that hawthorn may be useful as a treatment for angina (chest pain due to insufficient blood flow to the heart) and may also decrease the heartbeat rate, preventing the heart from becoming overworked. Many natural healers believe that hawthorn can keep an aging heart pumping like a young one!

Horsetail

FACTS

Horsetail is a bamboolike plant that lives in marshes which has been used for hundreds of years by herbal healers as a treatment for rheumatoid arthritis. This herb is also a mild diuretic; it is used by homeopathic physicians as a remedy for urinary problems and enlarged prostate. There is a growing interest in herbs such as horsetail these days due to the aging population and the rise in age-related ailments such as arthritis and prostate problems.

THE RIGHT AMOUNT

Horsetail is available as tablets or capsules at natural food stores. Take up to 3 tablets or capsules daily. Some studies show that very high doses of horsetail have been toxic to livestock. However, the low doses recommended here should not have any adverse affects.

POSSIBLE BENEFITS

Rheumatoid Arthritis • Gold shots are a traditional remedy for rheumatoid arthritis. Horsetail has been shown to absorb minute quantities of gold that are dissolved in water. Some herbalists believe that the gold residue in horsetail may be the reason why some people find it effective against the joint pain and stiffness associated with arthritis.

Hair Enhancer • The Meskawki Indians fed horsetail to their ponies to improve the gloss of their hair. Horsetail is rich in silica, a mineral that is reputed to add shine and strength to hair. In fact, it is used in many shampoos and conditioners. Silica is also used to strengthen nails.

Legumes

FACTS

Legumes (dried beans and peas) are a mainstay of many diets around the world, although not in the United States. Rice and beans is a staple south of the border; *pasta e fagioli* (pasta and beans) is standard fare in Italy. Maybe not so coincidentally, people who live in countries where legumes are a major part of their cuisine have substantially lower rates of cancer and heart disease.

Legumes include all kinds of beans, ranging from kidney to navy to lentil to black beans. All legumes are pretty much the same nutritionally, although there are some slight variations in fiber content and caloric value. Legumes are an excellent source of protein; however, most lack certain essential amino acids that are found in meat (soybeans are the exception—they contain all eight essential amino acids that cannot be produced by the body). The amino acids that are missing in legumes are present in grains; therefore, by eating legumes with a grain such as rice, you can create a meal containing all eight essential amino acids.

THE RIGHT AMOUNT

I recommend eating at least three legume-based meals weekly.

POSSIBLE BENEFITS

Cancer Fighter • Legumes contain many compounds that are believed to protect against cancer. Legumes are a good source of *isoflavones*, compounds that block estrogen receptors in some cells and by doing so may deactivate potent forms of estrogen that can trigger the growth of estrogen-dependent tumor cells. About 30 percent of all breast tumors are estrogen dependent.

Legumes are also rich in *protease inhibitors*, compounds that block the action of enzymes that can trigger cancer growth, and *phytic acid*, compounds that in animal studies have been shown to thwart the growth of tumors.

Legumes are an excellent source of *fiber*, substances in plants that are not digested and absorbed by the body. A diet high in fiber is believed to protect against some forms of cancer, particularly cancer of the colon. No one knows exactly how fiber helps to prevent cancer, however, one theory is that fiber moves food more quickly through the colon. As food is broken down into its basic components, potential carcinogens are released into the gut. Some carcinogens may be naturally occurring; some may be from insecticides or added in processing. If food is speeded through the gastrointestinal tract, there is less exposure to these potential cancer threats.

Lowers Cholesterol • A study at the University of Kentucky showed that legumes are powerful cholesterol busters. Eating 4 ounces of cooked beans daily (1 cup) can over time reduce cholesterol levels of over 200 milligrams per deciliter by as much as 20 percent!

Diabetes • As we age, we are much more likely to develop insulin resistance, that is, the body becomes less efficient at metabolizing or utilizing glucose (blood sugar). High levels of blood sugar are associated with diabetes, which increases the risk of heart attack, stroke, and other vascular problems. Many researchers believe that diet may help to prevent diabetes, or at least delay its onset in some people. Notably, foods that avoid a heavy concentration of sugar in the bloodstream at one time may be better than foods that force insulin to work overtime. Complex carbohydrates, the kind found in legumes and grains, are just what the doctor ordered. They burn slowly and steadily in the body (not like sweets, which burn very quickly), thus giving the insulin the time it needs to utilize glucose.

Lemongrass

FACTS

Lemongrass is one of many foods that is widely used in Asian cuisines but virtually nonexistent in American cooking. Also known as *citronella*, lemongrass adds a fresh, lemony flavor to food. It's not only delicious, but studies show that lemongrass oil may help protect against heart disease by lowering cholesterol.

Fresh lemongrass and lemongrass oil is sold in Asian markets and natural food stores. If using the whole plant, the lower part of the stalk is crushed and finely chopped. Lemongrass oil is used as a flavoring.

THE RIGHT AMOUNT

Use the plant or the oil in cooking whenever you can. Add one stalk of chopped lemongrass to stir-fry vegetables and other Oriental dishes. Many Oriental recipes call for lemongrass oil.

POSSIBLE BENEFITS

Heart Disease • Researchers at the University of Wisconsin gave men with high cholesterol 140 milligrams of lemongrass oil daily for 3 months. At the end of the study, 30 percent of the men experienced a 10 percent decrease in cholesterol. The researchers suspect that a compound in lemongrass decreases the synthesis of cholesterol from fats.

Licorice

FACTS

When Westerners think of licorice, they think of the licorice-flavored candy that contains little if any of the real herb. In China, however, licorice is the mostly widely used of all medicinal herbs. Five thousand years ago, licorice was immortalized in the famous *Shen Nung Herbal*. Today in China, licorice is highly regarded as a tonic and longevity herb. Recently, licorice's potential health benefits have attracted the attention of Western scientists; it is currently under investigation by the National Cancer Institute for its possible anticancer properties.

THE RIGHT AMOUNT

Take 1 capsule up to three times daily.

Caution: Licorice should not be used by people with high blood pressure.

POSSIBLE BENEFITS

Menopause • Licorice is frequently used to treat symptoms of menopause. Licorice contains a glycyrrhizin, a hormonelike compound that appears to help normalize hormone levels in women.

Cancer Fighter • Animal studies show that glycyrrhetinic acid (derived from glycyrrhizin) can block carcinogen-induced tumor growth. More studies are being done to determine if licorice is an anticancer herb.

Arthritis • Due to its anti-inflammatory action, herbal healers prescribe licorice to treat the swelling, aches, and pains of arthritis.

Antiulcer • Carbendoxolane, a compound found in licorice, has been used successfully to treat stomach ulcers.

Lignans

FACTS

People who live in countries where plant food is a mainstay of the diet, such as in Asia and Africa, have a much lower rate of many forms of cancer than people who live in Western countries where the diet is heavy in meat and light on fruits and vegetables.

For several decades, researchers have attempted to isolate the specific components in plant food that may help to prevent various diseases. Scientists have studied various vitamins, minerals, and fiber, the nondigestible food substance in plants that is not digested by the body. Each of these substances may play a role; however, some may play a greater role than others. In 1979, scientists discovered a compound in fiber called *lignans*, and today, many researchers believe that lignans may be responsible for much of fiber's protective effect.

Many studies have shown that lignans have anticarcinogenic, antiviral, and antifungal properties. They are also rich in phytoestrogens, hormonelike compounds that mimic the behavior of natural hormones in the body.

Flaxseed is the best plant source of lignans. However, wheat bran and rye also have these compounds. Smaller amounts of lignans can be found in many plants and vegetables.

THE RIGHT AMOUNT

Research on lignans is relatively new; therefore, we have no idea of the precise amount that is needed to prevent cancer. I recommend eating foods that are rich in lignans, such as grains, fruits, and vegetables. Bread made from flax is a particularly good source of lignans and can be found at many natural food stores.

POSSIBLE BENEFITS

Cancer Fighter • There are several theories on why lignans may protect against cancer. Studies have shown that vegetarian and semivegetarian women have a much lower rate of breast cancer than women who eat meat. Researchers have measured the amount of lignans and estrogen in the urine of vegetarian women and have found that their urine contained higher amounts of both estrogen and lignans than women who were not vegetarians. What was even more interesting was the fact that women who had breast cancer excreted much smaller amounts of lignans and estrogen in their urine than either vegetarians or meat eaters and had higher blood levels of estrogen. From these studies, researchers suspected that lignans had a protective effect against breast cancer.

Other studies have shown that lignans are converted into estrogenlike compounds in the body that mimic the behavior of estrogen. Some forms of naturally produced estrogen are believed to promote the growth of estrogen-sensitive tumors. Certain cells in the body have receptors that bind with estrogen. Lignans, which are chemically similar to estrogen, may compete with the more potent natural forms of estrogen for space on estrogen-sensitive cells. If natural estrogen has no place to bind, it becomes deactivated, thus losing its ability to promote the growth of tumors. Excess estrogen is excreted in urine.

Some researchers believe that lignans may also be protective against cancer of the prostate and colon.

Ligusticum

FACTS

Ligusticum (licidum or wallichii) is an important Chinese herb that is in hot demand in the West because of its reputation as an immune booster. This herb, combined with astralagus, reishi, and other immune herbs, is used by natural healers to strengthen compromised immune systems (as in the case of AIDS patients or cancer patients receiving chemotherapy).

Ligusticum is a highly revered herb in China and is used in a famous woman's tonic called Four Things Soup, which includes dong quai. (See p. 68.)

There are more than sixty species of ligusticum worldwide. In the southwestern United States, Native Americans have long used *Ligusticum porteri* to treat viral, fungal, and respiratory infections. In the United States, ligusticum is marketed as osha and can be found in most natural food stores.

THE RIGHT AMOUNT

Osha and ligusticum are sold as capsules and extract at natural food stores. Take 2 or 3 capsules daily, or 5 to 10 drops of extract in liquid two or three times daily.

POSSIBLE BENEFITS

Cancer Fighter • Many species of ligusticum have been shown to inhibit the growth of tumors in animals.

Cardiovascular • A stroke can occur if the flow of blood to the brain is impaired in any way. There have been many studies investigating ligusticum and its role in the prevention of stroke. Several animal studies performed in China show that ligusticum can promote circulation to the brain and prevent the formation of blood clots. When a stroke was induced in animal tests, ligusticum helped restore circulation to the brain, thus minimizing brain damage. In fact, one Chinese study involving 158 patients with transient ischemic attack (tiny strokes) showed that ligusticum was even more effective than aspirin in helping to resolve blood clots and improve blood flow to the brain.

In China, ligusticum has also been used to treat angina, a condition that is caused by a reduction in blood flow to the heart.

Lutein

FACTS

Lutein is a member of the carotenoid family, a group of six hundred compounds naturally occurring in fruits and vegetables (of which beta-carotene is the most well known). Carotenoids are believed to offer special protection against many different forms of cancer, and recent studies suggest that lutein may also be a cancer fighter. Carotenoids provide fruits and vegetables with their orange, red, and yellow colors. However, they are also found in green leafy vegetables, but they are hidden by the green color of chlorophyll.

Good sources of lutein are spinach; greens, such as collard, turnip, and mustard; broccoli; green peas; celery; and kale.

THE RIGHT AMOUNT

There is no recommended daily allowance for lutein; however, I recommend eating one serving of a lutein-rich vegetable daily.

POSSIBLE BENEFITS

Cancer Fighter • A recent study of twelve hundred people performed at the University of Hawaii found that people who ate foods high in lutein had a lower risk of lung cancer than those who ate lower levels of lutein. Researchers suspect that lutein's anticancer properties are due to its antioxidant action.

Population studies have linked a high intake of fruits and vegetables that are rich in carotenoids with a lower risk of cancers of the head, neck, lung, esophagus, and colon.

Lycopene

FACTS

Lycopene, a member of the carotenoid family, is a potent antioxidant that may prove to be one of the most important of all the phytochemicals.

Lycopene, which gives fruits and vegetables a reddish color, is found primarily in tomato, ruby red grapefruit, and red peppers.

THE RIGHT AMOUNT

Eat one lycopene-rich food daily. Lycopene (along with other phytochemicals) is now available in capsule form. However, the studies linking lycopene to a reduced risk of certain forms of cancer have all been done on food and not on supplements. Therefore, I still recommend getting your lycopene from food if you can.

POSSIBLE BENEFITS

Cancer Fighter • A handful of studies have linked low blood serum levels of lycopene to an increased risk of certain forms of cancer. No one is certain how lycopene may offer protection against cancer; however, most researchers believe that its antioxidant properties may play a role.

- A study at the School of Public Health and the University of Illinois at Chicago showed a link between lycopene blood levels and cervical dysplasia, a precancerous condition in women.
- Bladder cancer is the most common malignant tumor of the urinary tract and is prevalent among fifty- to seventy-year-olds. Recent studies have shown a link between low blood levels of lycopene and an increased risk of bladder cancer.

- Pancreatic cancer, one of the most lethal forms of cancer, primarily affects people between the ages of fifty and eighty. There are 28,000 new cases of pancreatic cancer each year, and the disease is very difficult to treat. Researchers speculate that lycopene may offer some protection against pancreatic cancer based on a recent study that showed that people with the lowest levels of lycopene had the greatest risk of developing pancreatic tumors.

Magnesium

FACTS

As minerals go, magnesium is hardly a superstar—few people think about whether or not they're getting enough magnesium in the course of a day. And yet, as we age, magnesium may prove to be one of the most important anti-aging minerals.

Magnesium is essential for calcium and vitamin C metabolism and also plays a role in the metabolism of phosphorus, sodium, and potassium. This mineral is important for converting blood sugar into energy and is necessary for effective nerve and muscle functioning.

In recent years, magnesium has been touted as an essential mineral for heart health, and recent studies suggest that it may also play a role in helping to prevent diabetes, especially later in life.

Good sources of magnesium include nuts, unmilled grains, seeds, apricots, dried mustard, curry powder, dark leafy vegetables, and bananas.

THE RIGHT AMOUNT

The National Research Council recommends 250 to 350 milligrams daily for adults. Magnesium is available in most multivitamin and mineral supplements and can also be purchased in the form of magnesium oxide supplements (250 milligrams of magnesium oxide = 150 milligrams of pure magnesium per tablet).

Chelated magnesium (a more digestible form of the mineral) and calcium supplements (with half as much magnesium and calcium) is an excellent source of both minerals.

People who drink heavily require extra magnesium.

Caution: Excess magnesium (over 1000 milligrams daily) can cause diarrhea. Over time, it can be toxic. Do not take a magnesium supplement if you have kidney disease.

POSSIBLE BENEFITS

Heart Disease • Epidemiological studies show that people who live in regions with high levels of magnesium in the soil and water have a lower rate of heart disease than the general population. Many other studies have shown that people who have heart attacks have a lower than normal level of magnesium in their body tissues. As far back as the 1950s, animal studies have shown that high doses of magnesium can actually reverse atherosclerotic plaques. Other studies show that magnesium decreases blood pressure and improves the flow of blood to the heart. It's logical to conclude that magnesium plays some role in protecting against heart disease, although the precise role is not known. Some researchers, however, believe that magnesium works in conjunction with calcium to prevent fatal arrhythmias, similar to calcium channel blockers.

In many hospitals, intravenous magnesium is routinely given to patients after they have a heart attack. The effectiveness of this treatment is still under debate. Several studies have shown that people who get intravenous magnesium after a heart attack have a significantly better survival rate than those who don't. However, a major U.S. study involving thousands of heart attack patients did not support magnesium's use post–heart attack.

Improves Glucose Handling • As people age, they are likely to develop insulin resistance, that is, they cannot use insulin efficiently to turn glucose into energy, thus blood glucose levels rise, which can lead to diabetes. According to a recent study at the University of Naples, magnesium supplements can improve glucose handling in older people with insulin resistance. Other studies have shown that magnesium supplements can reduce blood pressure and lower the risk of complications in patients who already have diabetes.

Melatonin

FACTS

Melatonin is a hormone secreted by the pineal gland in the brain during sleep. Melatonin is vital for the maintenance of normal body rhythms, especially the sleep–wake cycle, and appears to play a critical role in many other body functions. When I'm on the road, I use melatonin to help ease the symptoms of jet lag, when normal sleep patterns are disturbed by a disruption in the daylight–darkness pattern. Melatonin helps to normalize the body's circadian rhythm, which regulates sleep–wake cycles. Recently, melatonin has been successfully tested as a cure for insomnia.

The production of melatonin declines dramatically with age. Today, many researchers suspect that melatonin may be a natural anti-aging hormone.

THE RIGHT AMOUNT

Synthetic forms of melatonin are sold in natural food stores in tablet or capsule form in 3-milligram strength. A faster-acting sublingual tablet, which is placed under the tongue, is also available. Take 1 to 2 tablets or capsules about 1½ hours before bedtime. If using the sublingual form, take them 45 minutes before going to sleep. Occasional use preferred. (Do not drive or operate heavy machinery after taking melatonin.)

POSSIBLE BENEFITS

Longevity • In 1987, Walter Pierpaoli, M.D., Ph.D., and his colleagues at the Biancalana-Masera Foundation for the Aged in Ancona, Italy, showed that adding melatonin to the drinking water of mice during darkness prolonged the life span of the animals by more than 20 percent (about six months longer than average). The researchers speculated that melatonin may help reduce stress and improve the function of the immune system in animals and, perhaps, in humans. Other animal studies have shown that the removal of the pineal gland (which produces melatonin) can result in an acceleration of the aging process. In a review article published in *The International Journal of Neuroscience* (Vol. 52, 1990, pp. 85–92), psychiatrist Reuven Sandyk of the Department of Psychiatry of Albert Einstein College of Medicine in New York stated, "There is evidence from both experimental animal and human studies to suggest that decreased melatonin functions may accelerate the aging process and thus support the notion that melatonin may function as an anti-aging hormone."

Some researchers speculate that melatonin may be an antioxidant, that is, it prevents cellular damage associated with aging by thwarting the action of free radicals. Others feel that melatonin may slow down aging by controlling the timing of the release of certain hormones, proteins, and neurotransmitters (chemicals that help nerve cells communicate with each other).

Insomnia • Disruption in sleep cycles is a common ailment among older people, and many scientists have suggested that a reduction in melatonin may be responsible. In fact, recent studies show that melatonin may be a potent sleep aid. Researchers at Massachusetts Institute of Technology in Boston have shown that melatonin can induce sleep in young volunteers within 5 or 6 minutes. Volunteers given a placebo took 15 minutes or more to fall asleep. In addition, those taking the melatonin slept twice as long as those taking the placebo. Scientists hope that melatonin may prove to be a safe, nonaddicting sleep agent.

Breast Cancer • Several studies have linked a higher rate of breast cancer to both women and men who are in professions where they are exposed to low-frequency electronic magnetic fields (EMFs). Researchers were puzzled by this finding and were not certain how or even if EMFs played a role in cancer. However, one recent study showed that exposure to EMFs can reduce the pineal gland's ability to produce melatonin at night. Test tube studies have shown that melatonin can inhibit the growth of breast tumor cells; therefore, some researchers now suspect that low blood levels of melatonin may promote the growth of breast tumors. Although these findings are interesting, as of yet, scientists caution that the case of EMFs and melatonin is far from closed and much more research is needed.

Menadione (Vitamin K)

FACTS

When *Earl Mindell's Vitamin Bible* was first published in 1979, little was known about menadione, also called vitamin K, except that it was essential for the synthesis of proteins involved in proper blood clotting. Nearly two decades later, however, vitamin K is attracting the attention of researchers worldwide because of the possible role it may play in helping to prevent osteoporosis. In fact, at the U.S. Department of Agriculture's Human Nutrition Research Center at Tufts University, there is a special laboratory devoted to investigating the relationship between vitamin K and aging.

Vitamin K is formed by intestinal bacteria. It is also found in green leafy vegetables, alfalfa, egg yolks, safflower oil, soybean oil, kelp (seaweed), and fish liver oil.

THE RIGHT AMOUNT

The recommended daily allowance for vitamin K is 80 micro-grams for men and 65 micrograms for women. I recommend taking a supplement of 50 to 100 micrograms daily. Do not exceed 500 micrograms daily. According to researchers at Tufts, older people may require higher levels of vitamin K due to a decreased rate of absorption.

People on long-term antibiotic regimens may develop a vitamin K deficiency.

Caution: People taking blood thinners should not take vitamin K unless under the supervision of a physician.

POSSIBLE BENEFITS

Osteoporosis • Several studies have shown that vitamin K supplements may help reduce the loss of calcium in urine, thus preventing the thinning of bones. For example, in one Dutch study presented at the New York Academy of Sciences special meeting on vitamins in 1991, researchers noted that a vitamin K supplement reduced urinary excretion of calcium in post-menopausal women and was particularly effective in stemming the loss of calcium among fast losers of calcium. Previous studies have linked a low level of vitamin K to an increased risk of fractures.

Milk Thistle

FACTS

Milk thistle preparations are popping up in natural food stores and are already extremely popular in the United States. Since ancient times, the seeds from this weed have been used to treat many different ailments including digestive disorders. However, today milk thistle is fast becoming known as the "liver herb."

Milk thistle contains silymarin, a compound that belongs to

the flavonoid family. Flavonoids are antioxidants and help protect cells from free radicals, unstable oxygen molecules that can cause dangerous mutations.

THE RIGHT AMOUNT

Milk thistle is available in capsules. Take 175 milligrams three times daily.

POSSIBLE BENEFITS

Liver Disease • The liver is the most complicated organ in the human body. It performs many vital tasks including the production of bile, which is necessary for the breakdown of fat and the storage of glycogen to fuel the muscles. The liver also produces other important substances such as clotting factors (so we don't bleed to death), blood proteins, and more than one thousand different enzymes. One of the liver's most critical roles is the detoxification of drugs and poisons, such as alcohol, which may be taken externally or produced internally. Injury to the liver can be life threatening. Inflammation of the liver is called *hepatitis* and can be caused by drug toxicity and viral infection. Many studies have shown that milk thistle has a strong therapeutic effect on the liver, protecting it from damage inflicted by toxins and disease. In fact, in Europe, milk thistle has been used as an effective treatment for viral hepatitis and cirrhosis of the liver (a condition often caused by alcohol abuse). Many people take milk thistle daily as a liver tonic to strengthen and protect this important organ.

Monounsaturated Fat

FACTS

Fat has become a dirty word lately, especially for people who are concerned about health and longevity, but eating monounsaturated fat may actually help you live longer. Studies show that in countries such as Italy and Greece, where the diet is rich in monounsaturated fat (mainly olive oil), the incidence of heart disease is a fraction of what it is in the United States.

There are three kinds of fats: saturated, polyunsaturated, and monounsaturated. The degree of saturation is determined by the number of hydrogen molecules: the more hydrogen molecules, the more saturated the fat. Saturated fat is believed to promote the formation of plaque, which can lead to atherosclerosis.

Olive, canola, and avocado oils are excellent sources of monounsaturated fat. Nuts such as almonds, peanuts, and walnuts are also rich in monounsaturates.

THE RIGHT AMOUNT

I believe that people should consume no more than 20 percent of their daily calories in the form of fat of any kind. (The American Heart Association recommends no more than 30 percent fat from daily calories, which I believe is too high. The late Nathan Pritikin and Dean Ornish, M.D., recommend no more than 10 percent, which I feel may be too difficult to adhere to.) Therefore, it's important to watch fat intake, even if it's "good" fat.

Use 1 to 2 tablespoons of olive or canola oil in your salad or cooking daily.

If you eat nuts, keep the portions small.

POSSIBLE BENEFITS

Heart Healthy • Although monounsaturated oil doesn't necessarily lower total blood cholesterol levels, it does raise the levels of high-density lipoproteins, or "good" cholesterol. High levels of high-density lipoproteins are associated with lower rates of heart disease.

Recently, Israeli researchers found that olive oil was less prone to oxidative damage than polyunsaturated oil. Oxidative damage of blood lipids is believed to be a major cause of atherosclerotic lesions that can lead to a heart attack or stroke. Olive oil in particular is also high in vitamin E, an antioxidant that helps prevent heart disease and cancer.

Diabetes • A handful of studies suggest that monounsaturated fat may be beneficial for diabetics.

Longevity • Other studies have linked consumption of monounsaturated foods—notably nuts—to a longer life span and a dramatically lower rate of heart attack. In fact, a major study of 26,000 members of the Seventh Day Adventist Church showed that those who ate almonds, peanuts, and walnuts at least six times a week had an average life span 7 years longer than the general population.

PERSONAL ADVICE

Keep in mind that fat in any form contains 9 calories per gram (as compared to 4 calories per gram for carbohydrates and protein). As beneficial as monounsaturated fats may be, a little goes along way.

Motherwort

FACTS

As its common name implies, motherwort has a long tradition of being used to treat problems of the female reproductive system. The Latin name for motherwort is *Lenonurus cardiaca*, and as that name implies, motherwort is also known as a heart healthy herb.

Motherwort contains compounds that can cause uterine contractions. For thousands of years, motherwort has been prescribed by herbal healers to bring on delayed menstruation or to speed up childbirth. However, today it is gaining popularity as a menopause aid.

THE RIGHT AMOUNT

Take 10 to 20 drops of motherwort in liquid up to three times daily, or drink 1 cup of tea.
Caution: Do not use this herb during pregnancy.

POSSIBLE BENEFITS

Heart • Motherwort is a mild sedative. It helps control palpitations and rapid heartbeat due to anxiety. It also temporarily lowers blood pressure. This herb is frequently used to treat anxiety related to the physiological changes that can occur during menopause.

Bloating • During menopause, women often retain water due to hormonal swings. This herb is a mild diuretic that can help relieve some of the discomfort due to bloating.

PERSONAL ADVICE

If you are experiencing rapid heartbeat or palpitations, check with your physician or natural healer. It could be a sign of a more serious problem.

Niacin (Vitamin B₃)

FACTS

If you have high cholesterol or have had a heart attack, this vitamin could save your life.

Niacin works with two other B vitamins, thiamine and riboflavin, in the metabolism of carbohydrates. It is also essential for providing energy for cell tissue growth. The body produces niacin from tryptophan, which is abundant in milk and eggs. Recent studies suggest that as people cut back on high-fat and high-cholesterol foods, such as milk and egg products, they may become deficient in niacin.

In recent years, niacin has gained fame as a potent cholesterol-lowering agent.

THE RIGHT AMOUNT

The recommended daily allowance for women is 15 milligrams and for men, 19 milligrams. High doses—the kind prescribed to cut cholesterol—can result in unpleasant side effects such as flushing and itching. If you are using niacin to lower cholesterol, I recommend the "no flush" niacin supplements with inositol hexanicotinate. Supplements are available in 50- to 1000-milligram-dose tablets or capsules. Usually, between 800 and 1200 milligrams daily are needed to lower cholesterol. However, you can reduce the niacin dose by taking it with chromium: take 100 milligrams of niacin with 600 micrograms of chromium daily.

Caution: High levels of niacin can interfere with the control of uric acid, bringing on attacks of gout in people who are prone to this disease. In addition, niacin may interfere with the body's ability to dispose of glucose and may promote liver abnormalities. Therefore, I recommend using niacin under the supervision of a physician. (Given the side effects of some of the other cholesterol-lowering drugs, niacin is relatively safe.)

POSSIBLE BENEFITS

Heart Disease • In 1975, the Coronary Drug Project, a major study, reported that niacin could dramatically reduce cholesterol levels and, even better, could cut the rate of second heart attacks by 30 percent. A 15-year follow-up study comparing niacin to clofibrate, another cholesterol-lowering drug, found that even though both agents lowered cholesterol, patients who had taken the niacin had significantly fewer heart-related deaths than those who had taken the clofibrate.

Other studies confirm that niacin can lower both cholesterol and triglycerides and can raise the level of high-density lipoproteins, or "good" cholesterol.

Cancer Fighter • There's some evidence that niacin may offer some protection against cancer. In a recent study, scientists
at the University of Kentucky's Markey Center tested the effect
of niacin deficiency on human and animal cells. Cells that were
deprived of niacin began to show signs of malignant changes
that could lead to cancer. More studies need to be done on the
role of niacin in cancer.

Nitrosamine Blockers

FACTS

Nitrosamines are cancer-causing compounds that are formed
during normal digestion. Nitrosamines can occur when nitrites,
a commonly used food preservative, or nitrates, a naturally occurring chemical in food, combine with amino acids. Nitrosamines can destroy DNA, which can lead to cancerous
changes in cells. Several years ago, researchers at Cornell University reported that certain foods, such as tomatoes, green peppers, strawberries, pineapples, and carrots, can prevent the
formation of these troublesome nitrosamines. Initially, scientists
believed that vitamin C was the primary nitrosamine blocker in
these foods. However, in a recent article in *Agriculture and Food
Chemistry,* Cornell University food scientists reported the discovery of two other compounds in tomatoes—*p*-courmaric acid
and chlorogenic acids—that appear to be potent nitrosamine
blockers. This discovery has led scientists to believe that there
are probably other nitrosamine blockers in fruits and vegetables
that have yet to be identified.

You can't get these compounds in a pill or capsule—you
must eat fruits and vegetables. Cooking doesn't destroy these
compounds, and they are also present in juice.

THE RIGHT AMOUNT

There's no recommended daily allowance for nitrosamine blockers. Eat a wide variety of fruits and vegetables daily. I make it a point to eat a tomato or drink a glass of tomato juice daily.

POSSIBLE BENEFITS

Cancer Fighter • Researchers at Cornell University tested tomato juice on volunteers. After drinking the juice, the volunteers produced fewer cancer-causing nitrosamines. Although more studies need to be done, there is evidence that eating foods rich in nitrosamine blockers may help to prevent cancer.

PERSONAL ADVICE

Nitrites are added to cured meats such as bacon and hot dogs to prevent botulism and as a coloring agent. Try to buy nitrite-free products, which are available at many supermarkets and meat markets.

Nucleic Acids (DNA and RNA)

FACTS

DNA (deoxyribonucleic acid) and RNA (ribonucleic acid) are present in the nucleus of every cell in the body and are essential for the production of new cells, cell repair, and cell metabolism. As we age, cells begin to wear out and eventually die. When we're young, we grow new cells very quickly, but as we age, we replenish cells more slowly. Internally, our body systems begin to slow down, and externally, we begin to show signs of wear and tear. Some researchers believe that aging may be a result of a decline in the level or effectiveness of these important nucleic acids. The theory goes, if we replenish the lost nucleic acids, we may be able to halt or even reverse the aging process.

Good food sources of nucleic acids include Portuguese sardines (water packed), salmon, wheat germ, asparagus, mushrooms, and spinach. Nucleic acids are also available in supplement form at natural food stores.

THE RIGHT AMOUNT

Combinations of DNA and RNA are sold in tablet form at natural food stores. Take 1 to 3 tablets (up to 1500 milligrams) daily. I have been doing so for over thirty years.

Caution: Drink at least 8 glasses of fluid daily if you are taking nucleic acids in supplement form or are eating a diet rich in nucleic acids. RNA can raise uric acid levels, which may trigger gout in susceptible people. If you have a tendency to develop gout, do not take nucleic acids.

POSSIBLE BENEFITS

Longevity • A handful of studies suggest that nucleic acids may increase the life span of animals. For example, in one study reported in *The Journal of the American Geriatrics Society* almost two decades ago, five laboratory rats were given weekly injections of DNA and RNA, and five were untreated. The untreated mice died within 900 days; however, the treated mice lived between 1600 to 2250 days. Researchers also noted that the mice given nucleic acids looked healthier and were more alert than the other mice. More studies need to be done to confirm whether nucleic acids are truly a "fountain of youth."

There is anecdotal evidence, however, that nucleic acids may have a dramatic effect on humans. In his book, *Nucleic Acid Therapy in Aging and Degenerative Disease,* Benjamin Frank, M.D., reports on his experiences treating patients with nucleic acid therapy. Based on Dr. Frank's observations, patients given nucleic acid supplements showed a marked improvement in the color and texture of their skin, a reduction in age spots, and an increase in energy level.

Oat Bran

FACTS

Oat bran contains a compound called beta-glucan, a potent cho-lesterol-lowering agent. Beta-glucan is a form of soluble fiber.

Good sources of oat bran include oat bran cereal and high-fiber oatmeal. Instant oatmeal (the kind that cooks in the bowl) usually has less oat bran than regular oatmeal.

THE RIGHT AMOUNT

A bowl of oatmeal and an oat bran muffin daily can help reduce a high cholesterol level and keep normal cholesterol in check.

POSSIBLE BENEFITS

Heart Disease • There have been numerous studies docu-menting oat bran's ability to lower cholesterol. When combined with a normal low-fat diet, about 2 ounces of oats daily can re-duce cholesterol by 5 to 10 percent. Oat bran can also lower low-density lipoproteins, the "bad" cholesterol, and can raise high-density lipoproteins, the "good" cholesterol.

Diabetes • Researchers at the University of Kentucky have found that oat bran can help improve glucose and blood lipid levels in diabetics, helping diabetics reduce or eliminate their need for insulin.

Octacosanol

FACTS

Octacosanol is a natural substance present in small amounts in many vegetable oils. A popular commercially marketed form of octacosanol is made from wheat germ oil. Proponents of octacosanol contend that it is a treasure trove of phytochemicals that can increase energy, improve oxygen utilization, and even prevent heart disease. Octacosanol is an excellent source of another member of the anti-aging hot 100: vitamin E.

Good food sources of octacosanol include wheat germ, whole grains, and alfalfa.

THE RIGHT AMOUNT

Supplements of 1000 to 6000 micrograms per tablet are available at natural food stores. Take one daily.

POSSIBLE BENEFITS

Improves Stamina • Studies suggest that octacosanol may improve exercise performance in animals and humans. Octacosanol is believed to reduce oxygen debt, that is, it helps the body utilize oxygen more efficiently during times of stress. Therefore, if you use octacosanol, you're less likely to be huffing and puffing after a strenuous workout.

Heart Disease • Octacosanol contains plant sterols, compounds that have been shown to reduce cholesterol levels in animal and human studies. However, the high vitamin E content of octacosanol may also play a role in reducing cholesterol by preventing the oxidation of low-density lipoproteins, or "bad" cholesterol, which can lead to the clogging of important arteries.

Omega-3 Fatty Acids

FACTS

In the 1970s, scientists noticed an interesting phenomenon: although Eskimos consumed large amounts of fat daily, they had an exceptionally low rate of heart disease and cancer. But unlike Americans who also ate lots of fat—notably from meat and dairy—the predominant fat in the Eskimo diet was in the form of omega-3 fatty acids. Omega-3 is found primarily in marine plant life called *phytoplankton*, which is eaten by fatty fish, a mainstay of the Eskimo diet. On land, omega-3 is present in some plant food including flaxseed and purslane, a plant that is used in salads.

Since the 1970s, there have been hundreds of studies performed worldwide on omega-3 fatty acids. These studies have shown that omega-3 does indeed offer protection against heart disease and possibly many other ailments.

Omega-3 contains two polyunsaturated fats: decosahexaenioc acid and eicosapentaenoic acid.

Good sources include fish such as salmon, mackerel, albacore tuna, halibut, and sardines.

THE RIGHT AMOUNT

According to the National Heart and Lung Institute, eating as little as 1 gram of omega-3 fatty acids daily may reduce the risk of cardiovascular disease by as much as 40 percent. Omega-3 fatty acids are available in capsule form. Take 3 to 6 capsules daily.

Super eicosapentaenoic acid—a more concentrated form—is also available. Take three capsules daily.

Flaxseed oil capsules are another source of omega-3 fatty acids. Take 1 or 2 capsules (1000 milligrams) daily with meals.

However, fatty fish is the best source of omega-3 fatty acids. In fact, studies suggest that the whole fish may be more effective than simply taking an oil supplement.

Caution: Do not take omega-3 supplements if you are already taking a blood thinner (such as coumadin or heparin) or using aspirin daily without first consulting with your physician. Excessive amounts of omega-3 fatty acids may cause bleeding, which can result in hemorraghic stroke.

POSSIBLE BENEFITS

Heart Disease • Epidemiological studies document a lower rate of coronary artery disease among fish eaters among Greenland's Eskimo population and the Japanese.

Omega-3 fatty acids appear to have several positive effects on cardiovascular health. Omega-3 fatty acids are blood thinners and may help prevent the formation of blood clots that can lead to a heart attack. A recent study of fifteen thousand people in four communities in the United States demonstrated that an increased intake of fatty fish can make a positive difference in terms of cardiovascular health. In this study, researchers compared the level of clotting factors (proteins found in the blood that can contribute to the formation of clots) to the amount of fatty fish in people's diet. Those who ate even one additional daily serving of fish had lower levels of three clotting factors that have been implicated in the development of coronary artery disease. Those with the highest levels of omega-3 fatty acid intake had higher levels of a fourth protein, protein C, a natural anticoagulant.

Several studies have shown that omega-3 fatty acids can lower total cholesterol and triglycerides in people who also cut back on saturated fat. In a Danish study, pathologists who autopsied fatty abdominal tissue and coronary arteries of forty deceased people found a direct correlation between the amount of omega-3 fatty acids in the tissue and the degree of narrowing of the coronary arteries due to atherosclerosis. In other words, omega-3 fatty acids appear to prevent the formation of atherosclerotic plaque, which can hamper the flow of blood to the heart.

A recent animal study performed at Australia's Commonwealth Scientific and Industrial Research Organization in Adelaide investigated the effects of dietary fat on susceptibility to ventricular fibrillation, a potentially lethal heart arrhythmia. (Ventricular fibrillation may be responsible for as many as 250,000 deaths in the United States annually.) According to the study, animals who were fed fish oil were better able to withstand induced heart arrhythmias than animals fed sunflower oil. The researchers concluded that omega-3 fatty acids may help prevent heart arrhythmias in humans.

Stroke • A long-term Dutch study shows men who consumed more than 20 grams (about 0.67 ounce) of fish per day had a lower risk of stroke than those who ate less fish. This is believed to be the first reported finding between higher fish consumption and lower stroke risk.

Cancer Fighter • In numerous animal studies, omega-3 fatty acids have delayed the onset of tumors and decreased both the rate of growth, size, and number of tumors in animals in which cancer was induced. Interestingly enough, in similar studies, other forms of fat typically increased tumor growth.

Arthritis • Omega-3 fatty acids have an anti-inflammatory action in the human body, that is, they alter the biological pathways that trigger inflammation, which is responsible for the pain and stiffness of arthritis and other related conditions. In several studies, patients with rheumatoid arthritis reported a decrease in symptoms after taking omega-3 fatty acid supplements in addition to their nonsteroid antirheumatic drugs.

Diabetes • In a Dutch study of 175 older people (sixty-four to eighty-seven) for 3 years, those who ate fish were least likely to develop glucose intolerance, a common problem among older adults that can lead to diabetes.

Papain

FACTS

If you find yourself popping more and more antacids, you're not alone. As we age, our digestive system gets less efficient. As a result, indigestion is a common malady among people over fifty. Natural compounds such as papain, which is derived from pa-

paya, may help to quiet an angry gut. Papain contains two enzymes, papain and prolase, which help to break down protein.

THE RIGHT AMOUNT

Chewable papaya supplements are sold in natural food stores.
Chew 1 to 3 tablets ½ hour before eating.

POSSIBLE BENEFITS

Digestive Aid   •   In older people, indigestion is often due to
the inability of the body to produce enough hydrochloric acid
to break down food effectively. Although there has been little
scientific research in this area, anecdotal evidence suggests that
papain supplements may help improve digestion and reduce the
need for antacids.

PERSONAL ADVICE

If you're experiencing a great deal of gas or bloating, although
it's probably simple indigestion, it could be a symptom of another underlying problem. Check with your physician before
self-medicating.

Pectin

FACTS

Everyone has heard that an apple a day will keep the doctor
away. However, not everyone knows that pectin may be the reason why apples are so healthful. Pectin is a form of soluble fiber
found in fruits and vegetables. Recent studies suggest that
pectin may be a potent force against both cancer and heart disease.

Good food sources of pectin include apples, bananas, the
pulpy portion of grapefruit, dried beans, and root vegetables.

THE RIGHT AMOUNT

Try to eat some pectin-rich foods daily. If you have high cholesterol, consider taking pectin capsules, which are available at most natural food stores. Take 1 or 2 capsules after each meal. Pectin powder is also sold in natural food stores; sprinkle ½ ounce of pectin powder in your food. It is flavorless and adds body to yogurt, puddings, or fruit salads.

POSSIBLE BENEFITS

Heart Disease • Several forms of pectin appear to lower blood cholesterol levels. Researchers at the University of Florida gave twenty-seven people with high cholesterol either 3 tablespoons of powdered grapefruit pectin daily or a placebo. After 16 weeks, the group taking the pectin showed a 7.6 percent reduction in cholesterol and a 10.8 percent reduction in low-density lipoproteins, or "bad" cholesterol. The group taking the placebo showed no change. Although powdered grapefruit pectin is more potent than plain grapefruit, eating one or two whole grapefruits daily—not just the segments, but the pulpy portion between the segments—would probably also significantly lower cholesterol (in combination with a low-fat diet).

Carrot, which contains calcium pectate, also appears to be a cholesterol buster. In fact, according to the U.S. Department of Agriculture, eating two carrots a day may reduce total cholesterol levels by as much as 20 percent.

Eating two apples a day may keep the cardiologist away. A recent study showed that people who ate two apples daily can reduce total cholesterol by as much as 16 percent.

Cancer Fighter • Researchers at the University of Texas Health Science Center in San Antonio recently discovered that fiber may help to prevent colon cancer. The researchers fed laboratory rats a carcinogenic agent that predisposed them to develop colon cancer. One group of rats was fed a high-pectin diet, the other group was fed a normal diet. After 24 weeks, the group on the high-pectin diet had a significantly lower rate of colon cancer than those fed the regular diet. (In addition, the rats on the high-pectin diet had a 30 percent drop in choles-terol.) The pectin performed two roles: it increased the rate at which food passed through the gastrointestinal tract, which reduced the rat's exposure to carcinogens. Second, it bound with digestive bile, a derivative of cholesterol, thus reducing blood cholesterol levels.

Phytic Acid

FACTS

In the 1970s, researcher Denis Burkit published a now-famous study in which he showed that in third world countries where people ate a diet rich in plant foods, the rate of various forms of cancer was significantly lower than in the West. Dr. Burkit attributed the reduced rate of cancer to a higher intake of fiber, and soon Americans were loading up on bran and other sources of fiber. However, some researchers speculate that although fiber may be beneficial, the real hero may be phytic acid, a major ingredient in grains, nuts, and legumes (dried beans such as soybeans and lentils).

Phytic acid is an antioxidant; it protects cells against oxidative damage from free radicals or unstable oxygen molecules, which can cause mutations in DNA. Phytic acid is also a chelator, which means that it binds easily to metal, particularly iron. In the presence of oxygen, iron can create free radicals that attack DNA. Phytic acid can prevent this damage from occurring by binding with the iron, thus keeping it away from oxygen.

THE RIGHT AMOUNT

There is no recommended daily allowance for phytic acid. I recommend eating a diet rich in grains and legumes. Although nuts are an excellent source of phytic acid, they tend to be high in fat, so eat them sparingly.

POSSIBLE BENEFITS

Cancer Fighter • In several animal studies, phytic acid has
been shown to inhibit the growth of tumors, especially in the
colon. In one review of phytic acid published in *Free Radical Biology and Medicine* (Vol. 8, 1990) researchers noted that in populations where people eat high quantities of red meat, which is
rich in iron, "the simultaneous presence of phytate may act to
suppress iron-driven steps in carcinogenesis."

Potassium

FACTS

More than sixty million American adults have high blood pressure, which is a leading cause of heart attack and stroke. (High
pressure is characterized by a systolic pressure over 140, and a diastolic pressure over 90.) The older you are, the greater the risk
of developing this potentially lethal disease. There is strong evidence that dietary potassium intake may help to prevent high
blood pressure and may even be used to enhance the effect of
antihypertensive medications.

Potassium is an essential mineral that assists in muscle con-
traction and works with sodium to maintain the fluid and elec-
trolyte balance in body cells. Nerve and muscle function may
suffer when the sodium–potassium balance is off. Potassium is
also critical to maintaining a normal heartbeat. In cases of severe potassium deficiency, the heart can develop a dangerous
arrhythmia or irregular beat.

Potassium is found in fruits and vegetables and dairy products. Good sources include bananas, oranges, cantaloupe, dried
apricots, squash, and plain low-fat yogurt.

THE RIGHT AMOUNT

The Food and Nutrition Board of the National Academy of Sciences has estimated the minimum requirement for potassium for adults to be 2000 milligrams daily. Potassium is available in most high-potency multivitamin and multimineral preparations. Excess amounts (over 18 grams) can be toxic. (Ninety milligrams per tablet or capsule is the maximum dosage allowed by law. A banana contains 560 milligrams of potassium.)

If you consume large quantities of coffee, are taking diuretics, have severe diarrhea and/or vomiting, or have hypoglycemia (low blood sugar), you may be deficient in this mineral. People on very low calorie weight-loss diets may also have a potassium deficiency.

Caution: People with kidney disease should not take potassium supplement or consume foods high in potassium.

POSSIBLE BENEFITS

Lowers Blood Pressure • A recent Italian study reported in *The Annals of Internal Medicine* (115, 1991: 753–759) underscored the importance of eating a diet rich in potassium, especially if you have high blood pressure. Fifty-four patients with controlled hypertension were randomly assigned to one of two groups. One group was given advice aimed at increasing potassium intake through diet; the other remained on their usual diet. Potassium intake among both groups was checked monthly by referring to patient food dairies and urinary potassium excretion. At the end of the year, the group on the high-potassium diet found that they needed far less medicine to control their blood pressure than the group not eating potassium-rich foods. The researchers concluded "increasing the dietary potassium intake from natural foods is a feasible and effective measure to reduce antihypertensive drug treatment."

PERSONAL ADVICE

If you're taking medication for high blood pressure, don't discontinue it, but work with your physician to see if you can decrease your need for medication by increasing your potassium intake. Eating a banana and a baked potato daily can increase your potassium intake by 1200 milligrams.

Propolis

FACTS

Propolis is a by-product of honey. It is a resinous material made from leaf parts and tree bark that is used by honeybees to cement together their hives. For thousands of years, honey and its related products have been valued for their medicinal properties. Hippocrates used propolis to treat sores and ulcers. Nicholas Culpepper (1616–1654)—perhaps the most famous herbalist of all time—recommended propolis to be used externally on wounds. Modern herbalists use propolis to ease cold symptoms and soothe a sore throat. Recently, scientists worldwide have begun to recognize that propolis may not only be an effective treatment for minor ailments, but may help to prevent a very major one: cancer.

THE RIGHT AMOUNT

Propolis is available in many different forms. Honey is rich in propolis. Pure propolis is available in capsule form at natural food stores. Take 500-milligram capsules up to three times daily.

Propolis salve may be used externally on sores. Propolis lozenges (which have a pleasant, sweet taste) are good for a sore throat.

POSSIBLE BENEFITS

Cancer Fighter • For decades, proponents of natural foods have touted propolis for its anticancer properties. Recently, serious researchers have investigated these claims. Researchers at the American Health Foundation in Valhalla, New York, tested caffeic acid esters, a compound found in propolis, for potential use against cancer. In the study, rats were fed a potent carcinogen. Some of the rats were also fed caffeic acid esters from propolis. After 9 weeks, the rats given the propolis compounds showed significantly less precancerous changes in colon cells than the rats not fed the propolis. Based on this and similar studies, it appears as if propolis can inhibit the growth of cancerous cells in the colon. Other studies are needed to determine whether propolis is useful against other forms of cancer.

Anti-inflammatory • Propolis may be similar to aspirin in that it also blocks the enzymes that produce prostaglandins, natural hormonelike substances that can cause pain, fever, and inflammation.

Antiviral • Propolis is rich in bioflavonoids, substances that appear to help protect against viral invasion. Viruses are encased in a protective protein coat. Researchers believe that the flavonoids in propolis may inhibit an enzyme in the body that strips viruses of their protective coating, thus allowing the infection to spread to other cells. As people age and their immune system weakens, propolis may give the immune system a much-needed boost against common viruses that can cause colds and flu.

Prevents Gum Disease • Periodontal problems are common from middle age on. Very often, as people age, the gum line begins to recede, causing inflammation, bleeding, and infection. This can lead to the weakening of the bone structure in the mouth, which can result in tooth loss. Some researchers believe that the flavonoids in propolis not only reduce inflammation, but also strengthen the blood vessels in the gums, making them less prone to injury.

Protease Inhibitors

FACTS

Protease inhibitors are compounds that inhibit the action of certain enzymes that promote tumor growth. The National Cancer Institute is investigating protease inhibitors for their potential anticancer properties.

Protease inhibitors are abundant in legumes (soy beans in particular and other dried beans) and whole grains.

THE RIGHT AMOUNT

There is no recommended daily allowance for protease inhibitors. I recommend eating at least one food daily that contains protease inhibitors.

POSSIBLE BENEFITS

Cancer Fighter • Several animal studies have shown that protease inhibitors can inhibit the growth of cancer. For example, soybeans contain a unique protease inhibitor: the Bowman–Birk inhibitor (BBI), which has been shown to stop the spread of many different forms of cancer. For example, in rats fed a carcinogen known to induce colon cancer, adding BBI concentrate to their diet suppressed the formation of tumors in 100 percent of the animals. In another study of mice fed a carcinogen known to induce liver cancer, BBI suppressed the formation of tumors by 71 percent. The National Cancer Institute is now conducting human cancer prevention trials using BBI in people at high risk of developing cancer.

Psyllium Seed

FACTS

Ground psyllium seed is a popular cure for constipation, a problem that seems to be a common ailment among the older population. For years, doctors have recommended psyllium as a natural way to regulate bowel function in people with digestive disorders such as irritable bowel syndrome and chronic constipation.

In addition, psyllium is a highly effective and safe cholesterol-lowering agent.

THE RIGHT AMOUNT

I recommend a teaspoon to a tablespoon of psyllium daily in juice or water. Psyllium is sold in powder form in drug stores and natural food stores. In fact, psyllium is the active ingredient in over-the-counter medications such as Metamucil and Fibercon. Some psyllium products contains other herbs, including slippery elm bark and acidophilus, which can help ease some of the gas and bloating that can occur when you aren't used to psyllium. Check them out at your local natural food store.

Caution: Although it is rare, psyllium can cause allergic reactions in some sensitive individuals. If you are sensitive, talk to your physician before using psyllium. In addition, to prevent gas, drink 6 to 8 glasses of water daily.

POSSIBLE BENEFITS

Heart Disease • Several studies show that psyllium can lower blood cholesterol from high levels to safer levels. In one study, twenty-six men with cholesterol levels over 240 milligrams per deciliter were divided into two groups. (The range was 180 to 314 milligrams per deciliter.) One group was given 1 packet of Metamucil (3.4 grams) three times daily in water before each meal. At the end of 8 weeks, the average cholesterol level in the treatment group dropped to 211 milligrams per deciliter. The level of low-density lipoproteins, or "bad" cholesterol, also dropped substantially.

In another study by fiber expert James W. Anderson of the University of Kentucky Medical Service, forty-four people with elevated cholesterol levels were given either psyllium flake cereal or wheat bran flake cereal daily for 6 weeks. The results: the group eating the psyllium flake cereal had an average 12 percent drop in cholesterol, but the group eating the wheat bran had no change.

Quercetin

FACTS

Quercetin is a bioflavonoid, a group of compounds found in fruits and vegetables. Many bioflavonoids are now being studied for their ability to prevent disease.

Quercetin, an antioxidant, also may have antiviral properties when combined with vitamin C. Several studies suggest that quercetin may be a potent cancer fighter.

The best food sources of quercetin are yellow and red onions and shallots. High levels are also found in broccoli and zucchini.

THE RIGHT AMOUNT

There is no recommended daily allowance for quercetin. In addition, quercetin is also available in supplement form, often in combination with other bioflavonoids or antioxidants. The usual dose is 250 milligrams one or two times daily.

POSSIBLE BENEFITS

Cancer Fighter • In many studies, quercetin has been shown to block the action of a variety of natural and synthetic initiators or promoters of cancer cell development. In addition, quercetin appears to inhibit the growth of human tumor cells containing binding sites for type II estrogen, which may be responsible for some forms of cancer, including breast cancer.

Population studies have shown that people who eat a diet rich in onions and other allium vegetables have substantially lower rates of gastrointestinal cancers than people who don't. Scientists are not precisely sure why onion protects against cancer—they do contain many potentially beneficial phytochemicals—but high levels of quercetin may be a major factor.

Anti-allergy • An allergy is an inflammatory condition triggered by an allergen, any substance—either natural or synthetic—that causes an allergic antibody reaction in the body. In an allergic antibody reaction, the immune system mistakenly identifies a harmless substance as a dangerous invader and begins to produce chemicals against it, including histamine. Histamine is responsible for sneezing, an itchy nose, watery eyes, and some of the other unpleasant allergic symptoms. Studies show that quercetin prevents the release of histamine, thus inhibiting the allergic response. Interestingly enough, several other bioflavonoidlike substances are marketed as allergy medications. Quercetin may also be useful against asthma.

Reishi Mushroom

FACTS

Aging takes its toll on the immune system. As people age, their immune systems become less effective at identifying foreign agents and fighting against viruses and bacteria. As a result, they are more vulnerable to cancer, infections, and other related problems. Reishi mushroom, known for its powerful immune-stimulating properties, is one of the most revered foods in Japan.

THE RIGHT AMOUNT

Reishi is available as capsules at natural food stores. Take 1 capsule up to three times daily.

POSSIBLE BENEFITS

Immune Booster • Studies show that compounds found in reishi mushrooms can increase the activity of two types of immune cells that are necessary to fight against potentially troublesome organisms.

Cancer Fighter • Compounds found in reishi mushrooms inhibited the growth of tumors in laboratory mice, which suggests that they may play a similar role in humans.

Heart Disease • Studies show that reishi mushrooms can lower cholesterol and reduce blood pressure.

Resveratrol

FACTS

For centuries, people have been drinking to each other's good health over an alcoholic beverage. And since biblical times, alcohol, especially wine, has been used as a traditional medicine for a wide range of ailments. In recent years, scientists have noticed that moderate drinkers tend to live longer than teetotalers. In fact, in countries where a glass of wine or two is a routine part of a meal, such as France and Italy, the incidence of heart disease is much lower than in countries where wine is not consumed in such great volume. Puzzled as to why wine drinkers fared so much better than non–wine drinkers, scientists began to examine the chemistry of wine to see what, if anything, could be offering its beneficial effects. Japanese researchers recently identified an antifungal compound in grape skins called *resveratrol* that lowers the fat content in the livers of rats, thus lowering overall cholesterol. Many scientists believe that resveratrol may have the same effect on humans, which is why a drink or two of wine a day may keep the cardiologist away.

THE RIGHT AMOUNT

Drink 1 or 2 glasses of wine several times a week. If you are taking any medication, check with your physician before drinking any alcoholic beverage. Nonalcoholic wine is also available.

Caution: Too much wine counteracts any of its potential benefits. People who drink more than 1 or 2 glasses of wine per day are putting themselves at risk for developing cardiovascular and liver disease as well as other health problems. If you have a drinking problem, no amount of wine is safe for you.

POSSIBLE BENEFITS

Heart Healthy • Several major studies have confirmed that alcohol in general, and wine in particular, appears to protect against heart disease. A glass or two of wine can lower your blood pressure. Researchers recently discovered that resveratrol and other chemicals in wine are vasodilators, that is, they relax the blood vessels, allowing the blood to flow more easily.

Starting in 1978, a group of researchers at Kaiser Permanente Medical Center in Oakland, California, began a study to determine the effect of alcohol on coronary artery disease. The team collected information on 81,825 men and women. Over the next 10 years, the researchers monitored this group for deaths due to heart disease. The results: those who regularly drank alcoholic beverages had a lower rate of death from coronary artery disease, but those who drank wine had the lowest rate of all.

In yet other studies sponsored by the American Heart Association, people who consumed alcoholic beverages, especially wine, had up to 49 percent reduction in heart disease versus those who abstained.

Not only does alcohol appear to cut total cholesterol, but it also raises the rate of beneficial high-density lipoproteins (HDLs), or "good" cholesterol. People who drank at least 1 glass of wine daily have been found to have higher levels of HDL than non–wine drinkers. This is true for both men and women. In fact, for women, just 1 glass of wine daily is all it takes to raise HDLs; men require 2 glasses.

Riboflavin (Vitamin B$_2$)

FACTS

The primary function of this B vitamin is to work with other substances to metabolize carbohydrates, fats, and proteins for energy.

Riboflavin may also protect against certain forms of cancer and oxidative damage by free radicals.

People over fifty-five are at risk of developing a riboflavin deficiency, especially if they do not eat a well-rounded diet and do not take a vitamin supplement.

Good sources of riboflavin include no-fat or low-fat dairy products, eggs, and leafy vegetables. (Liver is also an excellent source of riboflavin. However, I don't recommend eating liver due to its high-cholesterol, high-fat content. Toxins—natural and synthetic—are also concentrated in liver.)

THE RIGHT AMOUNT

The recommended daily allowance (RDA) for riboflavin is 1.2 to 1.7 milligrams for adults. Riboflavin is included in most multivitamin supplements as well as in B-complex supplements. The usual dose is 100 to 300 milligrams.

Women who take estrogen need to take a B$_2$ supplement.

Riboflavin works best with vitamins B$_6$ and C and niacin.

POSSIBLE BENEFITS

Antioxidant • Riboflavin has antioxidant properties. It also works with the enzyme glutathione reductase to maintain glutathione, which fights against free radical damage. A particularly important role of riboflavin is to protect against oxidative damage during exercise when the demand for oxygen by the body increases.

Cancer Fighter • Low levels of this B vitamin may increase the risk of developing cancer of the esophagus, especially for people who chew tobacco or drink alcoholic beverages.

Healthy Eyes • Riboflavin can help to prevent damage to the cornea of the eye, which can result in cataracts.

Boosts Immunity • Riboflavin deficiency can decrease the number of T cells, an important component of the immune system. Low levels of T cells may increase the risk of developing cancer and other diseases.

For Active Women • Studies show that active older women may require higher levels of riboflavin than the RDA. Researchers at Cornell University recently studied the effect of riboflavin levels on exercise in women ages sixty to seventy. For 8 weeks, these women exercised for up to 25 minutes daily on a stationary bicycle. Half the group was given the RDA for riboflavin, the other half was given 150 percent of the RDA. Blood levels of B_2 dropped in the women who were given only the RDA. Researchers concluded that older women who exercise regularly may need extra riboflavin.

Saw Palmetto

FACTS

Native Americans ate the berries of the saw palmetto plant by the handful. Known by the botanical name *Serenoa repens*, naturopaths and herbalists in the United States and Europe have long used saw palmetto berries to treat problems of the genitourinary tract in both sexes. In fact, saw palmetto is a folk remedy for so-called honeymoon cystitis, a condition caused by too much sexual activity. This herb was also touted as an aphrodisiac. Today, in Germany, extract of saw palmetto is a leading treatment for benign prostate hypertrophy (enlarged prostate) and is reputed to be so successful that American doctors are taking a second look at this "archaic" medicine.

THE RIGHT AMOUNT

Saw palmetto is available in extract or capsule form at most health food stores and herb shops. Mix 30 to 60 drops in liquid daily, or take 1 to 3 capsules.

POSSIBLE BENEFITS

Prostate • In men, the prostate gland is a walnut-size organ surrounding the urethra, which is located at the neck of the bladder. By age fifty, most men develop a slightly enlarged prostate, a benign condition that can result in excessive urination, especially at night, or difficulty in passing urine. Benign prostate hypertrophy is believed to be caused by an excess buildup of testosterone, the male hormone, in the prostate. Excess testosterone is converted into dihydrotestosterone, a more potent form of the hormone that can promote cell growth, thus leading to the enlargement. Excess levels of testosterone are also believed to be linked to cancer of the prostate. Several scientific studies have shown that saw palmetto extracts can alter the biological pathways that lead to the conversion of testosterone to dihydrotestosterone. In addition, by preventing the more potent testosterone from binding to receptor sites on the cells, it may help rid the body of this potentially dangerous hormone.

Saw palmetto may not only help to prevent enlargement of the prostate, but has proven to be an effective treatment for this condition. In a 1984 study published in *The British Journal of Pharmacology*, 110 patients suffering from enlarged prostate were either given saw palmetto extract or a placebo for 30 days. Patients on saw palmetto experienced a significant reduction in symptoms, such as fewer nighttime urinations (down by 45 percent) and improved urine flow. Those on the placebo showed little change in their condition.

PERSONAL ADVICE

If you have discomfort or difficulty with urination or pass blood with your urine, check with your physician. Don't self-diagnose. However, if your physician confirms that you have benign prostate hypertrophy, try using saw palmetto to see if it helps. If you don't see any improvement within a month or so, talk to your physician about medication. Proscar, a relatively new drug, has been quite effective in treating an enlarged prostate. However, Proscar is quite expensive and may run up to several hundred dollars a year; saw palmetto extract costs a lot less and, in some cases, may work just as well.

Schizandra

FACTS

This highly prized Chinese herb is fast becoming a best-seller in the United States because of its reputation as a longevity herb and aphrodisiac. Since ancient times, schizandra has been favored among the wealthy Chinese. Until recently, this herb has been rare and expensive, but today it is widely available in China and the United States. Herbal healers have used schizandra to treat lung disorders, and recent studies show that extracts from this herb are effective against the bacteria that causes tuberculosis.

Similar to ginseng, schizandra is also believed to increase stamina and relieve fatigue. It is also used to treat stress and depression. According to one study, polo horses given schizandra performed better and showed better physiological responses to stress after taking the herb.

THE RIGHT AMOUNT

Schizandra is available in capsules at natural food stores. Take 1 to 3 capsules daily.

POSSIBLE BENEFITS

Liver • Animal studies have shown that this herb can help protect the liver from toxins, thus helping to preserve this vital organ.

Aphrodisiac • In China, schizandra is highly regarded as an aphrodisiac for both sexes. According to Ron Teeguarden, author of *Chinese Tonic Herbs*, "it relieves fatigue and is quite famous for increasing the sexual staying power in men." Teeguarden notes schizandra does no less for women, adding that it is reputed to cause "the female genitals to feel warm, healthy and extremely sensitive."

Seaweed

FACTS

Seaweed, also known as algae, is a primitive, plantlike organism that grows in the sea. Although seaweed is still considered exotic fare in the United States, it is a dietary mainstay in Japan.

Dietary seaweed is sold in the United States in Asian and natural food stores. There are several varieties of seaweed, or algae, differentiated by their color. Nori, a red seaweed, is used to wrap sushi. Popular forms of brown seaweed include kelp, wakame, arme, and kombu.

Traditional Chinese healers have used hot water extracts of seaweed to treat cancer. Not surprisingly, recent studies show that compounds in seaweed may protect against cancer.

THE RIGHT AMOUNT

There's no recommended daily allowance or study that specifies the correct amount of seaweed needed to prevent cancer. However, in Japan, where the cancer rate is a fraction of that in the United States, most people eat some form of seaweed daily. In fact, the estimated per capital intake of seaweed in Japan ranges from 4.9 to 7.3 grams daily (that's roughly ¼ ounce).

POSSIBLE BENEFITS

Cancer Fighter • Japanese scientists isolated several polysaccharides, potentially anticarcinogenic compounds, in seaweed. Fucoidin, one of these compounds, may prove to be a potent cancer fighter. Several studies show that these compounds in seaweed may have a dramatic impact on cancer. In one study, laboratory mice were injected with cancer cells. One group of mice received an extract from marine algae, the other group was given water without the extract. The life span of the treated mice was 37 percent longer than that of the control animals. Researchers speculate that the seaweed may somehow boost the body's immunological defenses against tumor growth. However, test tube studies also show that seaweed extract can prevent or slow down the growth of cancer cells outside the body, which suggests that it may also inhibit the growth of cells on its own.

Selenium

FACTS

It wasn't until the 1950s that researchers recognized that this mineral played a vital role in the human body. In recent years, selenium has become a superstar among minerals because of its reputed ability to prevent cancer and heart disease.

Selenium is an antioxidant. It works with glutathione peroxidase to prevent damage by free radicals. Selenium is also involved in the metabolism of prostaglandins, hormonelike substances used by the body in many different ways.

In the body, selenium detoxifies metals, such as arsenic and mercury, that would otherwise be lethal.

Selenium is synergistic with vitamin E, which means that the two combined increase the potency of each other.

Good food sources of selenium include garlic, onions, tuna, herring, broccoli, wheat germ, whole grains, sesame seeds, red grapes, egg yolks, and mushrooms. The selenium content in food varies from region to region due to differing levels of selenium in the soil.

THE RIGHT AMOUNT

The recommended daily allowance is 50 to 100 micrograms. I recommend 200 micrograms daily. Some cancer researchers feel that 300 micrograms per day is needed. Selenium can be toxic in high doses; therefore, do not exceed 300 micrograms daily. (Studies have shown that toxicity may occur at levels of 2400 micrograms daily for a prolonged period of time. However, I suggest that we err on the side of caution until we know precisely what levels are safe.)

POSSIBLE BENEFITS

Cancer Fighter • Population studies show that the rate of cancer deaths can be directly correlated to the selenium intake in food: people who eat the least amount of selenium have the highest rates of cancer. For example, in Japan where the daily selenium intake is 500 micrograms, the cancer rate is more than five times lower than it is in countries where the selenium intake is half that amount. Researchers have also found higher blood levels of selenium in healthy people as opposed to cancer patients.

Many animal studies confirm that selenium can prevent cancerous growths. Some studies show that selenium actually protects cell membranes from attack by free radicals that may explain its ability to ward off cancer.

Cardiovascular Health • Selenium may also protect lipids from oxidation, a process that may contribute to the formation of atherosclerotic lesions in the coronary arteries. Selenium may also help to prevent blood clots which can cause a stroke. Studies have linked a low selenium intake to a higher rate of both heart attack and stroke. In Colorado Springs, Colorado, which can boast the highest selenium soil content in the United States, the death rate due to heart disease is 67 percent below the national average.

Anti-inflammatory • Selenium appears to have some anti-inflammatory properties. In fact, selenium in combination with vitamin E has been used to treat arthritis in animal studies. Some people swear that selenium can help reduce the pain and stiffness of arthritis.

Male Potency • Men need this mineral! Selenium is necessary for sperm production. Almost half of a male's supply of selenium is concentrated in the testicles and portions of the seminal ducts adjacent to the prostate gland. Selenium is reputed to increase the male sex drive.

Sesame

FACTS

No reputable Asian chef would be caught without his or her bottle of sesame oil, a commonly used seasoning in the Orient. Asians may use sesame oil because of its delicate, nutty flavor. Westerners, however, may turn to sesame oil as a painless way to help prevent cancer and heart disease.

THE RIGHT AMOUNT

Sprinkle a few drops of sesame oil in stir-fry dishes.

POSSIBLE BENEFITS

Cancer Fighter • Sesame seeds and oil are an excellent source of phytic acid, an antioxidant that may prevent the kind of cellular damage that can lead to cancer. In addition, Japanese studies have shown that sesame oil may protect against colon cancer. In animal studies, sesame oil added to the diet of rats reduced the amount of bile acids in the feces. Bile acids are believed to produce cancerous changes in cells of the intestinal wall, which could cause colon cancer.

Heart Disease • Sesamin, a lignin from sesame oil, significantly reduced the amount of serum and liver cholesterol in rats fed a normal diet. Researchers speculate that sesamin may help keep cholesterol levels under control in humans.

Solanaceous Foods

FACTS

Mediterranean countries, such as Crete and Greece, have a much lower rate of heart disease and cancer than Western countries. Perhaps these countries can attribute their good health to their high intake of solanaceous foods. The solanaceous family, which includes tomatoes, eggplant, and peppers, is being investigated by the National Cancer Institute for its potential cancer-preventive properties. These foods are a mainstay of Mediterranean cuisine and are found in abundance in nearly every meal. Solanaceous foods are also an excellent source of vitamins, minerals, and fiber.

THE RIGHT AMOUNT

I recommend eating at least one serving of solanceous food daily. You can't get these critical phytochemicals in a vitamin pill; you must eat the whole food!

Caution: Some people with arthritis may find that peppers and tomatoes may aggravate their condition.

POSSIBLE BENEFITS

Cancer Fighter • Out of the fourteen possible phytochemicals known or believed to possess anticancer activity, the solanaceous family has seven of these important compounds including flavonoids, glucarates, carotenoids, courmarins, monoterpenes, triterpenes, and phenolic acids. Researchers believe that each of these compounds may intercede at various stages of cancer development. Some compounds may block a carcinogen that can initiate cancer, that is, a substance that alters a healthy cell, making it susceptible to cancerous growth. Others may block a cancer promoter, the substance that stimulates the altered cell to grow.

Soybeans

FACTS

For a book full of information about these wonderful legumes, see *Earl Mindell's Soy Miracle*. The National Cancer Institute is giving top priority to investigating the potential cancer-fighting properties of soybeans, and several studies have shown that soy may protect against heart disease. Anyone who wants to live longer should be eating this food.

The Japanese, who live longer than any other nationality on earth, eat lots of soy. In fact, by the turn of the century, 20 percent of all Japanese will be sixty-five or over as compared with about 13 percent of people in the United States. Some researchers believe that Japanese longevity may be due to the fact that the typical Japanese diet is rich in soy foods, products derived from soybeans. Tofu, a bean curd made from dried soybeans, and miso, a soup made from soy paste, are staples in the Japanese diet.

Ironically, the United States—not Japan—is the world's leading producer of soy. Although soy is not as popular in the United States as it is in Japan, soy-based foods are popping up in natural food stores and supermarkets across the country. Rich in protein, soy is an extremely versatile food that can be used in many different ways. Soy milk is used in formula for infants who are allergic to cow's milk. Rehydrated textured vegetable protein, a soy product sold in natural food stores, can be used as a substitute for ground beef in dishes such as chili or tacos. Soy flour can be used to make everything from muffins to pancakes. Tofu, which is flavorless and odorless, assumes the flavor of other foods and spices and can be made into everything from a frozen dessert resembling ice cream to a mock egg salad.

THE RIGHT AMOUNT

I recommend eating at least one soy product daily, and substituting soy milk for cow's milk. I make a soy milk shake for breakfast every morning.

POSSIBLE BENEFITS

Heart Disease • Recent studies show that adding soy to your diet may be one of the most effective ways to lower cholesterol. A group headed by researcher Susan M. Potter at the University of Illinois at Urbana-Champaign, tested the effects of soy protein consumption on twenty-six men with moderately high cholesterol. The men replaced 50 percent of their normal daily protein consumption with 50 grams of soy protein. The protein was baked into foods such as muffins, cookies, and breads. At the end of 4 weeks, each man had an average reduction in total cholesterol of 12 percent, thus reducing their risk of heart disease by 25 percent.

Although soy is not typically used as a cholesterol-lowering treatment in the United States, according to Dr. Potter, it is the primary cholesterol reduction treatment in Italy. Based on the study at the University of Illinois, it appears as if soy protein may be as effective a treatment as some of the medications that are prescribed for hypercholesterolemia, which have many dangerous and unpleasant side effects. If you have high cholesterol, you may want to talk to your doctor about trying a soy regime before taking medication.

Cancer Fighter • There are several compounds in soy that may help to prevent cancer. Soy contains phytochemicals called *lignans* and *isoflavonoids*, two compounds that are converted in the intestine into an estrogenlike substance called *ekuol*. Ekuol competes with a more potent form of estrogen, estradiol, for space on estrogen receptors on some cells. If the estradiol has no place to bind, it becomes deactivated. Many researchers believe that estradiol promotes the growth of tumors, especially in the breast. (Japanese women, who typically eat lots of soy, have a much lower rate of breast cancer than American women. In Japan, 6 out of 100,000 women will develop breast cancer in their lifetime versus 24 out of 100,000 in the United States.)

Soy may have a similar effect on the hormonal balance in men: American men are four times more likely to develop cancer of the prostate than Japanese men. Prostate cancer is believed to be caused by high levels of a potent form of testosterone, which may be deactivated by lignans and isoflavonoids. There may be other factors contributing to the disparity in cancer rates—Japanese men eat a diet that is much lower in fat and red meat—however, the phytochemicals in soy may also offer some protection.

Genistein is another compound in soy that is believed to be a potent cancer fighter. Genistein blocks angiogenesis, the process in which new blood vessels grow, thus literally "starving" malignant tumors from the nutrients needed to help them grow.

Menopause • In Japan, hot flashes and other unpleasant symptoms of menopause due to lower estrogen levels are a rarity. In fact, few Japanese women take estrogen replacement therapy, a common treatment for menopause in the United States. Soy researcher Herman Aldercreutz of the University of Helsinki suggested in a letter to *The New England Journal of Medicine* that the hormonelike properties of the phytochemicals in soy may be one reason why Japanese women have an easier time with menopause than American women.

Sulforaphane

FACTS

Sulforaphane is a *phytochemical,* a biologically active compound found in many cruciferous vegetables (e.g., broccoli, brussels sprouts, kale, and cauliflower) and also in carrots and green onions. According to researchers at Johns Hopkins School of Medicine, sulforaphane may be the most powerful natural anticancer compound discovered to date.

THE RIGHT AMOUNT

There is no recommended daily allowance for sulforaphane. I recommend two servings (2 cups) of sulforaphane-rich foods daily.

POSSIBLE BENEFITS

Cancer Fighter • Vegetables contain chemicals that promote the formation of different enzymes in humans. Some of these enzymes (phase I) are "bad guys": they actually convert benign substances into oxidants, which can damage a cell's DNA, thus promoting the risk of cancer. In response to the oxidant threat, cells can also make phase II enzymes, the so-called good guys who protect the cells' vulnerable genetic material from the bad guys. Many foods, such as hamburger, cause cells to create both good and bad enzymes. However, researchers at Johns Hopkins discovered that sulforaphane promotes the production of only phase II good enzymes, thus helping the body to ward off potential carcinogens. Although there may be other foods that also trigger the production of only phase II enzymes, the researchers suspect that sulforaphane may create even higher levels of good enzymes than these other foods.

In animal studies, sulforaphane has been shown to protect against cancer. In one study, scientists pretreated twenty-nine rats with a synthetic version of sulforaphane and then injected them with a carcinogen known to induce mammary tumors. The scientists then injected twenty-five other rats with the carcinogen without pretreating them with the sulforaphane. More than two-thirds of the group that did not receive the sulforaphane treatment eventually developed mammary cancers as opposed to only 35 percent of the group that received a low dose of sulforaphane. Out of the rats that received a high dose of sulforaphane, only 26 percent went on to develop cancer. More studies are needed to determine if sulforaphane will have the same effect on women.

Thiamine (Vitamin B$_1$)

FACTS

Thiamine, known as vitamin B$_1$, breaks down and converts carbohydrates into glucose, which provides energy for the body. Thiamine is necessary for the normal functioning of the nervous system, heart, and other muscles.

Gross thiamine deficiency will lead to beriberi, a life-threatening disease that commonly used to afflict sailors. Today, beriberi is rare; however, mild thiamine deficiency is common among older people.

Mild thiamine deficiency can lead to lack of energy, moodiness, numbness in the legs, mild depression, loss of appetite, and a general apathy among other symptoms.

Good food sources of thiamine include brewer's yeast, rice husks, unrefined cereal grains, sunflower seeds, pecans, lean pork, green peas, organic meats, most vegetables, and milk. However, thiamine is easily destroyed by exposure to light and heat.

THE RIGHT AMOUNT

The recommended daily allowance for thiamine for adults is 1.0 to 1.5 milligrams. Thiamine can be destroyed by alcohol; alcoholics and heavy drinkers are at risk of thiamine deficiency. Thiamine is usually included in B-complex supplements and multivitamins.

If you use antacids or aspirin on a regular basis, you may need extra thiamine.

Thiamine has no known toxic effects.

POSSIBLE BENEFITS

Heart Disease • Thiamine is essential for the normal function of the heart. Serious thiamine deficiencies may lead to potentially fatal heart arrhythmias and heart failure. Given the fact that heart disease is the number one killer in the United States and studies show that thiamine deficiency is not uncommon among the elderly, it's critical for older adults to maintain normal thiamine levels.

Antistress • In times of physical or emotional stress, your intake of B vitamins, including thiamine, should be increased. In my experience, many people find that thiamine along with other B vitamins can help alleviate symptoms of stress such as mild depression.

Tocopherol (Vitamin E)

FACTS

A physician friend who is highly skeptical about all forms of vitamin supplements recently confessed that she is beginning to have second thoughts about vitamin E. "I've noticed that among my older patients, those who take vitamin E are the most together, healthiest people in my practice," she said. "It finally dawned on me that there must be something to this vitamin E."

A lot of people, many of them M.D.s, have reached the same conclusion. Sales of vitamin E have soared, and it is now enjoying superstar status among its fellow micronutrients. However, vitamin E is no overnight success; it took more than 70 years for the medical community to begin to take it seriously.

Vitamin E was first discovered in 1922 when researchers noticed, quite by accident, that rats could not breed without it. They dubbed this substance *tocopherol*, from the Greek "to bring forth in childbirth." They are actually eight different types of tocopherol, of which alpha-tocopherol is the most effective.

Vitamin E is a fat-soluble vitamin, which means that unlike water-soluble vitamins, it is not excreted in the urine, but stored in the liver.

Vitamin E is potent antioxidant; it has been dubbed the body's first line of defense against lipid peroxidation—that means it protects polyunsaturated fatty acids in the cell membrane from free radical attack.

Vitamin E is found in vegetable oils, whole grains, sweet potatoes, wheat germ, brown rice, nuts, and other foods.

Vitamin E is synergistic with selenium (another Hot 100 antioxidant), which means that the two combined greatly enhance each other's potency.

THE RIGHT AMOUNT

The recommended daily allowance for vitamin E is 8 to 10 international units; however supplements usually come in 100-international-unit strength. I recommend at least 400–800 international units of vitamin E daily. (With this vitamin, 1 international unit is equivalent to 1 milligram.)

Caution: Do not take vitamin E if you are taking a blood thinner such as aspirin or have vitamin K deficiency. If you've had a bleeding problem in the past, talk to your physician before taking vitamin E.

POSSIBLE BENEFITS

Heart Disease • In the 1970s, two Canadian physicians, Drs. Wilfred and Evan Shute, promoted vitamin E as a weapon against heart disease in their best-selling book, *Vitamin E for Ailing and Healthy Hearts.* Most cardiologists ridiculed the notion that a mere vitamin could be a powerful heart medicine. They're no longer laughing. Several recent studies have shown that a link between daily vitamin E consumption and a lowered risk of heart disease in both men and women. In May 1993, *The New England Journal of Medicine* reported the results of an 8-year study involving more than 87,000 registered female nurses and a related study involving close to 40,000 male health professionals. In both studies, participants who consumed vitamin E supplements (of at least 100 international units or more) for a minimum of 2 years had a 40 percent lower risk of heart disease than those who derived vitamin E through diet alone. At first, researchers suspected that people taking vitamin E may be more health conscious and therefore have healthier habits, which could also account for the reduction in heart disease. However, even after factoring in lifestyle, the vitamin E supplement appeared to be the primary difference between the group who developed heart disease and the group who remained disease free.

In another study sponsored by the American Heart Association, researchers found that long-term supplementation with high doses of vitamin E (160 milligrams) decreased the susceptibility of low-density lipoproteins, or "bad" cholesterol, to oxidation by 30 to 50 percent. (When low-density lipoproteins oxidize, they may contribute to the formation of atherosclerotic lesions in arteries supplying blood to the heart and other vital organs. A heart attack occurs when blood supply is cut off from the heart.)

Vitamin E is also a natural blood thinner and may prevent the formation of blood clots. If a clot enters the bloodstream and lodges in an artery feeding the brain, it could result in a stroke; if the clot lodges into a coronary artery, it could result in a heart attack.

Many cardiac surgeons give coronary bypass patients high doses of vitamin E prior to surgery. A recent study of coronary bypass patients performed at the Mayo Clinic in Rochester, Minnesota, found that patients given 2000 international units of vitamin E prior to surgery had much lower blood levels of free radicals after surgery than patients who had not been given the supplemental E. They also found that patients who had been given additional vitamin E had normal blood levels of E following surgery, whereas the unsupplemented patients had lower than normal levels.

Cancer Fighter • There is growing evidence that vitamin E may protect against various forms of cancer. A study sponsored by the National Cancer Institute suggests that people who take a vitamin E supplement for a minimum of six months cut their risk of developing oral cancers in half. Factors known to increase the risk of oral cancers, such as alcohol consumption, smoking, and dietary habits, made no difference in the outcome. These findings are consistent with animal studies that showed that vitamin E reduced the effects of carcinogens on cheek cells in hamsters.

Another study performed at the Biodynamics Institute at Louisiana State University showed that vitamin E may protect humans against the harmful effects of chronic exposure to ozone in smog. The study suggests that vitamin E's potent antioxidant activity may guard against the biological damage inflicted by ozone on lung tissue.

Vitamin E may also help to prevent stomach cancer and other cancers of the gastrointestinal tract by inhibiting the conversion of nitrates, which are found in food, to nitrosamines in the stomach. Nitrosamines are potentially carcinogenic.

Diabetes • In a recent Italian study, daily vitamin E supplements (900 milligrams for 4 months) helped people with type II diabetes better use insulin. Type II diabetes—also known as adult- or late-onset diabetes—accounts for 90 percent of all cases of diabetes and occurs during middle age and beyond. People with this form of diabetes can develop dangerously high levels of glucose in the blood. Based on this study, vitamin E appeared to help maintain normal blood glucose levels. (If you have diabetes, check with your physician before using vitamin E or any other medication.)

Immunity   •   Studies have shown that older people with low blood serum levels of vitamin E are more vulnerable to developing infections. A recent study in *The American Journal of Clinical Nutrition* showed that short-term supplementation with high doses of vitamin E can enhance immune responsiveness in healthy individuals over sixty. In the study, thirty-two healthy older adults who were not taking any vitamin supplements or prescription medication were either given 800 milligrams of vitamin E daily for 3 days or a placebo. Based on blood and skin tests, those taking the vitamin E showed a dramatic boost in immune function. Those taking the placebo did not show any change. Considering the fact that immune function declines as we age, this is a particularly important finding.

Brain   •   Researchers at the Neurological Institute at Columbia University College of Physicians and Surgeons in New York gave patients with tardive dyskinesia (a neurological disorder that can result from long-term use of antipsychotic medications) vitamin E supplements along with antipsychotic medications. The group taking the vitamin E showed improvement in tremors and a reduction in anxiety and depression. Researchers are considering using antioxidant vitamins including E on patients with Parkinson's disease, another neurologic disorder that often affects the elderly.

Skin   •   For decades, vitamin E fans have claimed that if used directly on the skin, vitamin E oil can help prevent the signs of aging. A recent study suggests that vitamin E may reduce the severity of wrinkles. In the study, twenty middle-aged women were given a 5 percent strength cream of vitamin E to put on their skin daily. At the end of 4 weeks, the women showed a 50 percent reduction in the length and depth of crow's feet; although the wrinkles were still there, they looked better. However, many cosmetic creams that tout vitamin E as an ingredient actually contain very little E. Use only creams that list vitamin E or tocopherol near the top of the ingredient list, which means that it is a primary ingredient. Do not use the oil from the vitamin E capsule directly on the skin; it can cause irritation in many people.

Protects Against Muscle Damage • Although vigorous exercise is good for your heart, it may also promote muscle damage due to oxidation. (Remember, as you exercise, your body's demand for oxygen increases—the more oxygen, the greater the risk of oxidation.) However, according to a study at the Human Nutrition Research Center on Aging at Tufts University, a daily vitamin E supplement may help protect against free radical damage caused by working out.

Eyes • Researchers suspect that cataracts, which cloud the eye lens, may be caused by oxidative damage to the lens covering of the eye and that vitamin E may help protect the eye from this kind of damage. A recent study suggests that they may be right. Finnish researchers discovered that people with low blood serum levels of vitamin E (and also beta-carotene, another member of the Hot 100) were twice as likely to develop cataracts as those with higher levels.

Arthritis • Studies suggest that vitamin E supplements may relieve some of the symptoms of osteoarthritis. Arthritis has been associated with elevated levels of free radicals.

Anecdotal Evidence • Many people swear that vitamin E helps to prevent their hair from turning gray. Recently, an Ohio physician even wrote a letter to the *New York Times* describing how he and his patients keep their hair from turning gray by taking vitamin E. Although there's no evidence to prove that vitamin E helps to keep the gray away, I've heard it from enough people to make me wonder whether there's any truth to it.

Tretinoin

FACTS

Marketed under the name Retin-A, tretinoin, a form of topical vitamin A, was approved by the Food and Drug Administration over 20 years ago as a treatment for severe acne. Dermatologists observed that this cream not only helped rid their patients of acne, but it also appeared to help erase fine lines and wrinkles. By the late 1980s, tretinoin was being touted as a miracle cream, and it quickly became one of the most frequently prescribed topical medications. In recent years, tretinoin has been eclipsed by the growing popularity of alpha-hydroxy acids and other hot, new "cosmetceuticals." Tretinoin has its shortcomings: its effectiveness peaks after about 24 months of use. In addition, if you stop using it, the changes begin to fade. Despite these problems, tretinoin is still one of the most effective anti-aging skin products on the market.

THE RIGHT AMOUNT

Apply cream as directed by your physician.

Caution: Most users experience skin peeling or irritation at least initially. Tretinoin must be used in conjunction with a sunscreen because it makes the skin more prone to sun damage. High doses of oral vitamin A have been associated with birth defects. Although there is no evidence that topical vitamin A can cause similar problems, women who are pregnant or trying to conceive should not use tretinoin.

POSSIBLE BENEFITS

Skin Rejuvenator • As we age, skin tends to thin out and become dryer. Wrinkles develop when collagen and elastin, proteins in the skin that provide elasticity, begin to break down. Studies have shown that tretinoin can increase skin thickness, improve circulation, and increase collagen. (Collagen is the "glue" that holds cells together.) Tretinoin appears to help plump out the skin, erasing fine lines and wrinkles. After about 6 weeks of use, many people find that their skin looks pinker and fresher. (However, tretinoin is ineffective against deep wrinkles.)

Turmeric

FACTS

Turmeric is an herb that adds flavor and color to many foods, including curry powder and sauces. In the West, turmeric has been used primarily as a spice. In Asia, however, this herb has a rich medicinal history. Westerners are just beginning to discover this herb's potential as a longevity booster.

Turmeric is a "heart healthy" herb that may help prevent heart disease. It is also a natural anti-inflammatory.

THE RIGHT AMOUNT

Turmeric is available in capsule and tablet form. Take 1 to 3 capsules or tablets daily.

POSSIBLE BENEFITS

Heart Disease • Studies show that turmeric can lower blood cholesterol levels. Turmeric stimulates the production of bile by the liver. Cholesterol is a component of bile, thus, when the liver produces bile, it utilizes excess cholesterol.

Turmeric also prevents the formation of dangerous blood clots that can lead to heart attack or stroke. In fact, as Daniel Mowrey noted in his book, *Next Generation Herbal Medicine*, people who live in countries where curry is frequently eaten have a much lower level of thrombosis (blood clots) than people who live in Western countries.

Arthritis • Traditional healers have used turmeric to reduce the inflammation and pain associated with arthritis. Based on anecdotal evidence, I believe that some people may find that turmeric may indeed help control arthritis.

Umbelliferous Vegetables

FACTS

In an article that appeared in *Food Technology*, Alegria Caragay, Ph.D., an advisor to the Designer Food Program for the National Cancer Institute (NCI), wrote, "Within the last decade, as research into the relationship between diet and cancer has proliferated, so, too, has the body of data from both epidemiological and animal studies that indicates vegetables, grains, and fruits may contain certain cancer-preventing substances." In the article, Dr. Caragay noted that umbelliferous vegetables were at the top of the NCI's list of foods with potentially important anticancer properties. In fact, the NCI is pouring millions of dollars into researching these foods.

Umbelliferous vegetables include carrots, celery, and parsnips.

THE RIGHT AMOUNT

Umbelliferous vegetables contain six important phytochemicals that may help prevent cancer and heart disease. You can't get these compounds in a pill, you must eat the whole food. People who want to live longer and live healthier should make sure that umbelliferous vegetables are included in their diets.

POSSIBLE BENEFITS

Cancer Fighter • Umbelliferous vegetables contain compounds that can thwart the initiation and spread of cancer such as the following:

> *Flavonoids.* These compounds help protect cell membranes against oxidation and may deactivate potent hormones that can trigger the growth of tumors.
> *Carotenoids.* These compounds help protect cells against oxidative damage that can damage DNA.
> *Coumarins.* These compounds may block the action of car-

cinogens before they can damage healthy cells, which can cause these cells to mutate.

Phenolic acids. These compounds may block the action of hormonelike compounds called *prostagladins*, which can promote the growth of tumors.

Heart Disease • Umbelliferous vegetables are rich in antiox-idants—carotenoids such as beta-carotene, flavonoids, and phenolic acids. Studies have shown that people who take antioxidants daily have lower rates of heart disease than those who do not. Researchers believe that antioxidants may prevent the oxidation of low-density lipoproteins, or "bad" cholesterol, which may promote atherosclerosis, or hardening of the arteries.

Vitex

FACTS

Vitex, an herb that dates back to ancient times, is being redis-covered by a generation of modern women who are seeking a natural approach to menopause. Also called *chaste tree* or *chasteberry*, vitex was used by the early Greeks who believed that it could dampen sexual desire. According to *The New Age Herbalist*, in Italy the flowers of this plant are still strewn in the path of novices when they first enter the monastery or convent, presumably because of vitex's reputation as an anti-aphrodisiac. Folklore aside, there is no evidence that vitex has any effect whatsoever on libido; however, this herb does appear to have a positive effect on the female reproductive system and is used to treat a wide variety of "female complaints."

THE RIGHT AMOUNT

Vitex is available in capsule form at natural food stores. Take 1 capsule up to three times daily. Vitex is also included in many herbal formulas for women.

POSSIBLE BENEFITS

Menopause • Herbalists have traditionally used vitex to treat symptoms associated with menstrual problems such as premenstrual syndrome. Recent studies show that vitex is a *hormone regulator*. It increases production of luteinizing hormone, inhibits production of follicle-stimulating hormone, and may stimulate the production of progesterone. The overall effect of vitex is to prevent the kind of hormonal fluctuations that can cause some very annoying symptoms during menopause such as hot flashes and irritability.

Water

FACTS

Most of us take water for granted, and yet, we couldn't live without it for more than a few days. Water is involved in nearly every bodily process. In fact, water is the most abundant fluid in the human body, accounting for one-half to two-thirds of total body weight.

Nutrients and hormones circulate throughout the body via water. Water also improves kidney function, which tends to decline with age. In addition, water cushions or lubricates joints and prevents friction between bones and ligaments.

Water is also an excellent source of minerals such as calcium, magnesium, and selenium. The rate of cardiovascular disease is higher in areas with "soft water," that is, where the water contains low levels of minerals such as magnesium and calcium.

As we age, our sensation of thirst becomes somewhat blunted, which increases the risk of not drinking enough fluids.

Good sources of water include drinking water, juices, milk, fruits, and vegetables. Watermelon, lettuce, cucumbers, and celery are especially good sources.

THE RIGHT AMOUNT

I advise 6 to 8 glasses of water daily. Be sure to drink water even if you're not thirsty.

Caution: Unfortunately, not all water is pure and healthy. In some cases, water may be tainted with lead from old pipes. In other areas, high levels of chlorine and other potential toxins may make water unsafe. If you live in an area where the water is suspect, I recommend installing a home filtering system or using bottled water for drinking.

If you use a home filtering system, remember that it must be properly maintained and checked periodically. Activated carbon filters must be changed every few months or they can develop harmful contaminants. If you have a reverse osmosis system (which removes chemicals but not necessarily all inorganic contaminants), be sure to test it periodically because the filter can become tainted with bacteria. In addition, distillers, which are excellent for removing inorganic contaminants (but not quite as good for organic contaminants), must be descaled regularly.

Depending on processing techniques, not all bottled water is safe either. To ensure purity, try to use only water that has undergone the process of reverse osmosis, distillation, or a combination of reverse osmosis and deionization. Stick to well-known or national brands.

POSSIBLE BENEFITS

Prevents Constipation • Older Americans spend millions of dollars a year on laxatives. Drinking 6 to 8 glasses of water per day will help to increase intestinal motility and prevent constipation.

Weight Control • Instead of reaching for something to eat, try drinking a glass of water. If you're dieting, drink a glass or two of water before meals to curb your appetite. Water fills you up without filling you out.

Skin • As we age, sweat and oil glands, which moisturize skin, begin to slow down. The top layer of skin begins to thin, which makes it more difficult for skin to retain its natural moisture, resulting in drier, older-looking skin. In addition, if you don't replace fluid lost to urination and sweat, your body will pull fluid from other body cells, including skin cells. Drinking water can help your skin retain some of its youthful freshness.

PERSONAL ADVICE

If you're running a fever, you need to be sure to drink enough water. In addition, caffeine is a natural diuretic that can increase water loss. If you drink a lot of coffee, tea, or colas with caffeine, be sure to increase your water intake.

If you want to test your tap water for lead, the Environmental Protection Agency's Drinking Water Hot Line (800-426-4791) will refer you to a certified lab in your area. Most labs will send a kit in the mail. (Prices range from fifteen to thirty dollars.)

Wheat Bran

FACTS

All bran is not the same. Researchers are discovering that different kinds of bran perform different functions in the body. Some types of bran are particularly good at lowering cholesterol, others promote bowel regularity. Because of its unique properties, wheat bran may protect against two common forms of cancer: breast cancer and colon cancer.

Good sources of wheat bran include whole wheat bread and cereals. Wheat bran can also be added to hot cereal or baked foods or mixed in yogurt.

THE RIGHT AMOUNT

I recommend one or two servings of a food rich in wheat bran daily.

POSSIBLE BENEFITS

Breast Cancer   •   Higher levels of circulating estrogen is believed to be a risk factor for developing breast cancer. Recently, researchers at the American Health Foundation studied the effect of three different types of bran (oat, corn, and wheat) on the estrogen levels of sixty-two premenopausal women. Participants were randomly selected to receive either a wheat, oat, or corn bran supplement in the form of food. For each woman, the average daily fiber intake was increased from about 15 to 30 percent. After 2 months, the women taking the corn or oat bran showed no change in estrogen levels. The women eating the diet rich in wheat bran, however, showed significant reductions in serum estrone, a potent form of estrogen that may promote the growth of estrogen-sensitive tumors.

Colon Cancer   •   Colon cancer is one of the leading causes of death in the United States annually, accounting for more than sixty thousand fatalities. Although some forms of colon cancer may be genetic, most appear to be due to diet and environmental factors. A recent study at New York Hospital/Cornell Medical Center suggests that wheat bran may play an important in preventing this disease. In the study, fifty-eight people with precancerous polyps were divided into two groups. One group was put on a high-fiber diet rich in wheat bran cereal. The other group was given a low-fiber cereal. Most of the people eating the wheat bran experienced a reduction in the size and number of their polyps. There was no change seen in those on the low-fiber diet.

White Willow

FACTS

For thousands of years, the bark of this tree has been used to treat pain and fever. White willow bark contains salicin, a compound that provided chemists with the model for acetylsalicyclic acid—better known as aspirin. White willow is similar to aspirin in activity but is weaker. Unlike aspirin, which can cause stomach irritation, white willow also contains tannins, which aid in digestion.

THE RIGHT AMOUNT

White willow is available as capsules at natural food stores. Take 1 or 2 capsules every 3 to 4 hours as needed.

POSSIBLE BENEFITS

Arthritis • About 20 million Americans suffer from arthritis, which literally means inflammation of a joint. Arthritis is a common ailment, especially among older women. In fact, some 10 million women suffer from this problem. There are many different forms of arthritis, and symptoms may vary. However, typical symptoms include aches and pains in joints and connective tissue throughout the body. Aspirin and other anti-inflammatory medications are prescribed as the first line of defense against this disease. As good as these drugs may be, many have some very unpleasant and potentially dangerous side effects including gastrointestinal distress and bleeding. For many people, white willow bark works as well as aspirin in controlling pain but without the side effects.

PERSONAL ADVICE

Herbal medications may take longer to work than stronger drugs. Use this herb for 2 weeks to see if it helps control your symptoms.

Wild Yam

FACTS

Wild yam, often touted as the hot anti-aging herb of the future, has an interesting past. For generations, southern blacks have used the root of this plant to treat rheumatoid arthritis and colic. Female herbalists have routinely prescribed it for menstrual disorders including premenstrual syndrome and threatened miscarriage. In 1943, wild yam attracted the attention of mainstream medicine when a scientist extracted the female hormone progesterone from this plant. In fact, until 1970, this plant was the sole source of progesterone used in birth control pills. Today, this herb is primarily used to treat two conditions associated with aging: menopause and arthritis.

THE RIGHT AMOUNT

Wild yam is available in capsule form at natural food stores. Take 1 capsule up to three times daily; I do.

POSSIBLE BENEFITS

Rheumatoid Arthritis   •   Animal studies have confirmed that the steroidal saponins in wild yam have an anti-inflammatory effect and, therefore, may be useful in treating the pain and stiffness associated with a flare-up of rheumatoid arthritis.

Menopause   •   Wild yam is believed to regulate hormonal fluctuations that can cause unpleasant menopausal symptoms such as hot flashes, fatigue, and vaginal dryness. This herb is often included in herbal formulas designed to relieve menopausal symptoms.

Yohimbe Bark

FACTS

Since ancient times, different herbs and potions have been touted as aphrodisiacs. Few of these so-called aphrodisiacs have withstood serious scientific scrutiny with the exception of yohimbe. A compound extracted from the bark of the African yohimbe tree is a proven aphrodisiac that works well for many men. In fact, it is even prescribed by physicians under the generic name yohimbine or yohimbine hydrochloride to treat cases of male impotency.

THE RIGHT AMOUNT

Yohimbine is sold by prescription only and should only be used under the supervision of a physician. If you are a man suffering from impotency, talk to your physician about this drug.

A weaker form of this drug is sold under the name yohimbe bark at many natural food stores and herb stores. Yohimbe bark is available without prescription, but it is not as effective as yohimbine. Yohimbe bark is often included in male potency formulas with other aphrodisiacs. Take 1 to 3 capsules daily.

Caution: High doses of yohimbe can cause serious side effects in some cases. Yohimbe can lower blood pressure and should not be used by people with hypotension. In addition, yohimbe should not be used by people with medical problems unless it is under the supervision of a physician.

POSSIBLE BENEFITS

Impotency • Impotency is a widespread problem for men over forty. In a recent study that appeared in *The Journal of Urology* of thirteen hundred men between the ages of forty and seventy, at least half of the men questioned claimed to have had trouble keeping an erection within the past six months. Animal and human studies have shown that in many cases, impotency caused by either psychological or physical problems can be successfully treated with prescription strength yohimbine. For example, in one Canadian study, forty-eight men were either given a placebo or yohimbine over a 10-week period. Of those taking the yohimbine, 46 percent reported a positive response.

Zinc

FACTS

In the not too distant future, a whole population of aging baby boomers may view this common mineral with new respect. In the body, zinc performs many vital roles involving cell division, growth, and repair—all of which are functions that tend to slow down with age. Men in particular may become interested in zinc. There is a heavy concentration of zinc in the male prostate gland. Many people—myself included—suspect that zinc may help to prevent prostate problems in older men. Last but not least, recent studies suggest that zinc may be an immune booster and may even help to preserve vision in the elderly.

Marginal zinc deficiency is widespread in the United States among people of all ages, but especially among older adults. On average, women consume 70 percent of the recommended daily allowance (RDA) for zinc; men consume 90 percent.

Good sources of zinc include oysters, pork, liver, eggs, brewers yeast, milk, beans, wheat germ, and pumpkin seeds.

THE RIGHT AMOUNT

The RDA for women is 12 milligrams; the RDA for men is 15 milligrams. Zinc is available in multivitamin and multimineral preparations. Zinc gluconate and zinc picolinate appear to be the most easily tolerated. Supplements range from 15 to 60 milligrams daily. I do not recommend exceeding 50 milligrams daily. Very high doses of zinc (over 150 milligrams) may actually depress the immune system. Excess zinc may also impair copper absorption.

POSSIBLE BENEFITS

Immune Enhancer   •   Several studies have been done on the role of zinc deficiency in the immune function of older people. One recent study showed that zinc supplements (220 milligrams twice daily for 1 month) increased the level of T cells in people over seventy. (T cells help fight infection.)

Cold Fighter   •   Move over vitamin C—zinc may be a more potent cold fighter. In a study, seventy-three Dartmouth College students with colds were given zinc lozenges (zinc–gluconate–glycine) at the earliest stages of the illness. The lozenges reduced the duration of colds by more than 40 percent (from an average of 9 days to 5 days) and also greatly reduced the severity of cold symptoms. The students sucked on 2 lozenges every 2 hours, up to 8 per day. (Zinc lozenges should not be taken on an empty stomach because they can cause nausea.)

Vision   •   Macular degeneration, which causes a blur or blind spot in the field of vision, is a common malady of aging, which, in some cases, can be treated surgically. In one small study performed at Louisiana State University Medical Center, zinc supplements appeared to help control vision loss due to macular degeneration. In the study, 151 patients were given either 100-milligram tablets of zinc twice daily or a placebo. Those who were given the zinc showed in the words of the researchers "significantly less visual loss" than the placebo group. The National Eye Institute in Bethesda is embarking on a 6-year study to determine the role nutrition and supplements such as zinc may play in the progression of eye diseases such as macular degeneration and cataracts. Perhaps by the twenty-first century, we'll have some definitive answers.

Prostate   •   For years, I've been recommending zinc supplements to men with prostate problems. There are heavy concentrations of zinc in the male prostate gland, which manufactures prostatic fluid, in which sperm cells are mixed to make semen.

There is a great deal of anecdotal evidence supporting zinc's role in prostate health and male infertility. However, few scientific studies have been done. In fact, recently, in the *Nutrition Action Healthletter* published by the Center for Science in the Public Interest, there was an interesting letter to the editor responding to an article in the newsletter that had stated that there was no scientific evidence linking zinc intake to prostate health. In the letter, a California man pointed out that he was one of three brothers, all in their midsixties. One brother was a regular user of zinc for 30 years, the others were not. The two brothers who did not use zinc had developed enlarged prostates and even cancer; the zinc user had not. Coincidence? Maybe. But I've heard enough of these kinds of stories to make sure that I get enough zinc daily!

Up and Coming Supplements

Here are some potentially beneficial anti-aging supplements that are the focus of several research projects. I predict that you'll be hearing a lot more about them in the near future.

DEHYDROEPIANDROSTERONE

Dehydroepiandrosterone (DHEA) is a hormone that is produced by the adrenal glands. DHEA is abundant in the young, but in middle age, the supply begins to drop. By age fifty, most people produce only one-third of the DHEA that they did in their youth. By age sixty, DHEA levels are barely detectable.

Some researchers believe that the precipitous drop in DHEA makes people more vulnerable to many of the ailments that are often associated with old age, including two of the leading killers of both men and women: cancer and heart disease.

In one long-term study of men between the ages of fifty and seventy-nine, researchers found that those with the lowest levels of DHEA had the highest rate of heart disease. Other studies of healthy men suggest that DHEA supplements can cut cholesterol, reduce body fat, increase muscle mass, and relieve depression. Animal studies have shown that DHEA supplements can thwart the growth of artificially planted tumors in elderly mice. In addition, DHEA can help improve memory, at least in laboratory mice, and may even make it easier to lose weight.

DHEA may sound like a wonder drug but like other forms of hormone therapy, it has its downside. In very high doses DHEA can cause the overproduction of sex hormones and liver enlargement. In women, DHEA can have an androgenic effect, which means it can produce some unwanted side affects such as a growth spurt in facial hair. Human studies are being conducted to determine what levels of supplemental DHEA are safe for humans and whether DHEA is truly a life extender. Dr. Arthur Schwartz, a biologist at Temple University and a leading authority on DHEA, advises people to avoid supplements until some of these questions are answered, but other proponents of DHEA feel that it is safe in low dosages.

DHEA is available only by prescription.

HUMAN GROWTH HORMONE

Human growth hormone is released by the pituitary gland until age thirty and is closely related to the stages of development. Levels of growth hormone are high in the fetus, decline during early childhood, and surge again during adolescence. (Interestingly enough, the greatest amount of growth hormone is released just before deep sleep, which could explain why adolescents seem to need so much sleep, and why children seem to grow in their sleep.) After age thirty, however, the levels of human growth hormone sharply decline and in some older persons, production seems to shut down altogether. As the level of growth hormone declines, so does body function. In fact, low levels of growth hormone have been associated with a drop in muscle mass, an increase in body fat, diminished immunologic response, a loss of appetite, and a reduction in kidney function. Some researchers have speculated that supplementing growth hormone in aging people may reverse some of these negative effects.

In 1990, Dr. Daniel Rudman of the Medical College of Wisconsin and the Milwaukee VA Medical Center assembled twenty-one healthy men, ages sixty-one to eighty-one, with one thing in common: unusually low levels of growth hormone. Twelve of the subjects received growth hormone injections over a 6-month period; nine did not. Those who received the injections had a 14 percent reduction in body fat and a 9 percent increase in muscle mass. Many of the subjects on the hormone claimed that they felt better than they had in years, and growth hormone was quickly lauded as the "fountain of youth." Once the hormone was discontinued, however, the subjects quickly returned to their original state.

So why isn't everybody popping growth hormone pills? In the United States the only medically accepted use of growth hormone is to supplement it in growing children with documented low levels. Growth hormone is available in many countries outside of the United States, and many clinics abroad are dispensing the stuff with a free hand. However, most scientists agree that more research needs to be done before growth hormone can be used by the general population. Growth hormone has some potentially hazardous side effects including cancer, arthritis, carpal tunnel syndrome, diabetes, and enlargement of the head. It can also cause swelling and headaches, even at low levels. The National Institutes of Health is funding several studies on growth hormone to determine whether it works as well as it appears, if it can be used safely, and the optimum dose.

RU-486

RU-486, or mifepristone, has gained notoriety as the so-called abortion pill. In fact, until recently, it was banned in the United States due to an extensive lobbying effort on the part of anti-abortion forces. This drug works by blocking key hormones necessary to sustain a pregnancy, including progesterone and stress hormones known as glucocorticoids. Many researchers worldwide believe that RU-486 may prove to be a real life saver.

One French study showed that RU-486 shrank tumors in 25

percent of women with advanced breast cancers. (Progesterone can stimulate the growth of tumors; therefore, any drug that can block the action of progesterone may also help prevent the growth of tumors.) More studies are being done in the United States and abroad to determine whether RU-486 could be used in the treatment or prevention of breast cancer.

Other studies suggest that RU-486 may have broader application as a general anti-aging drug. For example, in one study sponsored by the National Institute of Child Health and Human Development, RU-486 was an effective treatment for Cushing's syndrome in six out of ten children given this drug. This study caught the eye of longevity researchers primarily because the symptoms of Cushing's syndrome (which include a rapid decline in immunity, osteoporosis, and loss of muscle) closely resemble a speeded-up version of the aging process. Research is underway investigating RU-486 as a treatment for osteoporosis, high blood pressure, and adult-onset diabetes among other maladies associated with aging.

Words of Wisdom

Want to live to be one hundred and five? Follow the advice of the Delany sisters, authors of *Having Our Say: The Delany Sisters' First 100 Years.* As of this writing, Sarah L. (Sadie) Delany is one hundred and six and her sister A. Elizabeth (Bessie) Delany recently died at one hundred and four. According to the Delanys, the secret to their longevity is a combination of diet and exercise. They did yoga exercises daily and ate a clove of garlic chopped up and swallowed whole every morning with a teaspoonful of cod liver oil. In addition, the Delany sisters wrote, "We eat as many as seven different vegetables. Plus lots of fresh fruits. And we take vitamin supplements: Vitamin A, B complex, C, D, E, and minerals, too, like zinc. And Bessie takes tyrosine when she's a little blue."

Chapter 3

Living Well: A Guide to Preventing Common Ailments of Aging

Listed in this chapter are the common ailments afflicting older adults and ways that they can be prevented or treated.

Alzheimer's Disease

About 4 million Americans have Alzheimer's disease, an irreversible form of dementia that is characterized by the slow but steady destruction of key areas in the brain that control reasoning and memory. Symptoms include memory loss, the inability to speak, and difficulty in processing information. In most cases, Alzheimer's is a late-onset disease. About 10 percent of Americans over age sixty-five have Alzheimer's disease, and nearly half of those diagnosed are over eighty-five. However, about 5 percent of all Alzheimer's cases occur in people as young as forty.

Although we are quick to label any form of senility as Alzheimer's disease, in reality, there are many different types of dementia that can affect the elderly and can be caused by a wide range of factors including overmedication, stroke, poor blood flow to the brain, and even depression. In contrast, Alzheimer's is marked by specific brain abnormalities, notably, clusters of injured brain cells called *plaques,* which are believed to be responsible for the loss of memory and other behavioral abnormalities. The cause of Alzheimer's is still unknown, although it appears to be linked to certain genes. According to researchers at Duke University, people who inherit a gene that is responsible for producing a protein called Apo-E4 are four times more likely to develop Alzheimer's late in life. If they inherit the gene from both parents, the risk is doubled. (In addition, these people do not produce enough of two other proteins, Apo-E2 and Apo-E3.) However, not everyone who has these genes will get Alzheimer's, and not everyone with Alzheimer's has these genes. Other researchers believe that the culprit is actually a protein piece called *beta-amyloid peptide,* which lies at the center of the brain plaques. They suspect that this protein could be responsible for destroying brain cells.

There is no cure for Alzheimer's, and to date, drug treatments for Alzheimer's have been disappointing. However, there is strong evidence that there are simple steps that can be taken to delay the onset of Alzheimer's or to lessen the severity of the symptoms.

EARL'S RX

Use It or Lose It • Many studies have shown that people with the highest degree of education have the lowest rates of Alzheimer's disease. These results were initially chalked up to the fact that better-educated people tend to be more affluent, and more affluent people tend to take better care of themselves. However, recent research into the inner workings of the brain show that a lifetime of intellectual stimulation may have a far more profound effect. A child's brain is constantly producing new brain cells, but as we age, production of cells begins to fall off. Until recently, scientists believed that the mature brain followed a steady course of decline, but animal experiments have proved this theory wrong. Studies on rats have shown that learning new tasks can actually stimulate the production of *dendrites*, threadlike appendages at the end of brain cells called *neurons*, which helps cells communicate with each other. The growth of dendrites didn't just occur in young animals, as might be expected, but surprisingly in older animals as well. Scientists speculate that human adults who are constantly challenged by intellectual pursuits may actually be building a bigger store of dendrites than people who are not faced with intellectual challenges. Thus, it's possible that when people with a reserve of dendrites develop Alzheimer's, which slowly destroys a portion of their brains, they may not experience as severe symptoms as people with less education—and presumably fewer dendrites.

I'm not suggesting that anyone who has not attained a Ph.D. will get Alzheimer's disease. Education is not just about degrees; it's about staying interested in the world, learning new skills, and accepting new challenges at any age. Make a concerted effort to "grow your dendrites"—study a new subject, learn a new language, take up a new sport, or try your hand at painting or sculpting.

Limit Your Exposure to Aluminum • Some studies have shown high concentrations of aluminum—up to fifty times higher than normal—in some parts of the brains of Alzheimer's patients. This has led some scientists to speculate that aluminum, one of the most abundant metals on earth, may in some way be responsible for causing this disease. However, many researchers dismiss the aluminum connection, citing as evidence studies that show that people who live in areas with high levels of aluminum in their water supply do not suffer a higher rate of Alzheimer's than usual. In addition, critics of the aluminum hypothesis point out that half of all cookware used in the United States is made with aluminum, and if aluminum caused Alzheimer's, the disease would be more prevalent than it is.

Frankly, nobody knows what link, if any, exists between aluminum and Alzheimer's disease. In fact, the higher levels of aluminum found in some studies may simply be a result of the disease, not the cause. Nevertheless, I advise people to err on the side of caution. While it's impossible to avoid aluminum altogether—aluminum is present in natural sources such as fruits and vegetables and small amounts may leach from aluminum cookware into food—it is possible to avoid ingesting high doses of the metal. For example, many commonly used over-the-counter drugs such as antacids and buffered aspirin are high in aluminum. In fact, if you are a regular user of either of these products, you could be ingesting up to 5000 milligrams of aluminum daily! Many deodorants are also high in aluminum; aerosol antiperspirants may be particularly bad because anything inhaled through the nasal passages is more readily absorbed by the brain. (Fortunately, there are some excellent herbal deodorants sold at natural food stores that do not contain aluminum.) Until we know for certain that aluminum is harmless, I recommend avoiding products with a high aluminum content.

L-Carnitine • L-Carnitine (see p. 49) is a nonprotein amino acid that is found in heart and skeletal muscle. It's primary job is to carry activated fatty acids across the mitochondria—the so-called powerhouse of the cell—providing heart and skeletal cells with energy. The brain tissue of mammals is a rich source of carnitine. Some studies suggest that L-carnitine may be effective in slowing down the progression of Alzheimer's disease. Several European studies have reported that a daily supplement of L-carnitine (about 2 grams daily) can slow the mental deterioration typical of this disease. (Dietary intakes of L-Carnitine average 100 to 300 milligrams daily in the United States.) However, U.S. researchers did not report good results from a major trial testing L-carnitine on Alzheimer's patients. However, since L-carnitine is also excellent for the heart, I see no reason not to use it.

Control Stress • Learning how to cope with stress, and getting help when you are feeling overwhelmed may be the best preventive medicine against Alzheimer's. Several studies have shown that chronic stress can hamper the performance of cells in key parts of the brain, resulting in Alzheimer's-type symptoms such as memory loss and impaired mental capabilities. The damage occurs in the hippocampus, the portion of the brain essential for memory and learning. In animal studies, researchers have proven that prolonged stress can increase the signs of aging in the brain, and many suspect that the same may be true for humans. During stressful situations, people produce cortisol, a stress hormone that revs the body up, giving them the physical and mental stamina to withstand the extra pressure. Researchers at McGill University recently found that people with higher levels of stress hormones in their blood did not perform as well on tests of attention and memory as people with lower levels. In fact, older people with lower levels of stress hormones fared just as well as young people in cognitive tests, while those with higher stress hormone levels got scores up to 50 percent lower.

Some researchers believe that people become more susceptible to the ill effects of stress hormones as they age. In some cases, people may produce too much stress hormone, which could cause damage to brain cells. Interestingly, stress hormone levels have been found to be higher and more difficult to control in Alzheimer's patients.

A Word About Estrogen • Some studies have found that hormone replacement therapy may help prevent Alzheimer's disease in women. For example, researchers at the University of Southern California have found that women who take estrogen replacement therapy after menopause cut their risk of getting Alzheimer's disease by more than 40 percent, and if they do get it, they have much less severe symptoms. Other studies have shown that estrogen can increase the growth of dendrites and triggers the production of choline acetyltransferase, an enzyme that helps carry signals among neurons. However, before popping an estrogen pill, keep in mind that another major California study has found that estrogen has little, if any, effect on the incidence or course of Alzheimer's. In addition, estrogen replacement therapy is not without risk; women who take estrogen increase the odds of getting cancers of the breast and uterus. In addition, estrogen can be dangerous for women with certain medical conditions, including high blood pressure, clotting problems, and migraine headaches.

Garlic • French researchers recently reported that aged garlic extract appeared to slow down brain deterioration in aged laboratory rats with an Alzheimer's-type disease. In addition, the garlic normalized the brain's serotonin system; if the serotinin system malfunctions, it can cause depression. Although we don't know whether garlic will work as well on human brains, I feel that since garlic offers so many other benefits, it is wise to include it in your daily diet or take a garlic supplement.

Arthritis

Arthritis, which literally means the inflammation of a joint, is a general term used to described about 125 different conditions. The term *arthritis* encompasses a wide range of ailments ranging from osteoarthritis, the so-called wear and tear arthritis associated with advanced age, to gout, a painful condition caused by high blood levels of uric acid, to lupus, an autoimmune disease that primarily affects women. Due to the aging of the population, arthritis is a growing problem in the United States. According to a recent study by the Centers for Disease Control and Prevention, by the year 2020, nearly one in five Americans will suffer from some form of arthritic disease (as compared to one out of six today).

In this section, I will talk about the two most common forms of arthritis: osteoarthritis and rheumatoid arthritis.

Osteoarthritis

Also known as *degenerative joint disease,* osteoarthritis affects about 16 million Americans and usually strikes after age forty-five. Osteoarthritis is characterized by swollen joints, achiness, and stiffness or pain in the hands, spine, hips, or knees. It is caused by a gradual wearing away of the cartilage, the sponge-like material that cushions the ends of the bones, preventing them from rubbing together. In some cases, an injury to a bone or joint will cause osteoarthritic changes.

Bone X rays of most people over fifty will show some signs of osteoarthritis, and although it can cause some discomfort, it is rarely crippling. In fact, researchers suspect that people with severe osteoarthritis may have a genetic form of the disease. There is no cure for osteoarthritis; as of yet, we don't know how to stimulate the body to regenerate cartilage. And for most people, aspirin or its herbal counterpart, white willow bark, or acetaminophen may be all that's needed to control the occasional bouts of pain. However, there are several things that people can do to prevent osteoporosis from becoming a problem.

EARL'S RX

Lighten Up • The knee is typically the first area in the body to be affected by osteoarthritis, which in severe cases can impair mobility. Numerous studies have shown that overweight people are at greater risk of developing arthritic knees than normal-weight people.

Get Physical • Exercise may be the best preventive medicine against developing arthritis. Researchers suspect that exercise may help to retain cartilage by increasing the flow of blood to knee joints and other crucial areas, which is necessary to nourish cells. Walking, swimming, cycling, and rowing are excellent choices for most people because they move joints in a safe way. Sports such as tennis, basketball, and soccer, which require pivoting and sudden moves, may be riskier in terms of injury. Contrary to common belief, even a high-impact aerobic exercise such as running may be beneficial (but only for people who do not have osteoarthritis). Researchers at Stanford University studied the knee X rays of fifty men and women who ran about 3 hours a week. Some members of the study decreased their activity while others increased or maintained their time running. At the end of 2 years, researchers did not find any problems in the X rays of the most active group that would suggest that running had worn down cartilage.

At one time, people with osteoarthritis were advised to avoid the stress and strain of exercise. We now know that was precisely the wrong advice. For example, in a study conducted at the Hospital for Special Surgery and Columbia University, researchers found that people with osteoarthritis of the knee who followed a supervised walking program experienced improved mobility and decreased pain as compared to those who remained inactive. However, osteoarthritis sufferers should beware of any activity that further stresses already vulnerable knee and ankle joints. Running, jogging, and sports that require a lot of pivoting, such as skiing and basketball, may cause more harm than good. So what's left? According to the Arthritis Foundation, the solution may lie to the East: tai chi, a form of martial arts based on gentle, flowing movements, can provide a good workout without overworking the joints. In fact, the Arthritis Foundation is offering classes in tai chi. For more information on safe ways to exercise, call the national office (800-283-7800) or your local chapter.

Avoid Injuries • Warm up before exercising; warmed-up joints are less likely to be injured. Stretching limbers up muscles and tendons and improves joint mobility; in other words, it primes you for your workout. Take a stretch and tone class at your local Y or consult with a sports medicine specialist. Most importantly, don't overexert yourself if you're tired—that's likely to make you accident prone.

Become safety conscious. A little thought ahead of time can help to avert common injuries such as slipping on ice in the winter or falling in the tub that can damage cartilate and begin a downward spiral of pain and inactivity. Wear solid low-heeled boots or shoes outdoors. Be sure that your bathroom is designed for safety—more falls occur in the bathroom than anywhere else in the house. Repair lose or broken steps or anything else around the house or workplace that could promote injury.

Dietary Tips • Some people find that certain foods may aggravate their arthritis. Obviously, if you consistently feel worse after eating a particular food, try eliminating it from your diet and see if you improve. In addition, some people may find the nightshade vegetables (e.g., potatoes, tomatoes, peppers, and eggplants) to be irritating.

Antioxidants • Some researchers believe that degenerative diseases such as arthritis are caused by damage inflicted by free radicals, highly unstable oxygen molecules that can, among other things, promote premature aging. A daily antioxidant supplement including vitamins and minerals such as beta-carotene, vitamins C and E, and selenium may help to prevent or slow down arthritic changes.

Herbal Remedies

Ashwaganda • Part of the traditional Indian system of medicine called Ayurvedic, ashwaganda has been shown to reduce pain and stiffness caused by osteoarthritis. Ahwaganda is sold in natural food stores in tea and capsule form.

Boswellin Cream • Also from the Ayurvedic healing tradition, this greaseless cream contains extracts of *Boswellia serrata* plant, vitamin E, capsaicin, and methyl salicylate.

Cayenne Creams and Ointments • Creams and ointments containing cayenne pepper can help reduce pain by stimulating the production of endorphins, the body's own natural painkiller. Many are sold over the counter at drug and natural food stores.

Licorice • This herb stimulates the production of two steroids: cortisone and aldosterone, which can help relieve pain and inflammation (Aldosterone raises blood pressure; therefore, licorice should not be used by people with high blood pressure.) Licorice is available in tea and capsule form.

Rheumatoid Arthritis

About 2.1 million people in the United States—two-thirds of them women—suffer from rheumatoid arthritis, a condition that causes painful inflammation in the joints and can result in severe disability. Unlike osteoarthritis (which is caused by the wearing away of cartilage), rheumatoid arthritis is characterized by a glitch in the immune system that causes it to attack the collagen, which lines the membranes of the joint. No one knows the cause of rheumatoid arthritis, although some researchers suspect that an initial infection may be responsible for throwing the immune system out of whack, which triggers the autoimmune reaction. In addition, there appears to be a genetic tendency to develop rheumatoid arthritis. Although rheumatoid arthritis can strike young women, most cases of rheumatoid arthritis occur between ages forty and sixty.

If you have rheumatoid arthritis, you should be under the care of a physician or knowledgeable natural healer. Although there is no cure, there are many treatments available today that can help relieve pain and discomfort. In addition to conventional treatments, which range from anti-inflammatory medications such as aspirin or ibuprofin to antibiotics to immunosuppressor drugs, here are some alternative treatments that may help.

EARL'S RX

Gamma-linolenic Acid • Gamma-linolenic acid (GLA), which is found in evening primrose oil and borage seed oil, is an omega-6 fatty acid that is similar to the omega-3 fatty acids found in fatty fish. Natural healers have long prescribed evening primrose oil to treat rheumatoid arthritis. A recent study performed at the University of Pennsylvania found that a

daily dose of 1.4 grams of GLA could significantly reduce symptoms such as pain and joint swelling in patients with rheumatoid arthritis. Capsules of evening primrose oil and borage seed
oil are available at natural food stores.

Omega-3 Fatty Acids • Several studies have confirmed that
many people with rheumatoid arthritis have shown improvement after taking supplements of omega-3 fatty acids. Omega-3
fatty acids contain compounds that can inhibit the inflammatory response in the body.

Chicken Cartilage • Chew on some chicken bones! According to a study performed at Boston's Beth Israel Hospital,
chicken cartilage protein, which is found in chicken bones, can
help relieve the symptoms of rheumatoid arthritis. In the study,
one group of patients drank a solution made from chicken collagen in a glass of orange juice daily, whereas the other group
drank a placebo. Out of the chicken collagen group, four patients went into complete remission, and the others had a significant reduction in symptoms. In the placebo group, however,
none of the patients went into remission, although a small
group (four out of thirty-one) said they felt better, which researchers attributed to the "placebo effect."

Dietary Tips • There is also some evidence that a low-fat
diet may help to relieve symptoms such as pain and stiffness. In
a study conducted by Loma Linda University in California,
rheumatoid arthritis patients were given instructions on diet
and stress reduction several times weekly for a 5-week period.
The participants cut their daily calories by about 30 percent and
reduced their fat intake to about 10 percent of their daily caloric
intake. After 3 months, the group experienced vast improvement in the amount of stiffness and discomfort.

Other studies have shown that arthritis sufferers who eat a
vegetarian diet can find relief from their discomfort. Researchers can't say whether meat actually contributes to
arthritic flares or whether it's the increased intake of fruits and
vegetables that alleviates the symptoms.

Some rheumatoid arthritis patients have found that certain

foods may trigger a flare, and studies confirm that rheumatoid patients often develop allergic reactions to many foods. According to recent studies, rheumatoid patients often show signs of sensitivity to foods such as corn, wheat, bacon, oranges, milk, and oats. However, researchers are not sure whether food sensitivities actually contribute to arthritis. Eliminating dairy products and nightshade vegetables such as tomatoes, potatoes, bell peppers, tobacco, and eggplant may help your condition.

Herbal Remedies •

Horsetail • This herb contains minute quantities of gold, which may be effective against joint pain and stiffness. It is sold in tea and capsule form in natural food stores.

Propolis • Found in honey, this substance blocks enzymes that produce prostaglandins, hormonelike substances that can cause pain and inflammation. Propolis is sold in natural food stores.

Turmeric • This herb, which is used in curry powder, is a natural anti-inflammatory.

Wild Yam • This herb contains steroidal compounds that have an anti-inflammatory effect. It is available in tea and capsule form and is used in many herbal arthritis formulas.

Yucca • This native American herb is a long-time favorite for treating rheumatoid arthritis and is sold in natural food stores in tea and capsule form.

Cataracts

A cataract is a cloudy or opaque covering that grows over the lens of the eye, which can cause partial or total blindness. In rare cases, cataracts may be due to a genetic problem. In most cases, however, cataracts are a result of cellular damage to the eye lens inflicted by ultraviolet light or oxidation. Cataracts are very common among older people; it is estimated that as many as 50 million people worldwide are cataract sufferers. In fact, in the United States alone, over 1 million surgeries are performed each year to remove cataracts. According to the Nutrition and Cataract Research Laboratory at Tufts University, if we could postpone the formation of cataracts by 10 years, the United States could save more than $1.5 billion annually.

EARL'S RX

Cover Your Eyes • To protect against ultraviolet (UV) light, wear sunglasses outdoors, not just in the summer, but all year long. Be sure to buy sunglasses that specifically promise to block 99 to 100 percent of UVA and UVB rays. Not all sunglasses are effective; check with your eye doctor to see which glasses are right for you. In addition, a hat with a wide brim can block about 50 percent of UV light. (It can also help prevent wrinkles.)

Needless to say, avoid unnecessary exposure to UV light, such as tanning salons (which may also promote skin cancer).

Eat Your Fruits and Vegetables • According to researchers at the Human Nutrition Research Center at Tufts University, older adults with cataracts reported eating significantly fewer servings of fruits and vegetables than those who were cataract free. In fact, those who ate fewer than three and a half servings of fruits and vegetables daily had a fivefold greater risk of developing senile cataracts than people who ate more. This is not surprising, considering the fact that other studies have shown that people with cataracts have lower blood levels of carotenoids and vitamin C, compounds that are abundant in fruits and vegetables.

Take Your Vitamins • Antioxidants such as vitamin C, beta-carotene, and vitamin E may help prevent against oxidative damage that can lead to the formation of cataracts. For example, in one study performed at the U.S. Department of Agriculture's Human Nutrition Center on Aging at Tufts University, when vitamin C was added to the diets of guinea pigs, their eyes showed less oxidative damage after exposure to UV light than pigs who were not given the vitamin.

Other vitamins and minerals may also play a role in preventing cataracts. In a landmark study conducted by the National Eye Institute and the Chinese Academy of Medicine in Beijing, researchers gave more than 2100 Chinese adults (ages forty-five to seventy-four) in a malnourished population of Linxian either 2 Centrum multivitamin and mineral tablets and 25,000 international units of beta-carotene daily or a placebo. After 5 years, the vitamin takers were 43 percent less likely to have nuclear cataracts (cataracts that form in the center of the eye) than the placebo group.

In a second test, more than 3200 Linxian residents were given 2.3 milligrams of riboflavin and 40 milligrams of niacin daily. After 5 years, those who took the vitamins were 50 percent less likely to develop nuclear cataracts than those who didn't take the vitamins. Researchers speculate that riboflavin may have helped prevent cataracts because it is involved in the production of glutathione, a potent antioxidant in the eye lens.

Coronary Artery Disease

Heart disease is a national epidemic—it is the number one killer of men and women in the United States. When we talk about heart disease, we're really talking about coronary artery disease (CAD), a condition in which the arteries bringing blood to the heart become clogged or obstructed with a yellowish, waxy substance called *plaque* (the condition is known as *atherosclerosis*). If the arteries become too narrow, the flow of blood and oxygen to the heart will become severely impaired, which can lead to a heart attack.

Some people are more CAD-prone than others due to such factors as age, genetics, or lifestyle. The risk of developing CAD increases with age; about 55 percent of all heart attacks occur after age fifty-five. Before age fifty-five, men have a higher rate of heart disease, but postmenopausal women quickly catch up to men. Race is another risk factor. African-Americans have a higher rate of CAD than whites. People with a parent or sibling who has had a heart attack before age fifty-five (age sixty-five for women) are automatically put in a higher risk group for CAD. And in addition to immutable risk factors such as sex, age, and race, there are other more controllable risk factors that are equally important, including smoking, obesity, sedentary lifestyle, diabetes, high blood pressure, and high blood cholesterol levels. Few people are risk free. In fact, according to a recent study by the Centers for Disease Control and Prevention, more than 80 percent of all American adults have one or more risk factors for CAD. But take heart—even if you have one or more risk factors, it doesn't mean that you're going to have a heart attack. Although you may have no control over your genes or your race, you can control many of the other risk factors and, by doing so, can dramatically reduce the odds of developing CAD.

EARL'S RX

Caution: If you have a heart condition or are taking medicine for a heart problem, do not use any herbs, drugs, or supplements without first checking with your physician or natural healer.

Up in Smoke • Up to 40 percent of CAD deaths each year are believed to be due to smoke-related problems. Given the fact that smoking has also been associated with an increased risk of developing many different forms of cancer, by now, even the Marlboro Man knows that it's time to "butt out." But what you may not know is that secondhand smoke from someone else's cigarette may be inflicting damage to *your* heart. Researchers at New York University Medical Center have shown that exposure to secondhand smoke can accelerate the formation of plaque deposits in the arteries of male chicks. In fact, according to the study, the smoke-exposed chicks had plaques that were significantly larger than non-smoke-exposed chicks. Although no one knows whether human arteries behave quite the same way, it makes good sense to reduce your exposure to cigarette smoke.

Hold the Hostility • According to researchers at the National Institute on Aging and the University of Maryland, angry, hostile people are at greater risk of developing heart disease, especially if "they are arrogant, argumentative, surly, and rude." My hunch is that these people are also carriers, inflicting damage on their families and anyone else they come in contact with. If you find yourself losing control, seek professional help.

Know Your Numbers • Blood cholesterol levels should be maintained at under 200 milligrams per deciliter. High-density lipoproteins (HDLs) or "good" cholesterol, should be 35 or above. The low-density lipoproteins (LDLs): HDLs ratio should be 3:1 but should never dip below 4:1. For example, if the LDL level is 120, then HDLs should be 40. Eating a diet in which less than 25 percent of your daily calories is derived from fat will help maintain a low cholesterol. In addition, watch your intake of saturated fat (primarily from animal products) and polyunsaturated fat from foods such as margarine, which contain *trans*-fatty acids that can raise blood cholesterol levels.

Foods that are rich in fiber, including oat bran, psyllium, and pectin, which is found in grapefruit, can help lower total cholesterol.

Keep track of another type of blood lipid: triglycerides. Elevated levels of triglycerides are a risk factor for heart disease. Women should maintain triglyceride levels under 200 milligrams per deciliter, and men should maintain levels under 400 miligrams per deciliter.

Boost Your HDLs • If your HDLs are low, there are some things that you can do to raise them:

- Exercise has been shown to raise HDLs, especially if you've been sedentary. A 2-mile walk four or five times a week at a moderately brisk pace may bring your HDLs up to speed.

- A glass of red wine daily has been shown to raise HDLs.
- An onion a day can raise your HDLs.
- Niacin (100 milligrams daily) taken with chromium (600 micrograms daily) can lower cholesterol and raise HDLs. (High doses of niacin can be toxic to your liver and should be taken only under the supervision of a physician.)
- Eating four or five smaller meals frequently throughout the day instead of the usual "three squares" has been shown to lower cholesterol and increase HDLs.

Take Your Antioxidants • Several studies have shown that people who take antioxidant supplements have lower rates of heart disease than people who don't. Antioxidants such as vitamin C, beta-carotene, vitamin E, and selenium help prevent the oxidation of LDL cholesterol, which is believed to contribute to the formation of plaque.

Many herbs, including basil, dill, mint, parsley, and rosemary, are excellent sources of antioxidants.

Aspirin • A recent study of 22,000 male doctors showed that those who took 325 milligrams of aspirin daily (the amount in one adult aspirin) had 44 percent fewer heart attacks than those who didn't. Talk to your physician or natural healer before using aspirin on a regular basis.

Pass on the Sugar • The American diet is high in sugary foods, and this may contribute to the high incidence of heart disease. According to a recent study, high levels of dietary fructose, a sweetener derived from corn that is a common ingredient in foods, can raise blood serum LDL levels. Ironically, many of the new low-fat or no fat-baked products on the market include fructose. Consume these foods in moderation.

Those Amazing Monos • People in Mediterranean countries eat a diet rich in monounsaturated fats (mostly from olive oil) and not so coincidentally have the lowest rates of heart disease in the world. Studies have shown that monounsaturated fats can reduce overall blood cholesterol and specifically can cut LDL cholesterol.

Monounsaturated fats combined with vitamin E may be a particularly potent way to attack LDLs. Researchers from the University of California, San Diego, La Jolla discovered that oleic acid (which is found in monounsaturated fat) and vitamin E prevented the oxidation of a particular type of LDL—the smallest, densest portion of the LDL particle. Studies have shown that the small, dense LDL is more susceptible to oxidative damage than the larger LDL particle. About 33 percent of all men and 15 percent of all women have LDLs that are predominantly small and dense and thus may be at greater risk of developing CAD. In the California study, eighteen healthy volunteers (nine men and nine women, ages twenty-two to sixty-one) were given 1200 milligrams daily of vitamin E. Six of the eighteen volunteers ate the normal American diet, which is high in saturated fats; six ate a diet high in polyunsaturated fats; and six ate a diet high in oleic acids. Blood samples from the three groups showed that the rates of LDL oxidation for both dense and larger LDL particles were lowest in the oleic-enriched group.

Omega-3 Fatty Acids • Found in fatty fish, omega-3 fatty acids have been shown to decrease blood cholesterol and triglycerides. Omega-3 fatty acids can also help prevent blood clots. Good sources include mackerel, salmon, albacore tuna, herring, and lake trout. Fish oil capsules are available at natural food stores.

Herbal Remedies • Several herbs can help prevent heart disease.

Capsaicin • Capsaicin from hot chilies can lower blood triglyceride levels. Pour on the hot sauce!

Gamma-linolenic Acid • Gamma-linolenic acid, which is found in borage oil and evening primrose oil, is an effective cholesterol-lowering agent.

Ginger • Ginger can help prevent the formation of blood clots, which can lead to a heart attack.

Ginseng • Ginseng can help lower cholesterol.

Green Tea • Several animal studies confirm that compounds in green tea called *catechins* can lower cholesterol. Not so coincidentally, Japanese men have the lowest rate of heart disease in the world, and Japanese women have the second lowest rate (second only to France).

Hawthorn • This herb has been used for centuries in Europe to treat heart ailments. Hawthorn is rich in bioflavonoids, which can help strengthen tiny blood vessels called *capillaries*, thus improving the flow of blood throughout the body. Animal studies have shown that this herb can increase the contractility of the heart muscle, strengthening the heart's ability to pump blood. In fact, in Europe, hawthorn may be prescribed along with the drug digitalis to regulate the heartbeat.

Oriental Mushrooms • Reishi and shiitake mushrooms can lower cholesterol and prevent blood clots.

Turmeric • This spice, which is used in curry powder, is a natural blood thinner.

Other Supplements

Coenzyme Q10 • Coenzyme Q_{10} is found in every cell in the body, and as we age, levels of this enzyme begin to fall off. Coenzyme Q_{10} helps facilitate the process that provides energy to cells and improves the circulation of blood. In Japan, Coenzyme Q_{10} is used to treat angina, chest pain caused by a diminished blood supply due to CAD. Coenzyme Q_{10} capsules and tablets are sold at natural food stores. I recommend 30 milligrams daily.

L-Carnitine • L-Carnitine is a nonprotein amino acid that is found in the heart and skeletal muscle and helps to carry fatty acids across the mitochondria of the cell, thus providing heart and skeletal cells with energy. Some researchers believe that a deficiency of this amino acid may increase the risk of having a heart attack. Studies have shown that L-carnitine can also lower cholesterol and triglyceride levels and raise HDLs. L-Carnitine capsules are sold at natural food stores. I recommend 1 gram (1000 milligrams) daily.

Colorectal Cancer

About fifty thousand Americans die of colorectal cancer (cancer of either the colon or the rectum) each year, making it the third leading cause of cancer deaths. Each year, about 160,000 new cases are diagnosed. About 10 percent of all cases of colorectal cancer are genetic: as of this writing, geneticists have identified at least two genes that are believed to be responsible for this disease and even more may be involved. However, more researchers believe that perhaps as many as 90 percent of all colorectal cancers may be due to environmental factors, such as diet and lifestyle. Although colorectal cancer is common in the West, it is rare in the third world.

The warning signs include rectal bleeding, blood in the stool, and a change in bowel habits. (If you experience any of these symptoms, contact your physician for further tests.)

EARL'S RX

Cut the Fat • A high-fat diet can indirectly promote the growth of tumors in the colon. During digestion, fat stimulates the release of bile acids by the gallbladder. The fat and bile then travel through the small intestine to the colon. In the colon, the bile is converted into chemicals called *secondary bile acids*, which over time can produce cancerous changes in the colon. The less fat consumed, the smaller the amount of bile that is produced, resulting in a smaller amount of potentially carcinogenic secondary bile acids.

Wheat Bran • Researchers have known for some time that a high-fiber diet appears to protect against colon cancer. However, recent studies suggest that wheat bran may be one of the most potent protectors. A study conducted at the American Health Foundation in Valhalla, New York, compared the effects of different dietary fibers on seventy-eight women. Each of the women ate three or four muffins daily containing either corn, oat, or wheat bran for 2 months (consuming about 30 grams of fiber daily). At the end of the study, researchers measured the level of tumor-promoting enzymes and bile acids in the intestinal tract of the volunteers and found that only the wheat bran decreased the concentration of these potentially hazardous compounds.

In another recent study at New York Hospital/Cornell Medical Center, fifty-eight people with precancerous polyps were divided into two groups. One group was put on a high-fiber diet rich in wheat bran cereal and the other group was given a low-fiber cereal. Most of the people eating the wheat bran experienced a reduction in the size and number of their polyps. There was no change seen in those on the low-fiber diet.

Eat Your Five a Day • A major 6-year study of the diets of more than 764,000 adults by the National Cancer Institute and the American Cancer Society confirmed that those who consumed the least amount of fruits and vegetables were the most likely to develop colon cancer.

Protease Inhibitors • Compounds found in legumes called *protease inhibitors* may help to prevent colon cancer. For example, soybeans contain a unique protease inhibitor: the Bowman–Birk inhibitor, which has been shown to stop the spread of many different forms of cancer, including colon cancer. For example, in rats fed a carcinogen known to induce colon cancer, adding Bowman–Birk inhibitor concentrate to their diet suppressed the formation of tumors in 100 percent of the animals.

Indoles • Indoles are compounds found in cruciferous vegetables including bok choy (Chinese cabbage), broccoli, cauliflower, and brussels sprouts. Some studies suggest that indoles may help prevent cancerous changes in the colon.

Aspirin • Based on a study of more than 635,000 people performed by the American Cancer Society, those who took aspirin were at significantly lower risk of dying from colon cancer. In fact, men and women who took aspirin at least sixteen times a month were 40 percent less likely to die from cancers of the digestive tract than those who did not. Talk to your physician about whether or not you should take aspirin.

Calcium and Vitamin D • Several studies have found a link between low calcium/vitamin D consumption and an increased risk of colorectal cancer. A major 19-year population study of more than 25,000 people in Chicago found that those who had an average daily intake of 1200 milligrams of calcium daily had a 50 percent reduced risk of the disease. Researchers suspect that calcium may bind with bile, thus preventing it from irritating the colon wall.

Exercise • A sedentary lifestyle has been linked to an increased risk of colorectal cancer. In one study, men who scored the lowest in terms of activity had nearly twice the risk of colorectal cancer as the most active men. Presumably, the same is true for women.

Constipation

Constipation is a very common problem among older adults. As we age, the digestive system slows down a bit, making it harder to break down food and eliminate waste. In addition, hormonal changes during menopause can cause occasional bouts of constipation in some women. And prescription drugs such as diuretics, painkillers, tranquilizers, and even antihistamines can promote constipation. However, very often diet and lifestyle are the main culprits, and making simple changes can help to keep you regular.

EARL'S RX

Exercise • I think that inactivity is one of the main reasons why older people (and many younger ones) suffer from constipation. Sitting at a desk all day or sitting in your car prevents your body from working well. You don't have to overdo it; a simple walking program could make a real difference.

Water • Drinking 8 to 10 glasses of filtered water per day will help to increase intestinal motility and prevent constipation.

Fiber • Insoluble fiber—the kind found in foods such as celery, wheat bran, legumes, and most fruits and vegetables—softens and bulks waste to help move it more quickly through the colon, thus helping to prevent constipation. Try to eat between 20 and 30 grams of fiber daily. However, it may not always be easy to get enough fiber from food alone. Therefore, I recommend taking *psyllium* daily. Simply add a teaspoon of psyllium to water or juice, and follow with 2 glasses of water. **(Caution: Psyllium can cause allergic reactions in some people. If you are allergic to different foods, check with your allergy specialist before using psyllium.)**

To prevent bloating and gas, add more fiber to your diet slowly: if you have a low intake of fiber, don't shock your system by dumping in the whole 30 grams in 1 day. Give yourself time to get used to the new foods. If you have a bowel disorder, check with your physician before adding fiber to your diet.

Diabetes

More than 14 million Americans have diabetes, a disease characterized by an excess amount of sugar in the blood and urine. Juvenile diabetes, which occurs during childhood, is caused by the failure of the pancreas to produce enough *insulin,* the hormone that breaks down glucose or sugar so that it can be utilized by body cells. Adult-onset diabetes is somewhat different. In this case, the body produces enough insulin; however, the insulin works less efficiently. The precise cause of diabetes is still unknown; however, in some cases, it may be triggered by a viral infection. There also appears to be a strong genetic component.

Most people don't think of diabetes as a disease of aging, but that's precisely what it is. Eighty-five percent of all cases of diabetes occur in people ages thirty-five and older. If untreated, diabetes can lead to serious complications including heart disease, kidney disease, stroke, and severe circulatory problems. Many diabetics require insulin shots and/or medication that stimulates the production of insulin by the pancreas. However, many diabetics are treated solely through dietary regulation and the careful monitoring of blood and urine sugar.

About one in four Americans have a genetic tendency to develop adult diabetes. Women are twice as likely to develop diabetes as men. However, there is strong evidence that a proper diet and lifestyle can prevent or delay the onset of diabetes.

EARL'S RX

Stay Trim • Obesity is a major risk factor for diabetes (as well as a host of other diseases including coronary artery disease, stroke, and several forms of cancer). Insulin is produced by special cells in the pancreas called beta cells. Beta cells in the pancreas manufacture and store insulin until a rising blood sugar level signals to them to release them. Over time, however, beta cells begin to wear out. It stands to reason that people who consume large quantities of food—especially sugar—may be using up their life's supply of beta cells quicker than others who consume smaller amounts of food.

High-Fiber Diet • Fiber-rich foods help lower insulin needs. A diet rich in legumes, whole grains, fruits, and vegetables may be your best defense against diabetes (and many other degenerative diseases).

Low-Fat Diet • A high-fat diet appears to hasten the risk of developing diabetes. In one study performed at the University of Colorado Health Sciences Center in Denver, researchers tracked the progress of 123 people with a impaired glucose tolerance, a condition that dramatically increases the risk of developing diabetes. The researchers found that people who ate the diets highest in fat were much more likely to develop diabetes than those who adhered to low-fat diets. In addition, in subsequent blood tests, people eating the lowest amount of fat had normal blood sugar levels.

Monunsaturated Fat • Recent studies suggest that increasing your intake of monounsaturated fat (found in olive oil, canola oil, and avocados) may help stabilize blood sugar levels. Substitute other forms of fat, such as saturated and polyunsaturated, with monounsaturates. Do not exceed 25 percent of your daily calories in the form of any fat.

Exercise • A study performed at the U.S. Department of Agriculture's Human Nutrition Research Center on Aging at Tufts University showed that regular aerobic exercise can lower people's risk of diabetes. Researchers studied eighteen older men and women who had above-normal glucose levels on a glucose tolerance test, which increases their risk of developing diabetes by tenfold. After 12 weeks of cycling on an ergometer 4 days per week, the eighteen volunteers increased their blood glucose clearance by 11 percent. In addition, the exercise appeared to improve the ability of their cells to respond to insulin.

Supplements

Chromium • Animal studies have shown that chromium, a trace mineral, can help the body use insulin more efficiently; therefore, less insulin is required to break down sugar. Human studies have confirmed that chromium can reduce blood sugar levels in people with elevated blood sugar. Chromium is found in broccoli, cheese, brewer's yeast, shellfish, and whole wheat English muffins. Chromium supplements are sold in natural food stores. Take 200 micrograms daily.

Magnesium • Older people often become insulin resistant, that is, their insulin does not work as efficiently as it should. Insulin resistance increases the risk of developing diabetes. Studies show that magnesium supplements can help older people improve their ability to metabolize glucose.

Vitamin E (Tocopherol) • A recent Italian study showed that daily Vitamin E supplements of 900 milligrams for four months helped people with adult-onset diabetes use insulin more efficiently, thus helping to normalize blood sugar levels.

Herbal Remedies • U.S. Department of Agriculture researchers used a test-tube assay of insulin activity to identify plants that may help prevent diabetes. Nine plants were found to improve insulin activity including sage, lavender, bearberry (*Uva ursi*), hops, and oregano. (All these herbs and spices are available in natural food stores.) Other potential herbal remedies for diabetes include the following:

Cinnamon • In test tube studies, this spice appeared to significantly increase the ability of insulin to metabolize glucose. Take 1 to 3 capsules daily or sprinkle 1 to 2 tablespoons of cinnamon on your cereal.

Fenugreek • Fenugreek seeds (used to flavor curry and chutney) contain many different compounds that can help prevent surges in blood sugar. Take 1 to 3 capsules daily.

Garlic • Sauté some garlic in that olive oil! Garlic contains an amino acid called S-allylcysteine sulfoxide, which in animal studies has been shown to significantly decrease blood sugar and cholesterol levels. Garlic is also available in tablets and capsule form. Follow the package directions.

Turmeric • The spice that gives curry its golden color, turmeric has been shown to enhance the activity of insulin in test tube studies. Take 1 to 3 capsules daily.

Digestive Disorders

As we age, our bodies produce less hydrochloric acid, which is essential for the digestion of food, especially fibrous meats, vegetables, and poultry. As a result, it is quite common for people over fifty to develop chronic indigestion, which is characterized by gas and bloating after eating. Typically, people with this problem self-medicate by popping over-the-counter antacids. However, that is precisely the wrong treatment, because antacids actually reduce the amount of acid. Thus, the problem worsens. If you have chronic indigestion, first check with your physician or natural healer for an accurate diagnosis: the symptoms could also be related to an ulcer or other medical problem. If your symptoms are due to a reduction in HCl, try the following natural remedies.

EARL'S RX

Eat Smaller Meals • Smaller, lighter meals are kinder on the digestive system than larger, heavier meals. Try to eat small amounts of lean meat, fish, or poultry accompanied by lightly cooked vegetables.

Digestive Aids • There are several over-the-counter digestive aids sold in natural food stores that may help break down food. *Bromelain* is an enzyme found in pineapple that can help digest food and absorb vitamins. It is often used with *papain,* an enzyme found in papaya that can help break down proteins. Both are sold at natural food stores in a chewable tablet form. Chew one 500-milligram tablet daily.

 Betaine hydrochloric acid (made from beets) can also help to get the digestive juices flowing. Take one or two 500-milligram tablets with food up to three times daily.

Herbal Teas • Several herbal teas are excellent for digestion problems. Anise, fennel, and peppermint teas (all sold at natural food stores) are particularly soothing for an agitated stomach.

Diverticulosis

Diverticulosis is a condition characterized by the formation of tiny pouches, or diverticula, in the wall of the colon. Diverticulosis is rare among children and young adults but quite common among people over forty. By age sixty, about half of all people have diverticulosis.

Diverticulosis appears to be a natural part of the aging process and is not serious. However, in rare cases, the diverticula can become inflamed, which can lead to intestinal obstruction. The more serious diverticulitis appears to be related to chronic constipation and straining during bowel movements.

EARL'S RX

Avoid Constipation • A diet rich in fruit, vegetables, and whole grains is usually all it takes to maintain regular bowel habits.

Gallstones

The gallbladder is a sac in which bile from the liver is stored. Bile is essential for proper digestion. Gallstones are solid masses that form in the gallbladder or bile ducts, which can cause inflammation and pain. Up until age fifty, gallstones are more common among women than men; however, at that time, men are equally vulnerable. People with liver disease may be more prone to developing gallstones.

There are three types of gallstones: cholesterol stones, those consisting of pure bile, and stones that are mixtures of bile, cholesterol, and calcium. In some cases, gallstones can be dissolved with drugs, but if not, surgery may be required to remove them. Chronic gallbladder disease may result in the surgical removal of the gallbladder, a cholecystectomy, which is the fifth most common operation performed in the United States each year. However, through diet and supplements, many people can successfully maintain a healthy gallbladder.

EARL'S RX

Low-Fat Diet • An excess amount of fat may result in the overproduction of bile by the liver, which could lead to the formation of gallstones.

Lecithin • Lecithin supplements may help to control cholesterol buildup and may help to prevent gallstones. Lecithin is sold in granule and capsule form at natural food stores. Take 1 tablespoon of the granules or 6 capsules daily.

Herbal Remedies

Dandelion • This herb—or weed, depending on your point of view—enhances liver and gallbladder function and has traditionally been used by herbal healers to treat ailments related to these organs. Interestingly, dandelion is a rich source of lecithin. Eat fresh dandelion in salads, or buy the capsules at natural food stores. Take 1 to 3 capsules daily.

Turmeric • Studies performed in Germany and India show that this spice may help to prevent gallstones, probably by enhancing the action of the liver and gallbladder. Use this spice in cooking or take a 300-milligram capsule up to three times daily.

Gout

Gout is a particularly painful form of arthritis caused by the accumulation of *uric acid,* a substance that is produced by the body from purines, compounds that are found in many different foods. Excess uric acid forms crystallike deposits in joints—typically in the large joint of one or both big toes—which can lead to arthritic-type swelling and pain. More than 2 million Americans suffer from gout; gout is much more common among men than women. After menopause, women are at a higher risk of developing this disease.

Gout tends to run in families. However, in some cases, the condition can be brought on by the use of diuretics and other drugs. Gout can be successfully treated with allopurinol (marketed under the names Lopurin and Zyloprim), which can control the rate at which the body produces uric acid. Other medications can speed up the rate at which the body disposes of uric acid in the urine. Although drug treatment has proven to be quite effective, eating too much of the wrong foods (and drinking too much of the wrong drinks) can still trigger a painful gout attack. If untreated, gout can cause permanent damage to the joints.

EARL'S RX

Watch Your Weight • Being overweight increases the odds of developing gout. Researchers at Johns Hopkins University tracked the health and weight of twelve hundred medical students for three decades. Those who had put on the most weight during early adulthood had a much higher incidence of gout than those who stayed trim.

Watch the Purines • Much of the misery of gout can be prevented by maintaining a sensible diet. People with gout should severely limit their intake of foods rich in purines, including mackerel, brains, anchovies, sardines, shrimp, scallops, and sweetbreads. Talk to your physician or natural healer about the right diet for you.

Watch the Booze • Alcoholic beverages—especially straight up on an empty stomach—can trigger an attack.

Do Drink the Water • Ten to twelve glasses of water daily can help flush the excess uric acid crystals out of the body.

Herbal Remedies • Many herbs have been used to help relieve the symptoms of gout.

Burdock root • This herb has been touted as a "blood purifier" because it can help control uric acid levels. Burdock is available in tea or capsule form at natural food stores.

Juniper Berries • Herbalists have used juniper berries to treat gout. This herb may help to prevent gout by normalizing levels of uric acid. (Ironically juniper berries are also used to make gin.) Juniper berry extract and capsules are available at natural food stores.

Gum Disease

Although Americans are getting fewer cavities thanks to the addition of fluoride in the water, gum disease, which can lead to the loss of teeth, is still very common in the United States. According to the 1985–86 National Adult Dental Health Study, nearly half of all adults had bleeding gums (a sign of inflammation), and 24 percent of all adults and 68 percent of all elderly people had significant periodontal attachments in their mouths, often due to tooth loss. Gum disease is usually caused by the accumulation of bacterial plaque near the gum line, which can cause gums to become inflamed. If the gingivitis progresses, it can destroy connective tissue and bones supporting the teeth. However, tooth loss is not an inevitable part of aging:

in most cases, gum disease can be prevented and teeth can be spared.

EARL'S RX

Oral Hygiene • I have difficulty believing that there are still people who are not flossing their teeth daily. It is one of the best ways to keep gum problems at bay.

Avoid Sugar • Sugar is the breeding ground for bacteria. Limit your sugar intake, and in particular, avoid washing your mouth with sugary drinks. Keep in mind that carbohydrates are converted into sugar in the mouth. Brush or rinse your mouth after eating.

Green Tea • Try washing your meals down with green tea! Green tea contains a compound that has an antibacterial action against *Streptococcus mutans,* the bacteria responsible for tooth decay, which can lead to gum problems.

Supplements

Calcium and Vitamin D • Animal studies show that low calcium intake can result in loss of the bone supporting teeth. Human studies show that Americans fall woefully short on this mineral. Be sure to eat calcium-rich foods or to take a calcium/vitamin D supplement daily.

Folic Acid • In human studies, folic acid supplements resulted in less inflammation of the gums in people with gingivitis. Take 400 micrograms of folic acid daily.

Propolis • Propolis, a by-product of honey, is a rich source of bioflavonoids, naturally occurring substances in food that may help to strengthen tiny blood vessels in the gums, thus helping to prevent injury.

Vitamin C Complex • Vitamin C is required for the formation of collagen in connective tissues and is necessary for the repair and maintenance of all body tissues, including the gums. Vitamin C complex includes several bioflavonoids, including rutin, which has been shown to be especially beneficial for gums. Take 1000 milligrams daily of calcium ascorbate.

Coenzyme Q10 • This works well for gum health. Take 30 to 60 milligrams.

Hearing Loss

Presbycusis, the age-related decline in hearing, can begin at around age twenty, when there is a gradual loss in high-frequency hearing. The loss is usually so subtle that it is hardly noticeable. However, by age sixty, there may be a noticeable loss of middle- and low-frequency hearing, making it more difficult to discern human speech. The extent of hearing loss largely depends on two factors: heredity and exposure to loud noises. However, atherosclerosis can also prevent the flow of blood and nutrients to the ear, which could also cause hearing loss.

EARL'S RX

Safeguarding Your Hearing • The best way to preserve your hearing is to avoid bombarding your ears with loud noises, which can actually cause permanent damage to the middle ear. The level of noise considered to be dangerous is 85 to 90 decibels—normal speech is usually 65 to 70 decibels. If you listen to loud music, work around loud machinery, or use many common items such as a lawn mower or vacuum cleaner, you could be exposing yourself to decibel levels that are unsafe. Impulse noise, such as loud explosions from firearms or firecrackers, are particularly dangerous. If you are in situations where you are exposed to loud noises, be sure to wear protective earplugs. They are sold in drugstores and sporting goods stores.

Hemorrhoids

Hemorrhoids are varicose veins in the anus and rectum. (For a full explanation of varicose veins, see p. 228.) Symptoms include pain and light rectal bleeding. (If you have any rectal bleeding, check with your physician. It could be a sign of a gastrointestinal problem or even colon cancer.)

Chronic constipation, pregnancy, or abdominal straining can cause hemorrhoids. In severe cases, surgery may be necessary. However, this is a problem that can usually be controlled through diet and the judicious use of supplements.

EARL'S RX

Avoid Spicy Foods • Hot pepper can aggravate existing hemorrhoids.

Fiber, Fiber, Fiber • The low-fiber diet typical of most Americans is the major cause of hemorrhoids. A diet rich in fruits, vegetables, and whole grains can help keep your bowels functioning normally, which will prevent the kind of straining that can result in hemorrhoids.

Vitamin E • For quick relief, place some vitamin E oil on a cotton ball or swab and apply to the affected area. (Some people are allergic to vitamin E oil. Be sure to try some oil on a small patch of skin and wait 24 hours. Watch for irritation or burning; if there is none, you can proceed with the treatment.)

Herbal Remedies

Butcher's Broom • A salve made from this herb can be applied directly to hemorrhoids. Butcher's broom products are sold in natural food stores.

Ginkgo • This herb helps to promote good circulation, which may help to prevent varicose veins, including hemorrhoids. Take 1 to 3 capsules daily.

High Blood Pressure

When blood is pumped through the heart, it flows through the large arteries into smaller arteries or arterioles. The walls of the arterioles can expand or contract, thus regulating the blood flow. Blood pressure measures the force of blood against the arterial wall. The top number, called the *systolic pressure*, measures the pressure of the blood flow when the heart is beating. The bottom number, called the *diastolic pressure*, measures the pressure of the blood flow when the heart is at rest. A normal adult blood pressure is around 120/80. High blood pressure is defined as a systolic pressure of 140 or above and a diastolic pressure of 90 or above. However, many studies show that a moderately elevated diastolic pressure (85 plus) may be a sign of a problem down the road.

Untreated high blood pressure is dangerous because it means that the heart is working harder than normal to pump blood, which can damage the heart, arteries, and kidneys. High blood pressure is a major risk factor for both heart attack and stroke.

In most cases, the cause of high blood pressure is a mystery. However, in about 5 percent of all cases, the problem can be attributed to an underlying physical problem such as a congenital heart problem, kidney abnormality, or tumor in the adrenal gland.

In the United States, blood pressure rises steadily with age. Men are more likely to develop high blood pressure at younger ages than women; however, by age sixty-five, women are at greater risk of developing high blood pressure than men. I want to stress that high blood pressure is not an inevitable part of aging. In some parts of the world, blood pressure remains relatively stable from childhood through old age. Many researchers believe that diet and lifestyle play a major role in helping to prevent high blood pressure.

There are numerous drugs that are prescribed to control

210 Earl Mindell's Anti-Aging Bible

high blood pressure. Although most work well, nearly all have some undesirable side effects ranging from excessive fatigue to impotency. However, there are many natural alternatives that may work as well in helping to control high blood pressure or even prevent it from happening in the first place. In addition, in many cases, simple changes in diet and lifestyle can reduce the need for medication.

EARL'S RX

Lose Weight • Being overweight increases the risk of developing high blood pressure. Often, a loss in weight is accompanied by a reduction in blood pressure.

Watch the Salt • Many people are salt sensitive, that is, excessive salt in their diet will cause an increase in blood pressure. The American Heart Association recommends limiting your salt intake to 2500 milligrams per day or 1000 milligrams per 1000 calories. In order to achieve this goal, you should probably not add additional salt to your food and steer clear of restaurants that serve highly salted food.

Exercise • A regular exercise program that requires aerobic activity, such as walking 2 miles daily or swimming laps, can help maintain normal blood pressure. In some cases, it can even lower blood pressure in people with high blood pressure.

Limit Alcohol • Drinking more than 2 ounces daily of an alcoholic beverage can increase the risk of developing high blood pressure.

Load Up on the Fruit • According to a study performed at Harvard Medical School, eating a diet high in fruit fiber can help prevent high blood pressure. In their study, the researchers tracked the diets of more than thirty thousand men and found that those who ate less than 12 grams of fruit fiber daily were 60 percent more likely to develop high blood pressure. The researchers found that fruit fiber was more effective in preventing high blood pressure than fiber from grains. Keep in mind, it may not be just the fiber that has a protective effect. Fruit also contains many different compounds, including some that may help to lower blood pressure.

L-Carnitine • L-Carnitine is a nonprotein amino acid found in the heart and skeletal muscle and has been shown to improve the flow of blood to the heart and reduce blood pressure. L-Carnitine is sold at natural food stores.

Mind Your Minerals

Calcium • A 13-year California study of more than 6600 men and women found that people who consumed 1000 milligrams of calcium daily reduced their risk of developing high blood pressure by 20 percent.

Garlic • Aged odorless garlic supplements can lower high blood pressure. Take 3 capsules daily.

Magnesium • A recent study sponsored by the Netherlands Heart Foundation showed that magnesium supplements were effective in controlling high blood pressure in women with mildly high blood pressure who were not on other medication. Six months of magnesium supplementation reduced the systolic pressure by an average of 2.7 and the diastolic pressure by an average of 3.4. Good food sources of magnesium include legumes, green leafy vegetables, whole grains, bananas, low-fat milk, and apricots.

Potassium • Several studies have shown that potassium can help reduce blood pressure. In fact, in one study of fifty-four patients with high blood pressure who were on medication, half the group was given information on increasing their dietary intake of potassium, and the other half was told to continue on their normal diet. At the end of the study, those patients eating the most potassium-rich foods required the least amount of medication to control their blood pressure. In addition, the patients eating the potassium-rich diet felt better and had fewer symptoms. Good sources of potassium include white potatoes, dried apricots, bananas, low-fat yogurt, and oranges.

Herbal Remedies

Astralagus • This herb, which is widely used in China, has been shown to lower blood pressure in animal studies. Astralagus capsules are available in natural food stores and herb shops.

Celery • Researchers at the University of Chicago discovered a compound in celery called 3-butylphthalide that can reduce high blood pressure in laboratory rats. Interestingly, celery is used by Asian healers to treat high blood pressure.

Dong Quai • Studies have shown that this Chinese herb can lower blood pressure in both men and women. Dong Quai is available at natural food stores in tea and capsule form.

Hawthorn • Human and animal studies have shown that hawthorn, a well-known cardiotonic, can reduce blood pressure during exertion. Hawthorn capsules and teas are sold at natural food stores and herb shops.

Motherwort • This herb is a mild sedative and can temporarily reduce blood pressure. It is available at natural food stores and herb shops.

Reishi Mushroom • Compounds found in this delicious mushroom, which is widely used in Asian cooking, can reduce high blood pressure. Reishi mushrooms are available at Asian markets and at better greengrocers.

Immune Weakness

Immunity is a highly complex system involving the interaction of armies of blood cells and proteins that protect the body against microorganisms (such as viruses and bacteria), other foreign substances, and cancer cells. As we age, our immune system becomes less efficient, making us more vulnerable to disease. At one time, it was believed that a weakened immune system was a natural part of the aging process. However, many researchers now suspect that nutritional deficiencies may be a major cause of immune problems in the elderly. Based on these studies, it appears that it may be possible to keep your immune system strong simply by maintaining adequate levels of crucial nutrients and by using appropriate supplements.

EARL'S RX

Beta-carotene • Several studies have shown a higher incidence of various forms of cancer among people with low blood levels of beta-carotene. One explanation is that beta-carotene is an antioxidant, which means that it protects cells against damage by free radicals, which can lead to cancer. However, recent studies suggest that beta-carotene has a specific effect on the immune system. In one important study, twenty-one HIV-positive patients were given very high doses of beta-carotene (180 milligrams, or 300,000 international units) or a placebo. After 4 weeks, the patients on the beta-carotene showed significant increases in several blood factors that fight infection, including T cells, an essential component of the body's defense system. Good sources of beta-carotene include apricots, cantaloupe, broccoli, sweet potatoes, and pumpkin. Beta-carotene is also available in supplement form. Take up to 25,000 international units daily.

Vitamin B₂ (Riboflavin) • Studies show that deficiencies in this B vitamin can decrease the number of T cells, which can impair immunity. Good food sources of riboflavin include low-fat milk, yogurt, beef, fortified breads and cereals, and green vegetables. It is also included in B-complex formulas and multivitamins. The recommended daily allowance (RDA) is between 1.3 and 1.7 milligrams. According to *The Surgeon General's Report on Nutrition and Health* (1988), a study of older people reported that more than one-third had low blood levels of riboflavin.

Vitamin B$_6$ (Pyridoxine) • Researchers have found that vitamin B$_6$ depletion in elderly people can result in a depressed immune system. Specifically, B$_6$ deficiency appears to impair the release of interleukin-2 and lymphocyte production, two important parts of the body's defense system. Good food sources include cantaloupe, cabbage, low-fat milk, and blackstrap molasses. B$_6$ is included in many multivitamins and B-complex supplements. The RDA for B$_6$ is 1.6 milligrams for women and 2 milligrams for men. Do not exceed doses over 2000 milligrams. I recommend 100 milligrams daily in a B-complex formula.

Vitamin C (Ascorbic Acid) • Several studies have shown that vitamin C can lessen the duration and severity of the common cold, attesting to its antiviral activity. It also appears to raise blood levels of glutathione, one of the most important antioxidants produced by the body, which also plays a role in immunity. The RDA for vitamin C is 60 milligrams. I recommend 1000 milligrams daily.

Vitamin E (Tocopherol) • A recent study published in *The American Journal of Clinical Nutrition* showed that vitamin E supplements can enhance immune response in healthy people over sixty. In this study, thirty-two healthy adults were given 800 milligrams of vitamin E for 3 days or a placebo. Those taking the vitamin E showed a dramatic boost in immune function but not those taking the placebo. Good food sources of vitamin E include whole grains, vegetable oils, avocados, wheat germ, and sweet potatoes. The RDA is 8 to 10 international units; however, I recommend a supplement of 400 international units daily.

Glutathione • Glutathione is an antioxidant produced naturally in the body. A recent study sponsored by the U.S. Department of Agriculture's Human Nutrition Research Center on Aging at Tufts University has shown that supplements of glutathione can dramatically improve immune function in older people. It not only enhanced the cell's ability to fight infection, but reduced inflammatory substances produced by cells. There is no RDA for glutathione. Take a 50-milligram capsule one or two times daily.

Zinc • According to recent studies, as many as 30 percent of all healthy people over fifty may be deficient in zinc, which could hamper immune function. Researchers at Wayne State University in Detroit gave 3 milligrams of zinc daily to thirteen zinc-deficient men and women. After 6 months, the participants showed signs of improved immune function, notably higher blood levels of thymulin, which is essential for the production of mature T cells. Good food sources include oysters, pumpkin seeds, lamb chops, brewer's yeast, poultry, fortified cereals, low-fat milk, and wheat germ. The RDA for zinc is 12 milligrams for women and 15 milligrams for men. To ensure an adequate amount of zinc, eat zinc-rich foods and take a supplement of 15 to 50 milligrams daily.

Herbal Remedies

Astralagus • Researchers at Texas Medical Center found that a purified extract of astralagus can stimulate T cells in cancer patients with impaired immunity. In addition, other studies have shown that astralagus can increase in the production of interferon, a protein in cells that fights against viruses. Astralagus is available in capsule form at natural food stores.

Echinacea • Several studies have shown that this herb can help the body ward off viral infections. Echinacea has been used to restore normal immune function in cancer patients receiving chemotherapy. It is a traditional Native American treatment for colds and flu. Echinacea is sold as capsules and extract at natural food stores.

Ligusticum (Osha) • Called ligusticum in the Orient and osha in the United States, this herb may boost the body's ability to fight against viruses. It was used by Native Americans to treat viral, fungal, and respiratory infections. Ligusticum or osha capsules and preparations are available at natural food stores.

Shiitake Mushrooms • Lentinen, a compound from shiitake mushrooms, may help activate the immune system and fight against tumor cells. The mushrooms are delicious to eat. Shiitake capsules are available at natural food stores.

Kidney Stones

The kidneys are bean-shaped organs that are located just above the waist. The primary job of the kidneys is to filter waste products from the blood. About 10 percent of all men and 3 percent of all women (usually over forty) will develop kidney stones, a condition that can interfere with normal kidney function and may damage the kidneys.

EARL'S RX

Calcium • Most kidney stones are made of calcium and oxalate, a compound found in many plants. Sources include spinach, tea, wheat bran, chocolate, nuts, and rhubarb. At one time, people with a tendency to develop kidney stones were advised to avoid both calcium and oxalate. However, a recent study suggests that that advice was wrong. In fact, calcium may actually help to prevent kidney stones. Researchers at Harvard School of Public Health studied the diet of more than fifty thousand middle-aged men. Much to their suprise, they found that men who consumed the most calcium were 34 percent less likely to develop kidney stones. The researchers concluded that calcium may have somehow prevented the absorption of oxalate.

Don't Load Up on Oxalates • Although you don't have to avoid foods high in oxalates, you should eat them only in moderation.

Potassium • Based on the same study of fifty thousand men, researchers found that men who ate the most fruits and vegetables had the lowest rate of kidney stones. The researchers speculated that since fruits and vegetables are rich in potassium, this mineral may play a preventive role in the formation of kidney stones.

Increase Your Fluids • Be sure to drink 8 to 10 glasses of filtered water or other nonalcoholic fluids daily. The Harvard

School of Public Health study found that men who drank the most fluids had a 30 percent reduction in risk of developing kidney stones.

Watch the Protein • A high-protein diet has been associated with an increased risk of developing kidney stones.

Macular Degeneration

The macula is a part of the retina that is responsible for central vision—the kind of vision required for activities such as reading fine print, sewing, or driving a car. Macular degeneration occurs when the macula is damaged, leaving a blind spot in the center of the visual field. Macular degeneration is the leading cause of blindness among adults over fifty. Laser surgery may help stabilize vision, but recent studies suggest that vitamins and minerals may help.

EARL'S RX

Pass the Collard Greens • A study performed at the Massachusetts Eye and Ear Infirmary in Boston suggests that a diet rich in spinach and other green leafy vegetables may help to prevent macular degeneration. The researchers compared the diets of 356 men and women (age fifty-five to eighty-five) with advanced macular degeneration to the diets of 520 men and women of the same age group who had some other form of eye disease. The researchers found that the people who ate the most carotenoid-rich food had a 43 percent lower risk of advanced macular degeneration than those eating the least carotenoids. In particular, two carotenoids, lutein and zeaxanthin, both found in spinach and collard greens, appeared to have the most potent protective effect. Interestingly enough, lutein and zeaxanthin form the yellow pigment in the macula of the eye. Although more studies must be done to determine whether these two carotenoids are truly effective against this disease, it makes good sense to include spinach and collard greens in your anti-aging diet.

Antioxidants • A complete antioxidant supplement consisting of alpha- and beta-carotene, vitamins C and E, and selenium, plus green tea and grapeseed extract should be taken daily.

Zinc • Preliminary studies suggest that zinc supplements may help to prevent macular degeneration. Take 15 to 50 milligrams of zinc daily.

Memory Loss

By age sixty, most people will experience some decline in short-term memory and alertness. Ironically, long-term memory may work better than ever; in fact, it may be easier to conjure up the name of a long-lost childhood friend than that of a recent acquaintance. Limited memory loss is not serious, and it is certainly not a symptom of Alzheimer's or senility. Nor is it inevitable that everyone will experience memory loss. In fact, some studies suggest that more than one-quarter of all elderly people perform as well on memory tests as younger people. However, there are several reasons why many older people may find their memory beginning to wane. An older brain may not produce the same quantity and quality of chemicals involved in memory function. The blood supply to the brain could be hampered by atherosclerosis or other circulatory problems. In some cases, medication could be interfering with brain function. Nutritional deficiencies have also been implicated as a factor in memory loss among the elderly. Emotions may also play a role. Some studies have even shown that undue stress can trigger memory loss in the elderly, and boredom and depression may also interfere with brain function. However, diet and supplements may help keep you smart and sharp.

EARL'S RX

Avoid High Blood Pressure • Older people with diastolic pressures over 90 (the bottom number) experience a decline in short-term memory loss, based on a study conducted at the University of Maine. In fact, the longer the person had high blood pressure, the worse the memory loss. However, once the blood pressure is normalized, the memory loss will not deteriorate any further.

Supplements

Vitamin B₁ (Thiamine) • Studies have shown that low levels of this B vitamin can cause subtle changes in brain function among older people that could contribute to memory loss. Good food sources of B₁ include brewer's yeast, unrefined cereal grains, pompano fish, sunflower seeds, ham, and peanuts. The recommended daily allowance for B₁ is 1.0 to 1.5 milligrams for adults. Thiamine is added to most B-complex supplements and multivitamins.

Folic Acid • This B vitamin may prevent memory loss by helping to maintain normal levels of homocysteine, an amino acid found in the body. According to a recent study performed by the Agriculture Research Service of the U.S. Department of Agriculture, researchers found a strong correlation between high blood levels of homocysteine and the loss of memory and the ability to learn that often accompanies depression in the elderly. Other studies have shown that folic acid supplements can normalize homocysteine levels in people with elevated levels. High levels of homocysteine have also been associated with an increased risk of heart disease. Good food sources include dark green leafy vegetables, sunflower seeds, wheat germ, liver, and peanuts. The recommended daily allowance for folic acid is 400 micrograms. Supplements are available at natural food stores.

Choline • The brain uses choline to make acetylcholine, a neurotransmitter that plays a role in memory function. As we age, we begin to produce less acetylcholine, or the acetylcholine that is produced is less efficient, which may be why many older people become forgetful. Some researchers believe that choline supplements can reverse this trend. Good food sources of choline include eggs, soybeans, cabbage, peanuts, and cauliflower. I also recommend phosphatidylcholine, which is actually the active ingredient in lecithin. Take 1200 milligrams daily.

Dimethylaminoethanol • Since the 1950s, this supplement has been dubbed "the smart drug" in deference to its reputed ability to enhance brain function. I recommend 130 milligrams in capsule or liquid form one or two times daily.

Herbal Remedies

Club Moss Tea • Researchers at the Shanghai Institute of Materia Medica recently reported that they had isolated natural compounds in club moss called *huperzine* A and *huperzine* B, which, according to animal tests, helped to improve learning, memory retrieval, and memory retention. (Huperzine A appeared to be the more effective.) Huperzine raised acetylcholine levels by inhibiting acetylcholinesterase, an enzyme that breaks down acetylcholine. Acetylcholine is a chemical found in the brain that is directly involved in memory and awareness. Drink 1 or 2 cups of brewed club moss tea daily. There are several different types of club moss; be sure that the tea is *Huperzia serrata* and not some other species of club moss. (The species of club moss native to the United States has not yet been studied, so there is no way of knowing whether it would be as effective.)

Ginkgo • Animal studies have shown that ginkgo increases the level of dopamine, which improves the body's ability to transmit information. Several human studies have shown that ginkgo can improve mental performance among elderly people who have shown deteriorating mental function. In addition, other studies have shown that ginkgo also improves the blood flow to the brain (and to other vital organs), thus providing the brain with oxygen and nutrients needed to function at peak capacity. Ginkgo is available in most natural food stores and even many drug stores. I recommend a supplement called Ginkgo 24. Take the 60-milligram capsules or tablets two or three times daily.

Sleep Disorders

Sleep disorders, ranging from insomnia to frequent night wakenings, are a major health problem in the United States, especially for people in their middle years and beyond. By age sixty-five, at least half of all Americans experience some form of sleep disorder according to the report *Wake Up America: A National Sleep Alert,* issued by the newly established National Commission on Sleep Disorders Research. Many sleep disorders begin during middle age. In fact, women past forty are at particular risk of developing insomnia, often due to menopausal discomfort.

Sleep disorders not only can severely hamper someone's quality of life, but can have a profoundly negative effect on health. Several studies have shown that lack of sleep can impair memory and make it difficult to concentrate, handle stress, and accomplish daily tasks. In addition, the fatigue caused by inadequate sleep can make you more prone to accidents.

Part of the nation's sleep problem stems from the fact that there are many myths about sleep, and one of the most prevalent is that the older you get, the less sleep you need. In reality, the experts say, if you needed 8 hours of sleep at twenty years of age, you still require the same amount of sleep at forty or even at eighty. And although older people may experience different patterns of sleep than younger ones, such as more frequent night awakenings, very often some of the more severe symptoms, such as chronic insomnia, may be caused by a physical problem such as sleep apnea or an emotional problem such as depression. It could even be something as simple as too much daytime napping or too little physical activity. However, as people age, they may simply accept a bad night's sleep as a way of life. They shouldn't. There are many things that you can do that may help to restore a normal sleep pattern. However, if self-help doesn't work, there are some excellent sleep–wake disorders clinics throughout the United States that have had excellent results. Here are some tips to help you get a better night's sleep.

EARL'S RX

Watch the Stimulants • From early afternoon on, avoiding drinking beverages containing caffeine that could keep you awake at nighttime. Caffeinated beverages include coffee, tea, and many colas and soft drinks. Chocolate also contains caffeine, so avoid eating a candy bar late in the afternoon or evening.

Ditto for cigarettes. I personally think that cigarettes should be avoided all the time; however, if you smoke, keep in mind that nicotine is a powerful stimulant. Try not to smoke too close to bedtime.

Pass on the Nightcap • A shot of booze may lull you to sleep, but it also makes you more prone to nighttime awakenings.

Get Enough Exercise, but Not Too Close to Bedtime • Daily exercise can leave you properly tuckered out at night. However, exercise can have a stimulating effect that can last several hours, so try to finish your exercise routine at least 2 to 3 hours prior to hitting the sack.

Sex • Sex is a natural relaxant that helps soothe the body and promote a good night's sleep. Orgasm triggers the release of chemicals by the brain that are natural pain relievers, which can help relieve any aches and pains that may be keeping you awake.

Avoid Sleeping Pills • Barbiturates can be habit forming and can cause dangerous interactions with other medications. Although it may be tempting to simply pop a pill, in my opinion, the risks far outweigh any advantages. In addition, there are numerous other remedies that work as well without any of the side effects.

Melatonin • Melatonin is a hormone produced by the pineal gland in the brain that helps to regulate sleep–wake cycles. Many scientists have suggested that a reduction in melatonin may be responsible for the disruption in sleep patterns experienced by many older people. The National Institute on Aging is sponsoring studies on the role of melatonin in controlling sleep and wakefulness. Preliminary results have been promising. Recently, researchers at Massachusetts Institute of Technology in Boston have shown that melatonin can quickly induce sleep in volunteers. I use melatonin when I travel to help adjust to different time zones. Take 1 to 2 (up to 5 milligrams) capsules or tablets about 1½ hours before bedtime. Occasional use is preferred. I prefer the sublingual (under the tongue) form. Take ½ hour before sleep; do not drive after taking melatonin.

Herbal Remedies

Chamomile Tea • I always end my day with a cup of chamomile tea. Chamomile has a relaxing effect on the body and is an old-time cure for insomnia. Chamomile tea is widely available at supermarkets and natural food stores. (Chamomile is a member of the daisy family, which also includes ragweed. If you are allergic to any members of the daisy family, avoid this herb.)

Hops • Hops, the flower used to brew beer, can be sprinkled on your pillow for a good night's sleep. Dried hops are available at natural food stores. It really works!

Lemon Balm • This pleasant-tasting herb has long been used to treat nervous tension and insomnia. It is available in tea form at natural food stores. Drink 1 cup daily.

Peppermint • This herb has a soothing effect on the body and may help to promote sleep. In addition, it is excellent for heartburn and stomachache, two conditions that can interfere with sleep. Peppermint tea is sold at supermarkets and natural food stores. Drink 1 cup at night.

Siberian Ginseng • Unlike other forms of ginseng that can cause sleeplessness in some people, Siberian ginseng (*Eleutherococcus senticosus*) is used by Chinese healers to treat insomnia. Siberian ginseng is sold at herb shops and natural food stores as capsules, teas, and extracts. Take 1 capsule up to three times daily or drink 1 or 2 cups of tea daily.

Skullcap • This herb is an old-time remedy for insomnia and muscle tension. It is available at natural food stores and herb shops as capsules and tea. Take 1 capsule up to three times daily, or drink 1 cup of tea daily, preferably toward evening.

Valerian • Herbal healers use valerian to treat insomnia due to anxiety-related problems. Valerian is sold at herb shops and natural food stores in capsule or tea form. Take up to 3 capsules daily, or drink 1 cup of tea daily.

Stroke

A stroke occurs when the brain is deprived of oxygen and nutrients due to the rupture or obstruction of the arteries supplying blood to the brain. Most strokes are caused by blood clots that form in the artery bringing blood to the brain or lodge there from some other point in the body. A minority of strokes are caused when a blood vessel on the surface of the brain ruptures and bleeds or when a defective artery in the brain bursts. The telltale signs of a stroke are sudden weakness or numbness in the face, arm or leg on one side of the body; loss or slurring of speech; difficulty understanding others; sudden and severe dizziness; or headaches. Stroke can result in permanent disability. About 10 percent of all strokes are preceded by transient ischemic attacks, so-called little strokes in which the symptoms disappear within a short time.

Stroke is the third leading cause of death in the United States. The incidence of stroke is directly related to age and sex:

men are three times more likely to suffer strokes than women. Thanks to growing public awareness about symptoms and risk factors, the rate of stroke has sharply declined in the United States. However, more than 500,000 strokes occur each year out which 145,000 are fatal. Sadly, I feel that many of these strokes could be prevented.

EARL'S RX

Watch Your Blood Pressure • High blood pressure is the major risk factor for stroke. (For information on how to control your blood pressure, see p. 209.)

Stop Smoking • If you smoke, you are twice as likely to have a stroke than a nonsmoker.

Maintain Normal Cholesterol • People with coronary artery disease are at an increased risk of having a stroke. High blood cholesterol will increase the odds of developing coronary artery disease.

Watch the Scale • Being overweight can increase your risk of high blood pressure, which in turn will increase your risk of stroke.

Protective Foods

Helpful Veggies • A study of 87,000 female nurses showed that eating lots of carrots and spinach can significantly lower a woman's risk of stroke and presumably a man's, too. Carrots and spinach are rich in antioxidants, including carotenoids, which may help prevent arteries from becoming clogged with cholesterol.

Citrus Fruits • Citrus contains coumarins, natural blood thinners, which may help prevent the formation of clots.

Something Fishy • A landmark Dutch study shows that men who eat more than 20 grams of fish daily (about two-thirds of an ounce) had a lower risk of stroke than those who ate less fish. However, don't go overboard on the fish: a previous study

226 Earl Mindell's Anti-Aging Bible

among Eskimos has shown that those who ate the most fatty fish (including mackerel, salmon, sardines, and albacore tuna) had the greatest risk of hemorrhagic strokes. To be on the safe side, stick to two or three fish meals per week.

Garlic • The "stinking rose," as it is sometimes called, contains a compound called *ajoene,* which is a natural blood thinner.

Supplements

Aspirin • Aspirin can prevent the formation of blood clots. Many doctors advise their patients to take a small dose of aspirin (1 baby aspirin) daily or every other day to prevent heart attack and stroke. (No one should take aspirin routinely unless under the supervision of a physician or natural healer.)

Selenium • Studies have shown that people who live in areas with the lowest level of selenium in the soil have the highest rate of stroke. Be sure to eat selenium-rich foods, including garlic, onions, red grapes, broccoli, whole wheat, and chicken. Selenium supplements are available at natural food stores. Selenium is often included in antioxidant formulas. (Doses of over 200 micrograms daily may be toxic.)

Vitamin E (Tocopherol) • Many studies have documented vitamin E's ability to prevent blood clots, which can help prevent stroke. Good food sources include olive oil, whole grains, avocados, sweet potatoes, and oatmeal. Vitamin E is available in supplement form at natural food stores. Take 400 to 800 international units daily.

Herbal Remedies

Ginkgo • This ancient herb improves circulation to the brain and can prevent the formation of blood clots. Ginkgo capsules are available at natural food stores.

Ginger • Ginger prevents "sticky blood," that is, it prevents blood cells from sticking together to form clots. Ginger capsules and teas are available at natural food stores. Ginger is widely used in Asian cuisines.

Ligusticum • Studies have shown that this Chinese herb can help resolve blood clots in patients with transient ischemic attacks and can help improve blood flow to the brain. Ligusticum is available in capsule or liquid form at natural food stores and herb shops.

Taste Loss

As we age, our sense of taste and smell begins to wane. By age sixty, there is usually a noticeable decline in the ability to taste food due to a reduction in the number of taste buds on the tongue. Although the loss of taste is not a medical problem, it can lead to one if it results in a loss of interest in eating, which can lead to malnutrition.

EARL'S RX

Zinc • A daily supplement of 15 to 60 milligrams of zinc gluconate may help to wake up your taste buds.

Check Your Medication • Certain drugs can interfere with the ability to taste food. For example, aspirin can increase sensitivity to bitter flavors, and several other medications such as Biaxin (a form of erythromycin) and tetracycline can cause a lingering aftertaste that can mask the flavor of food. If you're taking medication, check with your physician to see if it could be hindering your taste buds.

Try New Seasonings • Spice up your cuisine—and wake up your taste buds—with a wide variety of herbs and spices. Avoid using too much pepper because it can have a numbing effect on your taste buds.

Variety • Stimulate your taste buds by eating a variety of foods of different textures.

Varicose Veins

A vein is a blood vessel that carries blood back to the heart. (An artery is a blood vessel that carries blood away from the heart.) A series of valves help to push blood through the veins. However, as people age, the valves become less efficient, and skin supporting the veins can become less elastic. As a result, the veins can lose some of their tone, and blood can start to accumulate. After time, the veins can become distended, and varicosities can form. Typically the veins in the legs are most susceptible to becoming varicose, however, other affected sites can include the testes and the esophagus. Varicose veins are not only unsightly, but they can be quite painful.

In some cases, varicose veins are genetic; however, pregnancy, prolonged standing, or even excessive strain of the abdominal region can cause varicosities. Women are four times more likely to develop varicose veins than men, which suggests that hormones may play a role.

In severe cases, varicose veins can be surgically corrected. However, there are some things you can do that may help to prevent this problem.

EARL'S RX

Keep Moving • Although prolonged standing in one spot may cause blood to pool in the legs, exercise can improve circulation. A brisk walk or jog can actually help push the blood through the veins as well as tone up the leg muscles, which in turn help the valves work more efficiently.

Bioflavonoids • Rutin, a bioflavonoid, may help to prevent varicose veins by strengthening capillaries, which are tiny blood vessels. Bioflavonoid supplements are available at natural food stores.

Herbal Remedies

Ginkgo • This ancient herb is used to treat circulatory disorders, including varicose veins. It is rich in bioflavonoids, which may in part explain its beneficial effect on blood flow.

Butcher's Broom • In Europe, this herb is a popular treatment for varicose veins and related disorders. It is available as capsules or a salve that can be placed directly on the affected area.

Gotu Cola • Also known as centella, this herb has been used to treat inflammation and swelling associated with varicose veins. It is available as capsules at natural food stores.

Vitamin E (Tocopherol) • Vitamin E helps to circulate blood to your legs and other extremities. Take 800 to 1200 international units of the dry form in capsules or tablets.

Chapter 4

Just for Women

As more and more women enter their middle years, I am constantly asked about menopause, breast cancer, and other health-related issues of particular concern to women. In this chapter, I address some of these questions and discuss how women can stay healthy and vigorous for their entire lives.

Sexual Health

Between the ages of forty-five and fifty-five, most women enter into menopause, a time of life marked by profound hormonal changes. During this time, production of estrogen by the ovaries begins to decline, and menstruation becomes erratic and lighter and eventually begins to taper off. Once menstruation stops, the ovaries continue to produce estrogen, but at much smaller quantities. The word *menopause* actually refers to the last menstrual cycle; however, the entire process can take up to several years.

In the United States, the average age for menopause is 51, but heavy smokers can become menopausal up to 10 years earlier, and light smokers up to 3 years earlier.

Menopause affects women differently. Many women experience very few changes and suffer few of the unpleasant symptoms often associated with the "change of life." Others, however, may have a more difficult time adjusting to the sudden fluctuations in hormones.

Millions of American women are taking synthetic hormones (hormone replacement therapy) to help cope with menopausal symptoms. Hormonal therapy is not without risk, which I discuss later in this chapter. There are some tried and true natural alternatives that may ease some of the discomfort of menopause without any of the risk associated with hormone replacement therapy. Here are some common problems that women may experience during menopause and some natural remedies.

Bloating

Hormonal changes in menopause can cause the retention of water, which can result in premenstrual syndrome–type bloating. For some women, the bloating is mild. However, for others, it can be so severe that it is difficult for them to wear anything with a defined waistline.

EARL'S RX

Alfalfa • Also rich in phytoestrogens, the leaves of the alfalfa plant are an excellent diuretic. You can toss fresh alfalfa sprouts in salad, or the dried herb is available as capsules or tea. Take 3 to 6 tablets daily or drink 1 cup of tea daily. **(Caution: Alfalfa can aggravate lupus, an autoimmune disorder. If you have lupus or a lupuslike disease, do not use this herb.)**

Centella • Also known as gotu kola, this herb is a mild diuretic and has also been used to treat depression, another problem that can occur during menopause. Centella is available as capsules. Take 1 capsule up to three times daily.

Dandelion • Dandelion, which is also rich in phytoestrogens, is one of the best natural diuretics. The dried herb is available as capsules and tea. Drink 1 cup of dandelion tea daily or take 1 capsule up to three times daily. Dandelion leaves can also be added to salads. Dandelion is also abundant in potassium, a mineral that is often sapped from the body by synthetic diuretics.

Hawthorn • This herb is known as a cardiotonic because of its positive effects on the cardiovascular system. It is also a mild diuretic. It is available as capsules or tea. Take 1 capsule up to three times daily, or drink 1 to 3 cups of tea.

Other herbal diuretics include wild oregon grape or osha, burdock, nettle, chaparral, celery, and asparagus.

Caution: Many women use licorice root to relieve some of the symptoms of menopause. However, licorice can promote the retention of water and should not be used by women who are prone to bloating or those with high blood pressure.

Dry Mouth

The drop in estrogen can also result in less saliva production, which can create a dry, gritty feeling in the mouth.

EARL'S RX

Water • It seems obvious, but be sure to drink at least 6 to 8 glasses of water daily. Sip water throughout the day to keep your mouth and teeth moist. Chewing sugarless gum or sucking on sugarless candy may help.

Slippery Elm Bark   •   Cough drops made from this herb may also help to moisturize your mouth.

Synthetic Saliva Sprays   •   These sprays are sold over the counter and may also offer some relief.

Evening Primrose Oil   •   Two capsules (500 milligrams each) taken up to three times daily can help this condition.

If all else fails, there are several prescription products available that promote saliva formation that may be helpful. Talk to your physician about which one is right for you.

Fatigue

It is not uncommon for women to complain of excessive fatigue during menopause, which is most often due to hormonal changes. Some women may be awakened at night by hot flashes, others may have difficulty sleeping.

EARL'S RX

Suma   •   Many herbalists recommend the South American herb suma to treat fatigue. Also known as the South American ginseng, this herb is available at natural food stores. Take 1 to 3 capsules up to twice daily.

Hot Flashes

About half of all American women experience hot flashes during menopause. A *hot flash* is a sudden feeling of intense heat followed by sweating and sometimes chills. For some women, a hot flash can be a temporary nuisance, but for others, it can be debilitating. Hot flashes are caused by hormonal surges by the pituitary, which is trying to stimulate the production of estrogen by the ovaries. Stimulants such as caffeine and alcohol (which is also a depressant) may promote hot flashes.

EARL'S RX

Many women also have found that supplements of vitamin E (400 to 800 international units daily) and vitamin C (1000 milligrams daily) can help prevent hot flashes. In addition, there are other remedies that may help.

Ginseng • Ginseng, an herb that is rich in a plant form of estrogen, has been successfully used by herbalists to treat hot flashes. Ginseng is available in tea and capsule form. Drink 1 or 2 cups of tea daily, or take 1 to 3 capsules. I recommend American or Siberian ginseng; panax ginseng, which is commonly used in the Orient, may be too stimulating for many people and could cause insomnia. In rare cases, ginseng could cause vaginal bleeding. If you experience any irregular bleeding during menopause, alert your physician or natural healer, and be sure to tell her if you're using ginseng. Ginseng should not be used by people with high blood pressure or irregular heartbeats.

Dong Quai • This herb, which is highly prized in the Orient, is known as the female ginseng. It is mildly estrogenic in action and may help relieve hot flashes as well as other menopausal symptoms.

Vitex • This herb, used to regulate hormonal balance—unlike ginseng or dong quai, it is not estrogenic in action—is a very popular menopause aid. Vitex is available as capsules and in "change of life" herbal formulas for women. Take as directed.

Diet • Diet may also help. Interestingly enough, in Japan there is no word for *hot flash,* and its omission from the language reflects the fact that it is a rare symptom among Japanese women. Japanese women eat a diet that is rich in soy foods, such as tofu, tempeh, and soy milk, which are excellent sources of phytoestrogens, plant compounds that behave like estrogen in the body. Researchers speculate that these plant estrogens— although they are much weaker than real hormones—may help relieve some of the symptoms of menopause that are caused by a decline in the production of natural estrogen. Other foods that are rich in phytoestrogens include alfalfa, cherries, barley, apples, rye, potatoes, rice, wheat, yams, and yeast.

Deep Breathing • Deep breathing may also provide relief from hot flashes. In a recent study of thirty-three menopausal women experiencing hot flashes, slow, deep abdominal breathing appeared to cut their rate of hot flashes in half. The researchers suspect that the deep breathing may lower the arousal of the central nervous system, which usually occurs prior to a hot flash. Deep breathing can be used to prevent hot flashes or to try to ward one off if you feel a flash coming on. Simply take slow, relaxed breaths for about 15 minutes. Be sure you're really breathing from your stomach—your abdomen should fill up with air. Do this exercise twice daily.

Mood Swings

Similar to premenstrual syndrome, many women find that they experience mood swings, depression, or irritability during menopause, which are often caused by hormonal swings.

EARL'S RX

The herbs usually given for menopause, including dong quai, vitex, and ginseng, may help promote a feeling of energy and well-being. In addition, try the following remedies:

Vitamin B_6 • This vitamin is commonly used to treat depression or moodiness due to menopause. Take between 50 and 100 milligrams daily in supplement form. In rare cases, doses over 200 milligrams daily could be toxic.

Hops • This herb, which is rich in phytoestrogens, may soothe and help you to relax. It is especially good for women who may be bothered by insomnia. In the old days, people used to sprinkle hops with alcohol, put it in a pillowcase, and sleep on it. Today, hops are available as capsules. Take between 1 and 3 daily.

Ginger • A cup of ginger root tea is a nice pick-me-up.

Vaginal Dryness

The drop in estrogen can cause a thinning in the vaginal lining and a decline in vaginal lubrication. This can result in painful intercourse and makes the vagina more vulnerable to yeast and other infections.

EARL'S RX

Many women have found that vitamin E supplements (400 to 800 international units) can help prevent vaginal dryness. Here are some other things you can try.

Don Quai • Many women rely on dong quai for this and other menopause-related problems. Take 1 capsule up to three times daily.

Wild Yam • This herb is a rich source of plant hormones that may help prevent vaginal dryness. It is available in capsules. Take 1 up to three times daily.

Vaginal Moisturizers • There are many over-the-counter products that can help lubricate the vagina. To avoid potential irritants, be sure to buy one that is unscented.

Kegel Exercises • These simple exercises can help promote circulation to the vaginal lining and maintain vaginal muscle tone. Squeeze your vaginal muscles—it should feel as if you're trying to stop urinating midstream—hold in your muscles tightly for about 10 seconds, and then release. Repeat this exercise for up to 10 minutes twice daily.

Yeast and Urinary Tract Infections

The thinning of the vaginal and urethral lining make women more prone to yeast and urinary tract infections.

EARL'S RX

Lactobacillus acidophilus • This so-called friendly bacteria found in yogurt may help prevent yeast infections. If yeast infections are a problem, eat 2 cartons of yogurt daily (which is also a terrific way to get calcium) or take 2 acidophilus capsules ½ hour before or after meals three times daily.

Cranberry Capsules • These may help to prevent urinary tract infections. Take 2 capsules up to three times daily or drink 2 glasses of unsweetened cranberry juice daily.

Uva ursi • This herb is commonly used to treat urinary tract infections in women and men. Take 1 capsule up to three times daily to relieve symptoms.

Breast Cancer

Breast cancer is the second leading cause of cancer deaths among American women; lung cancer has the dubious distinction of being the number one cancer killer. In 1994, about 200,000 were diagnosed with this disease, and 46,000 died from it. Breast cancer is a very serious problem; however, the oft-quoted figure that one out of nine women will get breast cancer is somewhat misleading. The risk of developing breast cancer dramatically increases with age. Therefore, a twenty-year-old woman has a significantly lower risk of getting breast cancer than a forty-year-old, and a forty-year-old woman has a significantly lower risk of getting breast cancer than a sixty-year-old, and so on.

The incidence and mortality rate of breast cancer is much higher in western Europe and the United States than it is in Asia or Africa. For example, American women are four times more likely to die from breast cancer than are Japanese women. Yet, when Japanese women migrate to the United States, within one or two generations, their mortality rate from breast cancer is equal to that of the native population. Researchers speculate that breast cancer may be caused by environmental factors such as diet or exposure to cancer-causing chemicals.

Genetics may also play a role in breast cancer, but it appears to be a small one. Only about 6 percent of all cases of breast cancer are believed to be linked to heredity, which means that more than 90 percent of all cases of breast cancer occur in women who have no previous family history of this disease.

Why is the rate of breast cancer so high in the Western world? Is there anything a woman can do to reduce her risk? Although we don't have all the answers, there is some compelling evidence that diet and lifestyle may help prevent breast cancer.

THE LOWDOWN ON FAT

One obvious difference between the United States and countries such as Asia and Africa is diet in general and fat in particular. Our diet contains nearly two to three times the amount of fat as is eaten in less-developed countries. In particular, Westerners eat much more saturated fat, notably from dairy and animal products. In the human body, hormones are stored in fatty tissue. The female hormone estrogen has been shown to trigger the growth of estrogen-sensitive tumors in the breast and other parts of the body. (More than half of all breast tumors are estrogen sensitive.) Therefore, it's possible that a diet high in fat could result in more fat stores in the body and higher levels of hormones. In addition, in menopausal women, hormones produced by the adrenal gland are converted into estrogen by fat cells, which could explain why obesity is a risk factor for breast cancer among menopausal women.

Fat is also the storage site for many potentially dangerous carcinogens that we get from food and other sources that could also spur the growth of tumors.

Epidemiological studies, that is, studies of large populations, have shown a definite link between the consumption of fat and a higher rate of breast cancer among women. For example, in the United States, Seventh-Day Adventists, many of whom are vegetarians and consume less fat than the general population, have up to a 75 percent reduced risk of dying of breast cancer. In addition, animal studies have shown a direct correlation between a high-fat diet and the growth of breast tumors. However, human studies have been more ambiguous. In fact, a major study of nurses published in *The Journal of the National Cancer Institute* showed that there was little difference in the fat intake of women who developed breast cancer and those who did not. Critics of the study, however, contend that all the women in the study were eating too much fat—on average, over 30 percent of their daily calories—and that if women would reduce their fat intake to under 20 percent of daily calories, there would be a significant decrease in the incidence of breast cancer.

Another study revealed that out of a group of women with estrogen-sensitive tumors who have had mastectomies, those who ate a high-fat diet prior to surgery were more likely to suffer a relapse of breast cancer than those who ate leaner fare.

More research is needed to determine if a very low fat diet can significantly reduce the rate of breast cancer, and as of this writing, there are some studies exploring that question. However, given the fact that a high-fat diet has also been implicated in heart disease, diabetes, obesity, and a slew of other medical problems, I think it makes good sense to keep your daily fat intake to between 20 and 25 percent of daily calories.

ENVIRONMENTAL ESTROGENS

For more than a decade, scientists have known that certain chemicals and pollutants in the environment can disrupt normal biological processes in humans and animals. When these compounds are broken down in the body, they mimic the action of hormones such as estrogen. And similar to naturally produced hormones, these "chemical" hormones can trigger the growth of breast tumors and other cancers. Dichlordiphenyltrichloroethane (DDT), which was once widely used as an insecticide but was banned in 1972, is still causing trouble. DDT is broken down in the body to an even stronger compound, dichlordiphenylethylene. There is no evidence that DDT causes cancer, but studies have shown that women with breast cancer have significantly higher rates of dichlordiphenylethylene in breast tissue than women who are cancer free. DDT is not the only culprit. Other compounds that can have similar estrogenic effect in the body include ingredients in plastics, laundry detergents, and some other legal pesticides.

It's very hard to completely avoid many of these chemicals because they are ubiquitous in our environment. However, my philosophy is that you can try to avoid as much personal contact with these chemicals as possible. For example, to reduce pesticide exposure, eat only organically grown fruits and vegetables. Organic produce is available at natural food stores and many supermarkets. Although it costs a bit more, I think it's worth the difference. It's also wise to avoid saturating your lawn or garden with chemicals. Fortunately, there are many natural toxin-free lawn and garden products on the market that can do the job just as well. Check your local plant nursery, natural food store, or botanical gardens for information on environmentally friendly gardening techniques.

Try to avoid potential household toxins. Although we really don't know which, if any, of these products can raise the risk of developing breast cancer, I think it makes good sense to take some precautions. Avoid using aerosol sprays of all types; buy products that come in a pump bottle. Wear gloves when you're using cleansers to prevent skin contact. And avoid unnecessary products such as room deodorizers.

HORMONE REPLACEMENT THERAPY

Millions of women take a daily dose of synthetic hormones—estrogen and progesterone—to help alleviate some of the unpleasant symptoms and side effects of menopause. Studies show that in addition to preventing symptoms such as hot flashes, hormone replacement therapy can help prevent heart disease and osteoporosis. However, there is a downside to pumping your body full of synthetic hormones: women on hormones significantly increase their risk of breast cancer and uterine cancer. In fact, women age sixty to sixty-six on hormone replacement therapy have an 87 percent increased risk of breast cancer. At a recent meeting of the American Association for the Advancement of Science, Dr. Graham Colditz of Harvard Medical School asked an important question: should breast cancer be the price we pay for reduced risk of heart disease and bone fractures? His answer was no, and so is mine.

In the previous section on menopause, I detailed many natural and safe alternatives to hormone replacement therapy. I strongly advise women to think twice before doing anything that will increase their odds of becoming another breast cancer statistic.

ALCOHOL

There is a great deal of confusion about the possible link between alcohol and breast cancer. Some studies have shown that women who drink alcohol increase their odds of developing breast cancer. In fact, in a recent Spanish study of more than 760 women with breast cancer, there was evidence that even moderate drinking (1 or 2 drinks daily) increased the risk of developing breast cancer by 50 percent. However, other studies have not found any connection between drinking and breast cancer.

However, a recent study did find a connection between alcohol intake and estrogen levels. In a 1993 issue of *The Journal of the National Cancer Institute*, researchers reported that women who drank about 1 ounce of pure alcohol daily (roughly two average drinks) showed higher blood and urine levels of estrogen than when they abstained. Because estrogen can promote cellular growth in breast and reproductive tissue, this is a cause of concern, particularly for women who are at risk of getting breast cancer. Given this information, I feel that women with family histories of breast cancer should probably drink only very occasionally if at all. It's also advisable for women who are already taking synthetic estrogen in the form of birth control pills or hormone replacement therapy to think twice about ingesting a substance that will boost their estrogen levels even higher.

FIBER

Several studies have shown that a high-fiber diet reduces the risk of developing breast cancer. There are several reasons why fiber may offer some protection. For one thing, foods that are high in fiber, such as fruits, vegetables, and grains, tend to be low in fat. For another, these foods are also rich in phytochemicals that may help prevent the initiation and spread of many different forms of cancer. Finally, there is some evidence that a particular form of fiber—wheat bran—may help to lower the level of estrogen. In a study conducted by the National Health Foundation, premenopausal women were given 30 grams daily of either wheat bran, corn bran, or oat bran. After 2 months, only the women on the wheat bran showed a significant reduction in serum estrone and estradiol, two potent estrogens that are believed to stimulate the growth of breast tumors. Researchers believe that the estrogen binds with wheat fiber and is eliminated in the feces.

CANCER FIGHTERS

There are several other foods and supplements that are believed to have a protective effect against breast cancer.

Carotene • One study performed at the Department of Social and Preventive Medicine at the State University of New York at Buffalo, compared the diets of 439 postmenopausal women with breast cancer to postmenopausal women who were cancer free. The researchers found that the risk of breast cancer was highest among women with the lowest intake of carotene in their food. Although the study appeared to deal with only beta-carotene, it's important to note that foods that are rich in beta-carotene are also often good sources of alpha-carotene, lutein, and other carotenoids. Apricots, bok choy, pumpkin, carrots, and cantaloupe are excellent sources of carotenes.

Vitamin C • Several studies have linked a low intake of vitamin C with an increased risk of breast cancer.

Genistein • Found only in soy products, this compound has been shown to block the growth of breast cancer cells in test tube studies. Many people believe that the low rate of mortality from breast cancer among Japanese women is due to their high consumption of soy products. Tofu, soy milk, and soy protein is a good source of genistein.

Legumes • Legumes such as soybeans, lentils, and kidney beans are also believed to protect against breast cancer. Dried beans contain many anticancer compounds including phytic acid and protease inhibitors. They are also low in fat.

Lignans • Found in abundance in flaxseed and to a lesser extent in rye, lignans are hormonelike compounds that compete with the body's own estrogen for estrogen receptor sites on cells. By doing so, lignans deactivate potent estrogens that may trigger the growth of breast tumors.

Limonene • Found in the peel of citrus fruits, this compound has been shown to inhibit the growth of carcinogen-induced mammary tumors in rats and prevent new tumors from forming.

Omega-3 Fatty Acids • Found primarily in fatty fish, such as salmon, mackerel, and albacore tuna, studies have shown that omega-3 fatty acids can inhibit the growth of mammary tumors.

Quercetin • Studies show that this bioflavonoid can inhibit the growth of human tumor cells containing binding sites for type II estrogen, which may be responsible for some forms of breast cancer. Quercetin is abundant in red and yellow onions and shallots.

Sulforaphane • Found in broccoli and other cruciferous vegetables, sulforaphane promotes the production of anticancer enzymes in the body. In one study, rats were pretreated with either a high dose or a low dose of a synthetic form of sulforaphane and then given a carcinogen known to induce mammary tumors. Another group of rats were just given injections of the carcinogen. More than two-thirds of the group that did not receive the sulforaphane developed breast cancer, as opposed to 35 percent of the low-dose sulforaphane-treated group. Out of the high-dose sulforaphane group, only 26 percent developed cancer.

PERSONAL MAINTENANCE

There are no guarantees with cancer: you can do all the "right things," eat the right foods, take the right vitamins, and for some unknown reason still develop breast cancer. However, the earlier the stage in which breast cancer is diagnosed, the better the prognosis. Therefore, women should be vigilant about examining their breasts for lumps or signs of abnormalities at least once a month. If you don't know how, the American Cancer Society has some excellent pamphlets that can show you what to do.

Most women should have a baseline mammogram by age forty, and some should have one earlier depending on family medical history. By age fifty, women should have an annual mammogram. Be sure to get your mammogram at a facility that is accredited by the American College of Radiology.

Lung Cancer

Lung cancer actually kills more women annually than breast cancer. Although some cases of lung cancer may be genetic or even related to diet, in many cases, lung cancer is a self-inflicted disease, and cigarettes are the weapon of choice. Since women have started smoking, there has been a steady rise in the incidence and mortality rate from lung cancer. In fact, since the 1980s, mortality rates from lung cancer among women have increased 3 percent annually. Women smokers have more than five times the risk of developing lung cancer than nonsmokers.

I know it's not easy to quit. Cigarettes contain highly addictive substances that are designed to keep you coming back for more. However, keep in mind that it's not just your lungs that are in jeopardy. There is nothing that will age a woman faster than a cigarette. Women who smoke enter into menopause on average 2 years earlier than nonsmokers. They also are more prone to develop osteoporosis. In addition, they develop more wrinkles on their skin and look on average about 5 years older than nonsmokers.

Some forms of lung cancer are not related to smoking, and in these cases, dietary fat may be a major culprit. In a study conducted by the National Cancer Institute, researchers surveyed 1450 nonsmokers ages thirty to eighty-four. Out of this group, 429 had been diagnosed with lung cancer between 1986 and 1991. Based on this study, the 20 percent of the women who ate the highest amount of saturated fat had six times the risk of developing lung cancer than the 20 percent of the women who ate the least amount of saturated fat. Researchers aren't sure if fat per se is the "smoking gun" or whether fat was present in some other food, such as cooked red meat, which also contains potential carcinogens such as heterocyclic amines.

One interesting note: in this study, the women who ate the most beans (legumes) and peas had a 40 percent lower risk of lung cancer than those eating the least!

246 Earl Mindell's Anti-Aging Bible

Osteoporosis

Osteoporosis is caused by the thinning or wearing away of bone, which increases the susceptibility to breaks and fractures. Areas that are particularly vulnerable include the vertebrae, hips, and forearms. About four out of five of the 25 million Americans with osteoporosis are women, and the majority are menopausal. Small-boned white and Asian women are at greatest risk of developing this disease. Hispanic and African-American women are at the lowest risk.

Nearly 40 percent of all postmenopausal American women will suffer vertebral fractures, and in severe cases, some will develop a rounded back or dowager's hump. Osteoporosis is not merely an aesthetic problem: it can be very serious, even fatal. About 15 percent of all white women over fifty will fracture a hip sometime in their lifetime. About 20 percent of women hospitalized for hip fractures will develop medical complications such as pneumonia or blood clots that will result in their deaths. Osteoporosis is a growing problem. By 2030, the U.S. National Institutes of Health estimates that the rate of hip fractures will reach 400,000 annually, up from 300,000 in 1994.

Osteoporosis can also cause tooth loss due to bone deterioration in the jaw.

Losing bone is a natural part of the aging process and happens in both men and women. However, osteoporosis is the rapid loss of bone. During childhood and early adulthood, new bone is constantly being produced. Bone consists of several minerals including a large amount of calcium and phosphorus salts and smaller amounts of magnesium, zinc, iodine, fluoride, and other trace elements. By around age thirty, people develop their peak bone mass, that is, the production of new bone cells begins to slow down. In fact, after thirty-five, people begin to lose roughly 1 percent of their bone mass annually. After menopause, however, women begin to lose about 2 to 4 percent of their bone mass each year for up to a decade until it begins to level off. The rapid loss after menopause is attributed to a decline in estrogen, which is essential for calcium absorption. In fact, many menopausal women are given hormone replacement therapy (also known as estrogen replacement therapy, which has been shown to stem the rapid bone loss associated with menopause). However, hormone replacement therapy is a short-term solution. If a woman goes off hormones, as many do after 5 years, the rate of bone loss begins to accelerate. In addition, many women cannot take hormones in the first place.

Women who cannot or will not take hormones or who don't stay on hormones for their entire postmenopausal lives are not doomed to get osteoporosis. Osteoporosis is not an inevitable part of aging: with proper planning and intervention, it can be prevented. There are many things that a woman can do throughout her lifetime to keep her bones healthy and strong.

CALCIUM AND VITAMIN D

Several studies have underscored the need to get adequate amounts of calcium and vitamin D. Vitamin D is essential to help the body utilize calcium and phosphorus. Some forms of osteoporosis may be caused by a genetic inability to utilize vitamin D correctly, which adversely affects the body's ability to absorb calcium. In fact, researchers have recently isolated the gene that may be responsible for the malfunction in vitamin D absorption.

The recommended daily allowance (RDA) for vitamin D is 400 international units. (Vitamin D can be toxic at levels over 1000 international units daily. Do not exceed the RDA unless under a physician's supervision.)

The RDA for calcium is 800 milligrams for children up to 10, 1200 milligrams up to age 24, and 1000 milligrams for adults. Most adults consume roughly half the recommended amount. However, the National Osteoporosis Foundation recommends that postmenopausal women not taking estrogen replacement therapy should consume 1500 milligrams of calcium daily. There is even some evidence that 800 milligrams daily may be low for girls. In one study, adolescent girls consuming about

1600 milligrams of calcium were shown to develop significantly stronger bone mass than girls consuming less calcium. The researchers noted that the high-calcium consumers were not excreting excess calcium in their urine, which suggested that during adolescence when these girls were building their peak bone mass, the body was retaining the extra calcium. Although most experts do not recommend that parents give children more than 800 milligrams, it is imperative that children get the full RDA.

Even after peak bone mass is formed, calcium is needed to retain the bone you have. Many researchers believe that maintaining calcium levels during the thirties, forties, and fifties will help boost calcium stores, which women can draw upon in later years. There is also some evidence that increasing calcium levels during menopause may make a real difference. In one 1992 French study of 3270 women over age sixty-five, researchers gave half the group supplements of 1200 milligrams of calcium and 800 international units of vitamin D. The other half received a placebo. After about a year and a half, the vitamin-supplemented group had 43 prevent fewer hip fractures than the unsupplemented group. In addition, hip bone density increased in the supplemented group by 2.7 percent and actually decreased by 4.6 percent in the unsupplemented group.

Good food sources of calcium include low-fat or no-fat dairy products (one nonfat plain yogurt contains about 400 milligrams). However, many low-fat cheeses contain phosphate, which may interfere with the body's ability to absorb calcium; therefore, these foods are not a good calcium source. Other good food sources of calcium include tofu processed with calcium sulfate (434 milligrams per 4 ounces), sardines with bones (324 milligrams per 3 ounces), calcium-fortified orange juice (220 milligrams per 6-ounce serving), and broccoli (90 milligrams per 4 ounces, cooked). Calcium can also be obtained through supplements. There are many different types of calcium supplements; I recommend calcium citrate because it is the best absorbed. Supplements that contain calcium citrate contain less calcium per dose (about 200 milligrams) than some other forms of calcium, which means that you need to take more pills.

Calcium citrate should be taken on an empty stomach.

Beware of supplements made from bone meal, oyster shells, or dolomite; recent studies show that they may contain unsafe levels of lead.

Vitamin D is present in fortified daily products (1 cup of milk provides 100 international units) and fatty fish oils. Sunshine is also an excellent source of vitamin D, because ultraviolet rays stimulate certain skin oils to produce vitamin D. However, sunscreens and sunblocks may filter out the rays necessary to produce vitamin D. Therefore, it's important to expose your skin to sun without protective lotion once or twice a day for about 10 minutes. Limit your sun exposure to the very early morning (before 10 A.M.) or late afternoon (after 3 P.M.) when the sun is not at its strongest.

For many women, it may be necessary to supplement vitamin D during the winter when bone loss occurs at a faster pace than during the warmer months. In fact, according to a recent study, a supplement of 400 international units of vitamin D during the winter can reduce bone loss. Talk to your physician or natural healer about increasing your intake of vitamin D during the winter.

EXERCISE

A regular program of weight-bearing exercise may help strengthen bones. In fact, the lack of physical activity in our modern-day lives may be one of the major reasons why osteoporosis is on the rise. Studies show that human bones are actually getting weaker. For example, during the restoration of an old church in London, scientists compared the bone density of eighty-seven women buried in a church crypt from 1729 to 1852 to the bone density of postmenopausal women living today who were roughly the same age. The scientists discovered that the dead women had denser bones and appeared to have lost bone at a much slower rate than the contemporary women. The scientists were puzzled by the result but attributed the denser bones of the deceased women to the fact that they were probably much more physically active than women today. Without modern conveniences such as washing machines and cars, these women performed more physically demanding tasks. Studies have shown that weight-bearing exercise, such as walking, running, or jogging, can not only help build bone but will increase muscle mass, which can protect against fractures by absorbing the shock of a fall. (Swimming and cycling are not weight-bearing exercises.)

Combining calcium supplements with exercise may offer added protection. Researchers at Tufts University studied the effect of calcium and exercise on the bone density of thirty-six postmenopausal women. One group of women was given a high-calcium drink daily containing 831 milligrams of calcium, whereas the other group was given a low-calcium (41 milligrams) placebo. Each woman was told to include 800 milligrams of calcium in her diet. In addition, women were either assigned to participate in an exercise group (a 50-minute walk four times per week) or were told to refrain from any recreational activities. After 1 year, the researchers found that the women consuming the most calcium had a 2 percent increase in the femoral neck bone mineral density, whereas the placebo group had a 1.1 percent decrease. In addition, the exercise group showed a 0.5 percent increase in the bone mineral density of the spine, whereas the sedentary group experienced a 7 percent decline. This and other similar studies show that diet and lifestyle can make a significant difference in reducing the risk of osteoporosis.

MEDICATION

A drug called salmon calcitonin is one of two Food and Drug Administration–approved treatments for postmenopausal bone loss (estrogen is the other). Calcitonin is a hormone produced by the thyroid gland and is found in humans and many animals. Calcitonin helps to regulate the amount of calcium in the blood and by doing so indirectly affects the amount of calcium in the bone. Studies show that calcitonin can actually stop bone loss and is also used to relieve pain from fractures. Calcitonin may also stimulate new bone formation. Calcitonin is safe, but there may be some unpleasant side effects such as nausea. The real downside to calcitonin is that it must be delivered daily by injection; however, many people can do this on their own with little difficulty. In Europe, a nasal spray form of this drug is available, which may be sold in the United States within a few years. If you have osteoporosis and are not taking hormone replacement therapy, talk to your physician about using calcitonin.

OTHER BONE BUILDERS

There are other foods and supplements that may help to preserve bone.

Boron   •   Researchers at the U.S. Department of Agriculture found that a supplement of 3 milligrams of boron daily could double serum estrogen levels in women, which may help to prevent osteoporosis. Estrogen helps to retain adequate amounts of calcium and magnesium, which are needed to build strong bones. Good food sources of boron include dried fruit and grapes.

Soy Foods   •   Even though Japanese women are small boned, they suffer about half the number of hip injuries as American women. The fact that they may be more active physically may be one reason why they have fewer injuries. For example, Japanese women typically sit on the floor, and the action of getting up and down several times daily may help to develop their hip bones. However, their diet, which is rich in soy foods, may be another reason why they have stronger bones. Researchers at the University of North Carolina investigated the effect of genistein, which is found in soybeans, on the bone mass of rats who had their ovaries removed to eliminate their natural source of estrogen. Genistein is rich in plant estrogens, compounds that mimic the action of natural estrogen in the body. The study determined that genistein was able to prevent bone loss in rats almost as well as a synthetic form of estrogen. Although more studies need to be done, soy appears to be a bone-sparing food that American women should include in their diet. (Tofu made

252 Earl Mindell's Anti-Aging Bible

with calcium sulfate is a particularly good choice: it is abundant in both calcium and genistein.)

WATCH THESE BONE BREAKERS

Caffeine can hamper calcium absorption. In a 4-year study performed at the University of California of nearly one thousand postmenopausal women, researchers found that those who drank 2 cups of coffee per day or more suffered a significant drop in bone density. However, those who drank at least 1 cup of milk per day seemed to be protected from coffee's bone-breaking effect.

Smokers have a higher rate of osteporosis than nonsmokers. Yet another reason to kick the habit!

Alcohol can hamper the absorption of calcium, which will cause bones to become thin and brittle. Excessive drinking also makes you more prone to falling, which can result in a break or fracture.

Chapter 5

Just for Men

Men typically die younger than women. I don't believe that men are the "weaker sex," rather, men are more stoic about their health—they often ignore important symptoms and deal with health problems only when they absolutely have to (or when their wives force them to!). However, a new generation of men is taking a greater interest in health and fitness, and I believe this change in attitude may add years to the average man's lifespan. Here's some important information that every man should know about.

Sexual Health

Good health and great sex go hand in hand at any age, but it is particularly true for men once they reach middle age. As men approach the second half of life, hormonal shifts and other changes can alter sexual response. Hormone levels that control sexual arousal may dip. For example, many men showed a marked drop in testosterone production beginning around in their late forties. In Europe, this period is called *viropause,* and there are some similarities to the female menopause. Similar to female menopause, some men may experience minor symptoms resulting from hormonal fluctuations. Although men remain fertile, they may find that it takes longer to get an erection and they may have difficulty maintaining one at times. However, none of these factors should significantly impair a man's ability to enjoy sex.

There is no intrinsic reason why a man can't enjoy a vigorous sex life for his entire life. However, many men do not. According to the Massachusetts Male Aging Study, a recent groundbreaking study of men between the ages of forty and seventy, about half of the 1290 participants experienced some form of impotency. The researchers defined impotency as "the persistent inability to attain and maintain an erection adequate to permit satisfactory sexual performance." Most of the men experienced minimal or moderate forms of impotency. The risk of severe or total impotency increased threefold with age: 5.1 percent of all forty-year-olds complained of complete impotency versus 15 percent of all seventy-year-olds. But the researchers were quick to point out that in most cases, a persistent sexual problem was a sign of an underlying physical problem. In fact, 39 percent of the heart disease patients and 15 percent of the high blood pressure patients were completely impotent compared with less than 10 percent of the entire group. (In these situations, the impotency is often not due to the disease, but to the medication that is used to treat it, as I will discuss later.) Disregard for one's body also seemed to be a major culprit in promoting impotency. For example, for heart patients, smoking appeared to be the kiss of death for sex: those who lit up were three times more likely to be impotent than those who did not.

The study also revealed that the men least likely to complain of impotency were those with high levels of high-density lipoprotein, or "good" cholesterol. In addition, contrary to popular opinion, blood testosterone levels were not related to male potency. But another hormone was right on target: blood levels of dehydroepiandrosterone (DHEA), which is produced by the pituitary, were a good indicator of impotency. (For more information on DHEA, see p. 171.) In fact, men with the highest levels of DHEA were the least likely to be impotent. This doesn't necessarily mean that DHEA promotes sexuality; its effect on a man's sex life may simply be due to the fact that men with high DHEA levels are less likely to develop heart disease.

Many of the physical problems that can destroy a man's sex life are easily avoidable or can be successfully treated. The following section reviews some of the major causes of male impotency and ways to cope with them.

Poor Circulation

In order to maintain an erection, blood must flow freely to the penis. However, if the arteries delivering blood to the genitals become narrowed or clogged due to atherosclerosis, the blood supply will be impaired. This could explain why so many heart patients complain of impotency. Diabetics, hypertensives, and heavy smokers are also at great risk of damage to their vascular system, which could result in a poor blood flow to their genitals. Impotency is often the first sign of a circulatory problem in men.

EARL'S RX

A low-fat diet (with less than 20 percent of daily calories in the form of fat) is your best defense against clogged arteries. If you smoke, stop. Each and every cigarette you smoke inflicts slow damage to your vascular system, which will eventually result in circulatory problems. In addition, if you smoke, your partner may also light up. Smoking can impair a woman's vaginal lubrication, which will make having sex even more difficult.

If you are diabetic, be especially vigilant about maintaining normal blood sugar levels. There is evidence that high blood sugar can cause nerve damage that can contribute to impotency. The combination of cigarette smoking and diabetes appears to be particularly dangerous.

To improve blood flow throughout the body including to the sex organs, take a vitamin E supplement of 400 international units twice daily, morning and evening. (Do not take vitamin E if you are using a blood thinner.) In addition, the Chinese herb *Ginko biloba* has also been shown to improve circulation to the extremities. *Ginko biloba* is available in capsule form at natural food stores.

Alcohol

Although a drink or two may help you "loosen up," contrary to popular belief, alcohol actually inhibits erection and ejaculation in men. Heavy drinkers may damage their liver, thus impairing the production of sex hormones. In addition, chronic alcoholics may permanently damage nerves within their penis that are essential to maintain an erection.

Earl's RX • If sex is on your agenda, hold off on the alcohol until you're done. If you're a heavy drinker, talk to your physician about getting help to stop.

Drugs

Prescription and over-the-counter drugs can cause many sexual problems in men. Some medications, including those used to treat high blood pressure, depression, anxiety and even allergies, can sap sexual desire or cause impotency or difficulty with ejaculation. For example, some men on beta-blockers used to treat hypertension may experience what I call the "beta-blocker blues," a palpable loss in libido. In addition, men on antidepressant drugs such as amitriptyline hydrochloride (Elavil) may suffer a loss of libido or find that they have difficulty with ejaculation. Finally, some men may respond to certain medications with excessive fatigue: although they may be physically capable to have sex, they may feel too dragged out.

EARL'S RX

I don't want to panic men who may be on prescription drugs: these kinds of adverse reactions to drugs are relatively rare, affecting between 1 and 2 percent of users. However, if a man is experiencing impotency or other sexual problems and he is taking medication, he should check with his physician to determine if the medication could be causing the problem. Oftentimes, simply switching to another medication will solve the problem.

Caution: If you are on medication for heart disease, high blood pressure, or any other serious problem, do not discontinue your medication without first checking with your physician.

If you are hypertensive and suspect that your blood pressure medication is bringing you down, it may be possible to reduce your dose simply by adopting certain changes in your diet and lifestyle. Be sure to work closely with your physician or natural healer so that he or she can monitor your results.

If you're taking medication for a heart problem, keep in mind that fear may be hampering your sexual performance, not your medication. Many heart patients mistakenly believe that they cannot withstand the physical stress of sex. In most cases, this is simply not true. In fact, one recent study concluded that for most heart patients, having sex was no more dangerous than getting out of bed in the morning! Talk to your physician or natural healer about your fears.

Fatigue or Loss of Desire

If you simply can't summon up the energy or the interest to have sex, you need to reexamine your lifestyle. Are you getting enough sleep? Are you getting enough exercise? Are you eating a healthful diet? Are you knocking yourself out at night with a nightcap? Could you be suffering from a vitamin deficiency? Excessive fatigue could be a sign of depression or an underlying physical problem, so if you are constantly exhausted, you should consult with your physician or natural healer. However, very often, it's a sign of poor nutrition and poor health habits.

EARL'S RX

Vitamin A • Vitamin A helps produce sex hormones that are essential for sexual functioning. Eat foods rich in beta-carotene, which is converted into vitamin A as the body needs it. Take 10,000 to 15,000 international units of beta-carotene daily.

Vitamin B_6 • B_6 boosts the levels of hormone that regulates testosterone. Good food sources include brewer's yeast, wheat germ, cantaloupe, cabbage, and blackstrap molasses. A good multivitamin will contain B_6.

Manganese • This mineral helps produce two chemicals in the brain that heighten sexual arousal: dopamine and acetylcholine. Good food sources of manganese include nuts, whole grain breads, cereals, legumes, beets, and green leafy vegetables.

Zinc • Zinc is essential for the production of testosterone. (As I discuss later, it also helps to keep the prostate gland healthy.) Men should take between 15 and 50 milligrams of zinc daily.

Octacosanol • This natural food supplement, which is rich in wheat, wheat germ, and vegetable oils, is reputed to increase stamina and sexual performance in some men. Octacosanol is sold in capsule form in natural food stores.

Yohimbe • This herb is the only Food and Drug Administration–approved aphrodisiac on the market for men. The drug yohimbine is available by prescription only and has been shown to restore sexual potency in some men. The herb yohimbe, a much weaker version of the drug, is available in natural food stores and is included in many so-called male potency formulas. I recommend 500-milligram capsules up to two or three times daily.

Following my simple suggestions may help some men. However, any man who has a chronic problem with impotency should see his physician or natural healer. Fortunately, there are numerous medical treatments available for impotency including surgical penile implants. Don't suffer in silence, talk to your physician.

Prostate Problems

The prostate is a small walnut-sized gland located between the bladder and the penis, above the rectum. The prostate gland produces semen, the fluid that carries sperm. During childhood, the prostate is tiny; however, once puberty kicks in and testosterone levels rise, the prostate gland grows to adult size. The prostate gland remains stable until around age forty-five, at which time it often experiences a second growth spurt. By age sixty, most men have an enlarged prostate gland, a condition that is called *benign prostate hypertrophy* (BPH). As its name implies, in most cases, BPH is harmless, although it can be quite annoying. If the prostate gland becomes very swollen, it can push against the urethra and interfere with urination. In fact, in about 10 percent of all men, the first sign of BPH is urinary retention. Other symptoms include difficulty or straining during urination and frequent urination, especially at night. In severe cases, urine can gather in the bladder until it eventually backs up into the kidneys, causing kidney damage. About 10 percent of men with BPH will require corrective surgery; in fact, prostate surgery is the most common surgery performed on people over sixty-four.

Earl's RX • Some men may find that certain foods, such as caffeinated beverages, alcoholic drinks, and hot, spicy food, may aggravate their condition. Obviously, if you find certain foods or drinks to be irritating, your best bet is to avoid them. However, many men with BPH try to cope with their problem by drastically reducing their intake of liquids. This is not a good idea and could actually add to their woes by triggering a urinary tract infection. If you have BPH, consult with your physician or natural healer. Most men can be treated successfully with medication or with any number of herbal remedies that may relieve some of their discomfort.

In 1992, the Food and Drug Administration approved a new drug, finasteride, marketed as Proscar, for BPH. Proscar works by blocking the conversion of testosterone into a more potent form of the hormone that is believed to trigger prostate growth. Proscar works well for many men but is expensive and can cost up to one thousand dollars annually. A small number of men on Proscar experience impotency and decreased libido among other side effects. In addition, Proscar should not be used by people with liver problems.

Natural food stores are also filled with prostate remedies, some of which work well for many men. Natural remedies tend to work better in the early stages of BPH. The advantage of using a natural remedy is that it is inexpensive and can be purchased without a prescription. The downside of herbal remedies is that they are much weaker than the prescription drugs and may not work for everybody. On the positive side, however, they do not cause any known side effects. For many men, herbal remedies will do the trick. However, if the herbal remedy doesn't help, they can always switch to a stronger medication. Following are some popular remedies that may help men with BPH.

Saw Palmetto • Many herbal formulas for BPH contain extract from the berries of the saw palmetto tree. Native Americans ate saw palmetto berries as part of their diet. Natural healers have long prescribed these berries for urinary problems.

Several studies have shown that saw palmetto can increase

the flow of urine and reduce nighttime urination in men with BPH. In Europe, where most of the research on saw palmetto was conducted, this herb is an accepted treatment for BPH.

Some studies show that saw palmetto berry extract may work by preventing the conversion of testosterone to its more potent form, dihydrotestosterone. Compounds in the saw palmetto berry may block dihydrotestosterone's ability to bind to receptor sites on prostate cells, thus preventing the cells from growing. Take 1 to 3 capsules (540 milligrams) daily.

Pygeum • The bark of the pygeum plant has been used for prostate problems since the eighteenth century and is included in many modern herbal formulas. Pygeum contains phytosterols, compounds that have anti-inflammatory activity. Phytosterols block the production of prostaglandins, compounds that are involved in the inflammatory process. In addition, pygeum is a diuretic, which can help promote urination.

Pumpkin or Squash Seeds • A species of pumpkin or squash seeds grown in the Near East (*Cucurbita pepo*) is included in many herbal prostate formulas. *Curcurbita pepo* contain many beneficial phytochemicals including beta-sistosterol, an anti-inflammatory, and cucurbitacin, which may help facilitate urination by relaxing the sphincter (that regulates the flow of urine and increasing the tone of bladder muscles. Pumpkin seeds are also an excellent source of vitamin E and zinc.

Pumpkin seed oil is sold in natural food stores in capsule form.

Stinging Nettle • This herb is a a diuretic and anti-inflammatory. It is often in conjunction with the herbs discussed above to treat prostate problems.

Couch Grass • This mild diuretic is often included in many herbal combinations for BPH.

Zinc • Zinc plays a major role in the male reproductive system. There are heavy concentrations of zinc in the prostate gland. Zinc stimulates the production of testosterone, the male hormone that aids in men's capability for erection and ejaculation. A zinc deficiency may contribute to infertility. Zinc may also help to prevent BPH. Therefore, I advise men to take 15 to 50 milligrams of zinc daily and to eat foods rich in zinc, which include pumpkin seeds, oysters, cashews, nonfat dry milk, brown mustard, pork loin, round steak, and brewer's yeast.

CANCER OF THE PROSTATE

Cancer of the prostate is the second most common form of cancer in American men. (Skin cancer is number one.) In 1994, some 200,000 American men will be diagnosed with this disease.

Responsible for 35,000 deaths annually, prostate cancer is the second leading cause of cancer deaths among men, surpassed only by lung cancer. In the United States, the lifetime risk of getting prostate cancer is one out of eleven for white males and one out of nine for African-American men. The death rate from prostate cancer is steadily creeping upward by about 2 to 3 percent annually. African-American men are three times as likely to die from prostate cancer as white men, probably due to late diagnosis.

In most cases, if caught early, prostate cancer can be successfully treated by surgery or radiation therapy. In many older man (over sixty), however, the tumors are so slow growing that they may not need treatment at all. In these cases, the physician may recommend a policy of "watchful waiting" to see how the cancer progresses.

Because of the risk of prostate cancer, men over forty should have an annual physical examination that includes a digital rectal exam. In this exam, the physician inserts a lubricated finger into the rectum to palpate for any prostate irregularities or early rectal cancers. However, the digital rectal exam may not detect small tumors. That is why the American Cancer Society recommends that men over fifty also have an annual prostate-specific antigen (PSA) blood test. PSA is a protein produced by the prostate. High levels of PSA may be a sign of tumor growth.

All men should be aware of the warning signs and symptoms of prostate cancer. According to American Institute for

Cancer Research, men should report any of the following symptoms to their physicians.

- Any changes in urinary habits.
- Blood in the urine.
- Painful urination.
- Continuing pain in the lower back, pelvis, or upper thighs.

Keep in mind that having one or more of these symptoms does not mean that you have cancer. It could also be a sign of a urinary tract infection or another problem and should not be ignored. Even if it does turn out to be prostate cancer, the earlier the diagnosis, the better the prognosis.

In the United States, prostate cancer is relatively common, but not so in Asia or Africa. In fact, Japanese men have the lowest rate of mortality from prostate cancer in the world. Black men in Nigeria have a lower rate of prostate cancer than African-American men in the United States. Researchers suspect that diet and other environmental factors may contribute to the risk of dying from prostate cancer.

In one major study conducted at Harvard Medical School of 48,000 men, researchers found that diet may play a major role in determining who lives or dies from prostate cancer. In this study, researchers compared the diets of the 417 men out of the group who had been diagnosed with prostate cancer to those of the men who did not get this disease. The researchers found that diet did not appear to increase the odds of developing prostate cancer. However, among the men who developed this disease, a diet high in fat appeared to be a major risk factor in whether or not the disease emerged to a more advanced state. Animal fat in particular appeared to have a lethal effect on prostate cancer. Specifically, men who ate the highest amounts of red meat, butter, and chicken with skin fared the worst. However, eating skinless chicken, vegetable fat, or dairy products other than butter did not seem to have any adverse affect. From this information, researchers concluded that a particular form of fatty acid—alpha-linolenic acid found in animal sources— may be responsible for triggering tumor growth. It's interesting to note that other studies have shown that Seventh-Day Adventist men who follow a vegetarian diet have a much lower rate of prostate cancer than the national average. And even though Japanese men in Japan have an extremely low rate of mortality from prostate cancer, when they migrate to the United States—and presumably begin eating the typical American diet—their risk dramatically increases.

Another reason why Japanese men in Japan may be protected against prostate cancer is the fact that their diet is rich in soy foods such as tofu and soy milk. In my book *Earl Mindell's Soy Miracle,* I reviewed numerous studies that showed that many of the compounds in soy have potent anticancer properties. Soy is rich in phytoestrogens, hormonelike compounds that may deactivate the more potent hormones that can trigger tumor growth. One compound in particular, genistein, has been shown in test tube studies to inhibit the growth of prostate tumor cells. Genistein is now being tested on men in the United States who are in the early stages of prostate cancer to see if it can slow down the progress of the disease. Interestingly, autopsies of Japanese men reveal that their rate of prostate cancer is as high as that of American men. Most of them have small tumors in their prostates when they die; however, these tumors are not detected because they are so slow growing, they never develop into clinical disease. Studies will show whether or not genistein is the secret weapon against prostate cancer. Given the epidemic of prostate cancer in the United States, I recommend that men try to eat at least one serving (2 to 3 ounces) of tofu or soy food daily. I start my morning with a tofu shake. There are also powdered soy protein products on the market that offer a day's supply of genistein.

Other Male Concerns

HAIR TODAY . . .

Some men manage to keep a thick head of hair throughout their entire lives, but starting around middle age or even younger, most men experience hair loss that could eventually lead to balding. Healthy, young men lose an average of about 100 hairs daily, which are usually replaced by new growth. As men age, however, hair may tend to thin out and, in some cases, result in balding.

About two-thirds of all men have male pattern baldness, which is a genetic condition passed down by either parent. However, even if one of your parents is bald, it doesn't mean that your fate is sealed. The gene can skip a generation. However, the reverse is also true: even if your parents have thick, lustrous manes, you could still inherit the gene for baldness.

Male pattern baldness usually begins gradually, starting with a loss of hair at the front of the scalp at either side of the hairline or on the crown, the circular area on top. Hair loss can start as early as the teenage years, but more often than not, it begins during middle age.

Why so many otherwise healthy men lose their hair as they age is still very much a mystery. Some researchers believe that testosterone, the male hormone, may thwart hair growth by shrinking the hair follicle. Others believe that the hair follicle becomes clogged with sebum, a substance produced by the skin, which prevents nutrients from reaching the hair follicle, thus thwarting growth.

In some cases, hair loss may be caused by an underlying physical problem. For example, an underactive or an overactive thyroid can create a hormonal imbalance that can accelerate hair loss, but once the problem is corrected, the hair grows back. Cancer patients may suffer temporary hair loss after radiation or chemotherapy treatments. Sometimes rapid hair loss is a sign of an autoimmune disease called *alopecia areata*, which results in patchy bald spots on the scalp. However, hair loss due to alopecia is usually temporary in adults. In extremely rare cases, a severe vitamin deficiency may be the underlying cause.

For thousands of years, men have sought a cure for baldness. To this date, there is no tried and true cure for this problem. However, there are some treatments that may help some people.

A handful of men have had success with the drug minoxidil, marketed under the name Rogaine. Since 1979, minoxidil has been given orally to treat hypertension in patients in whom other drugs have not worked. Sold under the name Loniten, minoxidil had some scary side effects, including rapid heart rate, fainting, breathing difficulties, and the accumulation of fluid around the heart. Minoxidil had one other interesting side effect: physicians prescribing minoxidil noticed that it promoted hair growth on the scalp and other parts of the body including the hands, cheeks, and nose. Because minoxidil is a strong drug that could produce many dangerous side effects, it could not be prescribed orally to treat a cosmetic problem like baldness. However, researchers at Upjohn Company, the makers of minoxidil, devised a minoxidil–alcohol solution that could be applied directly to the scalp, thus eliminating many of the side effects associated with the oral form. In 1989, the Food and Drug Administration approved the external use of minoxidil, or Rogaine, to treat baldness.

No one is sure why minoxidil may help to grow hair. Some experts speculate that it works by stimulating the flow of blood to the scalp, which may stimulate the hair follicle. Others feel that minoxidil may counteract the balding gene in a cell, instructing hair follicle cells to grow although they may have been programmed to shut down.

How well does minoxidil work? Based on several studies, it appears that only a small number of men will experience noticeable hair growth. For many men, however, minoxidil will produce a disappointing fuzz or no results at all. For maximum result, minoxidil treatments should begin at the first sign of baldness. The solution must be rubbed into the scalp twice daily. If the minoxidil is discontinued, hair loss will resume.

Minoxidil is expensive; treatment can cost up to $100 dollars monthly. The usual dose is a 2 percent minoxidil solution; however, if the low dose fails, some physicians may prescribe up to a 5 percent solution.

Studies show that external minoxidil does not appear to produce any of the dire side effects of oral minoxidil. However, some physicians are still reluctant to give the drug to people with an existing heart condition. A small number of men who have used minoxidil complained of itching on the exposed areas, which was probably due to the alcohol.

There is one natural alternative to minoxidil that may or may not work for you, but it's a lot cheaper and you don't need a prescription. Jojoba (pronounced ho-ho-ba) oil, which is made from a desert plant, can also improve the blood flow to the scalp. After shampooing, massage a few drops of oil into your scalp and keep it on overnight. Be sure to avoid contact with your eyes, and if any irritation occurs, discontinue use. Shampoo out in the morning.

Diet and nutrition play a major role in how you feel, and how you feel is reflected in how you look. Although a healthy lifestyle may not prevent hair loss, it can help keep your remaining hair in peak condition. For a healthy, shining mane, be sure to eat foods rich in B vitamins. Brewer's yeast, wheat germ oil, raw and roasted nuts, and whole grain foods are packed with B vitamins.

As the baby boom generation grows up—the generation that turned long hair into a political statement—there is likely to be a frantic search for a cure for baldness. For example, researchers are investigating the possible use of Proscar, a drug designed to treat enlarged prostate glands, to treat baldness. Proscar works by keeping testosterone levels under control, which may help to reduce hair loss. One Canadian company is even experimenting with a machine that zaps the scalp with low-level electricity, which supposedly stems hair loss by stimulating the hair follicles.

When it comes to balding, men will try practically anything. Native Americans used to rub chili peppers on their scalp to stimulate hair growth. This is not as crazy as it sounds: similar to minoxidil, chili peppers stimulate blood flow to the hair follicles, allowing nutrients to flow freely. I don't recommend this treatment because chili peppers can be very irritating to the skin and eyes; however, it's interesting to note that the so-called hot new treatments of today are not really that hot or new.

SAVE YOUR SKIN

Skin cancer is the most common cancer to afflict men. Men are more likely to die from melanoma, the potentially lethal form of this disease, than are women. Not so coincidentally, men spend nearly twice as much time in the sun as do women and are four times less likely to use a sunscreen.

I can't stress this enough: if you are exposed to the sun, you must use a sunscreen of at least 15 sun protection factor (SPF) at all times. Make sure that the sunscreen offers broad-spectrum protection, which means that it filters out both ultraviolet A and B rays.

Keep in mind that sunscreens are not a panacea. Recent studies show that although sunscreens can help prevent basal cell and squamous skin cancers, both of which are highly treatable if caught early, they do not protect against the more serious melanoma. Try to avoid sun exposure during the "burning rays" of 10 A.M. to 2 P.M. However, if you spend a great deal of time outdoors, for example, if you work outside during the summer months, I recommend wearing sun-protective clothing. Dark clothing with a heavy weave offers the best protection; however, it's likely that it will also keep you uncomfortably warm. A summer-weight T-shirt offers protection equal to an SPF of 5 to 7 and only a 2 SPF when it is wet. Fortunately, there are some new lines of lightweight clothes that are specifically designed to offer additional sun protection. There are at least three manufacturers that claim their outerwear offers an SPF of 30. Look for sun-protective clothing at your local sporting goods store.

Don't forget to wear a hat. It not only offers additional protection for your face, but shields your scalp from the cancer-causing rays.

Men who feel that summer is just not summer without a tan should investigate using a self-tanning cream. In the past, these creams fell into disrepute because they turned the skin a sallow yellow color. However, the new creams produce a better result and in my opinion are a much safer alternative to a suntan.

SAVE YOUR BLADDER

It's conventional wisdom that people should drink between 8 and 10 glasses of water daily, and I know many active men who drink even more. Water helps prevent constipation, keeps the skin moist, and helps maintain the correct balance of fluids in the body. A recent study, however, showed that men who drink 14 or more cups of fluid daily of any kind—including coffee or fruit juice—face a two to four times greater risk of developing bladder cancer than men who drink around 7 cups. Further investigation showed that tap water—whether it was consumed in pure form or in fruit juice or brewed coffee—appeared to be the culprit. Researchers speculate that chlorine in municipal water systems may promote cancer. My advice: keep drinking water, especially in the hot summer months, but switch to bottled water or install a home filtering system.

Testosterone

At one time, researchers believed that the male hormone testosterone was the primary reason why men fell prey to heart disease at younger ages and had a shorter life span than women. However, recent studies suggest that testosterone may have been getting a bad rap. For example, one important study performed at Saint Luke's–Roosevelt Hospital Center in New York showed that contrary to previous assumptions, men with lower levels of testosterone were more likely to get heart disease than men with higher levels. In addition, men with higher testosterone levels had higher levels of high-density lipoproteins, or "good" cholesterol.

Testosterone levels tend to decline with age, and some researchers speculate that providing supplemental testosterone to men with low levels may help to ward off some age-related ailments. For example, studies have shown that testosterone supplements in older men may help to prevent osteoporosis, maintain muscle strength, control depression, increase sex drive, and even help to boost brain function. In fact, some researchers speculate that in the not too distant future, many older men may routinely take testosterone supplements much the same way that many menopausal women take estrogen replacement therapy. There is one downside to testosterone: similar to estrogen, it can stimulate the growth of hormone-sensitive tumors and may contribute to prostate cancer. My advice: as good as testosterone therapy may sound, proceed with caution.

Chapter 6

Getting Physical: The Power of Exercise

Since early times, men and women have been desperately searching for a fountain of youth—a magical pill or potion that could reverse the aging process. Fortunately, the search is over and the fountain of youth may be as close as your local gym. Study after study confirms the fact that exercise may be the one true way to turn back the clock. I'm not talking about becoming a marathon runner or an Olympic athlete; a moderate and consistent exercise program is all it takes to live longer, live stronger, and live better.

As we age, there are many physical changes that affect strength and appearance. For most people, by age forty-five, there is a noticeable decline in muscle mass and an increase in body fat. In fact, the typical sedentary adult loses up to 7 pounds of lean body mass per decade. There is also a decrease in bone density; bones get thinner and more prone to fracture.

Aerobic ability declines, which means that you may find yourself huffing and puffing more after exertion. There is also a loss of flexibility; you may feel stiffer and less supple. However, aging does not have to be a physical downward spiral. Many of these changes can be postponed, minimized, and even reversed by physical activity. In fact, experts say that a fit fifty- or sixty-year-old can actually be in better shape than a flabby thirty-year-old! In addition, exercise may help prevent many of the diseases that can cut life short.

Exercise: The Best Preventive Medicine

LONGEVITY

A recent study of ten thousand Harvard graduates ages forty-five to eighty-four showed that those who participated in moderately vigorous activities (such as tennis, swimming, jogging, and brisk walking) had up to a 29 percent lower death rate than the sedentary men. In fact, exercisers on average lived 10 months longer than those who did not exercise. Interestingly, even men who began exercising late in life (after age sixty-five) lived up to 6 months longer than couch potatoes.

In another study performed at the Institute for Aerobics Research and the Cooper Clinic in Dallas, researchers followed thirteen thousand men and women for an average of 8 years to determine whether there was any correlation between fitness levels and longevity. Based on the results of an exercise treadmill test, the group was divided into five levels ranging from the least fit to the most fit. The women in the least fit group had the highest mortality rate. However, women in the second lowest fitness group had nearly half the death rate of the least fit. Based on these findings, the researchers concluded that something as easy as taking a brisk walk daily could add years to your life.

HEART DISEASE

In the same study of ten thousand men in the previous section, those who exercised had a 41 percent reduced risk of heart disease than sedentary men. This is not surprising, considering that other studies have shown that regular exercise can decrease your total cholesterol, increase the "good" high-density lipoproteins, improve respiratory function, and lower your blood pressure. In another study conducted at the Laboratory of Cardiovascular Science at the Gerontology Research Center in Baltimore, researchers found that physical activity may retard the increased stiffness in arteries that often accompany aging. The scientists studied fourteen middle-aged long-distance runners who ran about 30 miles a week. They found that the runners had a greater capacity to dilate their coronary arteries than sedentary men of the same age, thus markedly increasing the blood flow to their heart. Researchers aren't sure how much activity is required to keep arteries from stiffening, but they do know that being sedentary is a sure way to speed up the process.

STROKE

In a 22-year follow-up of more then 5300 Japanese-Americans in the famous Honolulu Heart study, researchers found a strong association between a sedentary lifestyle and an increased risk of stroke. In inactive and partially inactive men between ages fifty-five and sixty-eight, there was a fourfold risk of hemorrhagic stroke (bleeding in the brain) and threefold risk of subarachnoid stroke (bleeding between the brain and the skull) when compared to active men.

Exercise also appears to protect women against stroke. Researchers at the University of Washington in Seattle investigated exercise intensity and early signs of cardiovascular disease in about twelve hundred women. The scientists found that the women who exercised the least were most likely to show signs of thickening of the inner and middle layers of the carotid arteries in the neck, which could increase the risk of stroke.

CANCER

Exercise appears to offer a protective effect against different forms of cancer. Many animal studies have shown that exercise can inhibit tumor growth. There's some evidence that increased physical activity may zap cancer cells in humans as well. For example, a recent study showed that men with sedentary jobs were 1.6 times more likely to develop colon cancer than those with more active jobs. Researchers speculate that physical activity causes an increased motility of the gastrointestinal tract and more frequent bowel movements, which limits exposure to potential carcinogens in stool.

There is also a link between exercise and lower rates of breast cancer. In a major study performed at the Harvard School of Public Health, researchers tracked the exercise habits of 5400 women graduates ages twenty-one to eighty. Based on the study, the more athletic the woman, the lower her risk of developing breast cancer. Other studies have shown that exercise can reduce estrogen levels; some forms of estrogen can trigger the growth of tumor cells.

IMMUNITY

Exercise may add some zip to your immune system. Exercise heats up the body much the same way a fever raises your temperature. When the body is warm, it triggers the production of pyrogen, a protein that is part of interleukin, a type of white blood cell that enhances immune function. Other studies suggest that exercise may reverse the drop in immune function that normally occurs with aging. Researchers at Appalachian State University in Boone, North Carolina, found that very fit women over seventy had immune systems that functioned as well as women half their age!

A word of caution: long-distance running may actually dampen your immune system. Studies show that runners are more prone to colds, flu, and upper respiratory ailments after participating in a marathon. Researchers suspect that overexertion may have a weakening effect on the body. Moderation is the key!

PREVENTING FRAILTY

Researchers are learning that exercise can keep you active and mobile at any age. According to a groundbreaking study conducted at the Hebrew Rehabilitation Program for the Aged in Boston, a carefully planned strength training program for the elderly can counteract muscle weakness typical of very old people. The study found an average 113 percent increase in muscle strength among the participants, which in many cases meant the difference between eating alone in their rooms and being able to walk to the dining room. On average, the exercisers experienced a 12 percent increase in walking speed and a 28 percent increase in stair climbing power. An added bonus: the people who exercised began to take part in more recreational and educational activities offered at the home, thus enriching their lives in other ways. Researchers suspect that if more older people participated in strength training programs, many could avoid the kinds of falls and injuries that force them into nursing homes in the first place. Other studies have shown that men as old as ninety showed a significant improvement in muscle strength after a mere 8 weeks of exercise.

MENTAL FITNESS

Flexing your muscles may strengthen your brain power. Researchers have documented that older people who do regular aerobic exercise perform significantly better on cognitive tests than their sedentary colleagues. One explanation could be that exercise improves blood flow to the brain.

MENTAL WELL-BEING

Exercise makes you happier. Physical activity increases the release of beta-endorphins, chemicals produced by the brain that are natural painkillers. Exercise also lowers your adrenaline level, which can reduce feelings of stress and anxiety.

OSTEOPOROSIS

Weight-bearing exercise can help slow down the loss of bone mass, which is particularly problematic in postmenopausal women. Researchers suspect that regular exercise could help women retain up to 5 percent of their bone mass—women on average lose up to 35 percent of their bone mass in the years following menopause. Beginning an exercise program before menopause will lay down a foundation of bigger and stronger bones.

Getting Started

TAKE THIRTY

Half of all Americans are sedentary, that is, they barely get any physical activity at all. Many people say that they'd like to exercise, but with their busy schedules, they simply can't find a chunk of time during the day to work out. In addition, many people were put off by exercise gurus who insisted that fitness could only be achieved by following a complicated and rigorous program. The good news is, they were wrong. According to the President's Council on Physical Fitness, all it takes to achieve a reasonable level of fitness is to exercise moderately for at least 30 minutes daily. It doesn't have to be in one continuous session—you can do a little bit of exercise throughout the day as long as it adds up to a total of 30 minutes.

Design an exercise program that works best for you. For example, it can be as simple as taking a brisk walk twice daily for fifteen minutes (or three walks for 10 minutes each). Or you can work out on an exercise bike for fifteen minutes in the morning before work and take a fifteen-minute walk after work. Have a back-up plan for bad weather. An indoor jogging track or shopping mall is a great place to walk or run on nasty days. Don't worry if you miss a day; as long as you exercise on most days, you're ahead of the game. Jogging, running, tennis, and swimming are also good choices. Or try something more exotic, such as fencing or martial arts. Many older people are discovering that studying tai chi can help build strength, grace, endurance, and confidence.

STRETCHING

In addition to the 30-minute activity program, I recommend that everyone do some simple stretching exercises at least three times a week for 15 minutes at a time to help maintain flexibility. It's not difficult: simply get down on the floor and gently stretch and flex every joint and bone in your body. Start with your toes and work your way up. Breathe slowly and deeply into the stretch, and stop if you feel any pain or discomfort. Even better, take a stretch and tone class at a health club or local Y. Even if you just attend one stretch class weekly, you can do the exercises at home on your own. There are also some excellent exercise videos on the market that include stretching and strengthening. One of my favorites is *Body Electric* with Margaret Richard. The videotape is fun and easy to follow. In addition, her show is featured on many public television stations and is a great way to start the day. *The Wellness Encyclopedia*, written by the editors of *The University of California, Berkeley, Wellness Letter*, includes a terrific section on exercise that provides specific information on working out at home.

STRENGTH TRAINING

Several studies have shown that strength training with weight can preserve flexibility, muscle, and bone in people well into their nineties. I don't recommend buying a set of weights and working out on your own; the chance of injury is too great. However, I do recommend learning how to use weights properly at a health club or Y. Hire a personal trainer to work with you for a few sessions so that you can learn how to use weights safely. In some cases, the facility may even provide new members with a few free sessions with a trainer. Be sure the trainer is accredited by the American College of Sports Medicine; there are many people out there claiming to be qualified exercise trainers but who have few qualifications.

HELPFUL TIPS

Find an exercise partner. It's more fun to have company, and you're less likely to slack off if another person is counting on you. It's also safer not to run or walk alone, but even with a partner, avoid walking in deserted areas. Be sure to wear reflective gear at night, especially if you're walking on a road that is used by cars.

If you have a heart condition or any other medical problem, check with your physician before beginning an exercise program.

Are You Getting Enough of What You Need?

Exercise places new demands on your body. Be sure that you are getting enough of these important vitamins and minerals.

CHROMIUM

Chromium helps to burn fat and regulate blood sugar. Combined with exercise, chromium can help build muscle. Many Americans are deficient in chromium. Good food sources include spices such as cinnamon, grape juice, brewer's yeast, broccoli, mushrooms, whole wheat, apples, and peanuts. Chromium supplements are sold in natural food stores. Take a 200-microgram capsule or tablet up to three times daily.

VITAMIN B$_2$ (Riboflavin)

This B vitamin helps the body release energy from food. Researchers at Cornell University found that the need for riboflavin increases with activity. Many studies show that older people do not get enough of this vitamin. Good food sources include low-fat milk, yogurt, lean beef, fortified breads and cereals, and green vegetables. Riboflavin is included in many multivitamins and B supplements. Take 50 to 100 milligrams daily.

VITAMIN E (TOCOPHEROL)

Although exercise offers many benefits, several studies have shown that vigorous exercise increases oxygen consumption, which may promote the formation of free radicals. Free radicals are unstable molecules that can destroy cells. However, antioxidants, particularly vitamin E, may help prevent this damage. In fact, studies also show that vitamin E supplements can help prevent muscle soreness that often occurs after a workout. It's difficult to get enough vitamin E from food alone. Therefore, I recommend taking 800 international units daily in the form of D-alpha-tocopheryl succinate (dry form).

POTASSIUM

Sweating can sap the body of important minerals including sodium, which most of us have enough to spare, and potassium, which can be replaced by eating potassium-rich foods. Fruits such as bananas, orange juice, and prunes are excellent sources of potassium. So are baked white potatoes and plain yogurt.

WATER

While you are exercising, take a few sips of water every 10 minutes or so. Don't forget to drink at least 2 glasses of water after working out.

ZINC

Increased physical activity can lead to a loss of zinc in sweat and urine. Zinc-rich foods include pumpkin seeds, oysters, low-fat milk, brewer's yeast, and lamb chops. Zinc is included in many multivitamins. Take 15 to 50 milligrams daily.

Chapter 7

Looking Good and Staying That Way

Nothing can make you look older than wrinkled, dried-out skin. But skin is not just for decoration: in reality, it is the largest organ system in the body and one of the most hardworking. Skin performs many critical tasks: it helps regulate body temperature; it enables the body to retain fluids; and it's the immune system's first line of defense against viruses, bacteria, and other foreign objects.

As we age, skin undergoes normal wear and tear. Fine lines and wrinkles may develop, which are caused primarily by a breakdown in *collagen*, the protein that is responsible for the support and elasticity of the skin. Gravity begins to pull the skin down, which can cause it to loosen and become flabby. The body produces less *sebum*, an oil that forms a protective coating on the skin, which can result in patches of dry, itchy skin. Cell regeneration slows down, which can leave the skin looking drab and tired. Perhaps the worst assault to skin is caused by exposure to ultraviolet (UV) light from sunlight, which can damage skin cells and cause premature aging and skin cancer.

Until recently, we believed that there was little that could be done to prevent the skin from showing signs of age. However, we now know that a combination of factors, including lifestyle, diet, supplements, and skin care products, can help skin maintain a youthful appearance and, more importantly, keep skin cancer free.

Getting Back to the Basics

Healthy habits are reflected in healthy, glowing skin. Before investing a lot of money in fancy products, try these simple things first.

BEAUTY IS FROM THE INSIDE OUT

Skin is made of cells, and cells need the proper nutrients to thrive. A careful diet including an abundance of fruits, vegetables, and fiber can help keep your body working well and your skin in top form. In addition, studies have shown that a low-fat diet (no more than 20 percent of your calories from fat) can reduce the risk of developing precancerous skin lesions (actinic keratoses) that can lead to nonmelanoma skin cancer, the most common cancer among white Americans. Vitamins and other supplements can also help. In particular, I recommend the following.

Earl's Rx for Beautiful Skin

RNA/DNA, 100 milligrams each daily
Superoxide dismutase and wild yams, 300 milligrams each daily
Cysteine, 500 milligrams
Vitamin C, 1500 milligrams
Biotin, 100 micrograms
Beta-carotene, 25,000 international units
Water, 6 to 8 glasses daily of filtered or bottled water

GET YOUR BEAUTY SLEEP

During sleep, our bodies secrete human growth hormone and other skin growth factors that may stimulate the production of collagen and the production of new skin cells. A chronic lack of sleep may take its toll on your complexion.

SMOKING

According to a report in *The New England Journal of Medicine*, smokers are more likely to appear at least 5 years older than nonsmokers. Smoking is associated with an acceleration in facial wrinkling, perhaps because smokers are constantly squinting their eyes to avoid smoke from their own cigarettes.

WATER

If you don't get enough fluids, your body will sap fluid out of body cells, which can leave them dehydrated. Dehydrated skin cells are more likely to have a dried-up, wrinkled appearance. The antidote is easy: drink 8 to 10 glasses of water daily. (A glass or two of juice is fine, but remember that many juices are laden with calories.)

284 Earl Mindell's Anti-Aging Bible

EXERCISE

Moderate exercise can relieve tension, and tension can add years to your face. A stressed-out twenty-year-old with "worry lines" on her forehead can look older than a relaxed and fit forty-year-old.

MAINTAIN NORMAL WEIGHT

Constant weight loss and gain can rob skin of its flexibility, resulting in sagging skin.

BE GENTLE

Don't tug or pull at your face. Cleanse gently with a cotton ball or soft washcloth, and pat dry. Loofas and grainy cleansers are often too rough for many people and should be used rarely on skin if at all. People with dry skin should avoid abrasive cleansers altogether.

Sun Protection

As far as your skin is concerned, UV light is public enemy number one. According to the American Cancer Society, about 700,000 new cases of skin cancer will be diagnosed this year, most of them due to sun exposure. Although most cases of skin cancer are not serious, more than 32,000 people develop malignant melanoma, which is potentially fatal. The bad news is, it appears that sunscreens and blocks do not protect against melanoma. Sun exposure can also accelerate the aging process. In fact, dermatologists blame as much as 80 percent of the skin damage associated with aging on exposure to the sun. As dangerous as the sun may be, I'm not suggesting that people spend their days indoors. However, be sure to follow these guidelines.

NO TAN IS A GOOD TAN

Until recently, the prevailing philosophy had been that if you gradually increased your exposure so that you didn't burn and wore a good sunscreen, it was possible to tan safely. We now know that there is no such thing as a good tan. Tanning is the body's response to injury; therefore, it should be avoided.

AVOID PEAK EXPOSURE

Do as my friend the dermatologist does: during the summer, he runs for shelter during the hours of 10 A.M. and 2 P.M., when the sun is the strongest. Confine your outdoor activities to early morning or late afternoon.

CHECK YOUR MEDICATION

Some medication, such as tetracycline, Retin-A, and even some diuretics, can increase sensitivity to the sun. If you're taking any medication, be sure to check with your physician before spending time outdoors.

WEAR SUNSCREEN

Wear a sunscreen with a sun protection factor (SPF) of 15 daily. Sunscreens come as high as 50 SPF, but many people may find these stronger screens to be irritating and not more effective than an SPF of 29. The SPF means that you can stay out in the sun that many times longer with the sunscreen on without burning than without it. Even if you use a waterproof sunscreen, always reapply sunscreen after swimming or sweating or at least every 2 hours. Apply your sunscreen at least a half an hour before going out in the sun; it takes time to soak into the skin.

A good sunscreen should protect against both UVA and UVB rays. UVB rays can cause wrinkling and damage to your skin. UVA, once believed to be safe, have also been shown to cause significant skin damage. For the best protection, use a broad-spectrum sunscreen that can reflect UV rays as well as absorb them. For example, some sunscreens contain titanium dioxide, a chemical that reflects UV light off the skin and is often used in so-called chemical-free sunscreens. (In reality, no sunscreen is chemical free; rather, the active ingredient sits on top of the skin and does not get absorbed.)

Many people may be allergic to some of the ingredients used in sunscreens. For example, PABA (*para*-aminobenzoic acid), a common ingredient, may trigger a rash of irritation in some people. In some cases, reflective sunscreen may be less irritating because it doesn't interact with the skin. Many brands of sunscreen now claim to be hypoallergenic, which means they are less prone to cause a rash or irritation. Others claim to be noncomedogenic or nonacnegenic, which means that they are less likely to clog pores. No matter what the manufacturer may claim, if you are sensitive to skin products in general, be sure to try a sunscreen on a small area of skin before using it all over your body. If the area remains irritation free for 24 hours, the product is probably safe for you. If in doubt, check with your physician.

If your skin dries out in the sun, be sure to use a sunscreen with a moisturizer. Aloe vera is still my favorite, and it is included in many sunscreens. It is also good to help heal skin after too much sun exposure.

Of course, it's critical to wear sunscreen in the summer when you're outdoors more; however, many dermatologists advise their patients to use sunscreens all year long, at least on their faces. In fact, many brands of makeup now include SPF protection. Using a foundation with a sunscreen is an easy way to make sure that your face is protected daily.

BRONZERS

There are several products on the market that can help you tan without ever stepping foot in the sun. These products contain dihydroxyacetone, which I'm told is harmless; however, I'm always reluctant to recommend chemicals, particularly if they haven't been used for that long a time. However, if you want a healthy glow, there's nothing wrong with using one of the new skin bronzers that are being marketed by several cosmetic companies. Although bronzers can make you look as if you've just stepped off the beach, they're a lot kinder to your skin. Some even offer UV protection.

PROTECTIVE CLOTHING

A dark T-shirt or slacks will help protect against UV rays. In addition, special SPF outdoor clothing is available at sporting good stores or through mail order.

SUNGLASSES

Sunglasses can prevent squinting, which can promote crow's-feet and fine lines around the eyes. (They can also protect against cataracts.) Be sure to buy sunglasses that offer UV protection.

Dry Skin

Dry, itchy skin is a common complaint among older people, especially in the winter. Dry skin is caused by a reduction in sebum, an oil that forms a protective coating on the skin, thus sealing in moisture. Although you can't replace lost moisture—as some advertisements for skin care products would have you believe—you can bolster the body's own protective seal by using products that reduce water loss from the skin's surface. There are numerous creams and potions on the market that can help seal moisture in. I recommend using fragrance-free, allergy-tested products that don't contain mineral oil, which can deplete the skin of vitamins. Aloe vera creams and lotions and jojoba oil (from the jojoba plant) are excellent for dry skin and are relatively inexpensive. In severe cases, your physician may prescribe a more potent moisturizer.

There are several new-generation moisturizers on the market that contain fancy-sounding compounds such as cholesterol isosterate, ceramides, hyaluronic acid, and fatty acids such as petrolatum and glycolic acid (fruit acids). Basically, despite the hype, these products are similar to traditional moisturizers in that they seal in moisture. However, some may work better than others. There's a wide range of prices among these product lines, and some of the cheaper ones sold at your local drug store may be just as effective as some of the products sold in fancy department stores. Keep in mind that a recent *Consumer Reports* study found that their testers often rated the cheaper skin products higher than the more expensive ones.

Avoid using harsh soaps: soap-free cleaners work well and are far less irritating for most people. Don't bathe or shower in very hot water. An oatmeal bath (Aveeno makes an excellent one) can offer instant relief for dry skin.

Dry heat in particular may sap needed moisture from your skin. Turn off the heat and wear a sweater, or use a humidifier, which can reduce dryness. However, make sure that you are scrupulous about maintaining and cleaning the humidifier because it could be a breeding ground for bacteria and fungi.

For severe dry skin, try taking 1 flaxseed oil capsule three times daily. Within a month, you should see softer, more supple skin.

Cosmeceuticals

Cosmeceuticals refers to a new breed of skin products that offer both therapeutic and cosmetic benefits. Unlike traditional makeups that merely cover up flaws and blemishes, cosmeceuticals contain biologically active ingredients that (at least according to their manufacturers) actually change the quality of the skin. Even skeptics agree that these new breeds of skin creams do have an effect on the outer layers of skin, at least temporarily. Tretinoin (marketed as Retin-A) was the first cosmeceutical. Although originally designed to treat acne, dermatologists noticed that Retin-A appeared to erase fine lines and peeled off the top layer of skin, leaving a pinkish, healthy glow. However, many patients found Retin-A to be very irritating, and it also caused excessive sun sensitivity. Nevertheless, Retin-A is now one of the most prescribed medications in the world. There are also a slew of other cosmeceuticals on the market, notably vitamin A derivatives, alpha-hydroxy acids, salicylic acid, and antioxidants.

RETINOL AND RETINYL PALMITATE

These nonprescriptive-strength vitamin A creams are being touted as antiwrinkle creams without the side effects of Retin-A. Many dermatologists are dubious that these creams are strong enough to be effective; however, they may work well for some people.

ALPHA-HYDROXY ACIDS

Alpha-hydroxy acids (AHAs), which include fruit acid, lactic acid, and glycolic acid, are actually exfolients, that is, they peel dead cells off the surface of the skin, making skin look smoother and less wrinkled. AHAs also help the skin to maintain moisture. Regular use of AHAs can give the skin a fresh glow. Unlike conventional face creams, AHAs are believed to work below the surface of the skin, dissolving the glue that holds the skin together. Over-the-counter products contain between 2 and 10 percent concentrations of AHAs. Dermatologists and plastic surgeons use much stronger concentrations of AHAs in facial skin peels. There is a great deal of controversy regarding the effectiveness and safety of these products. Not all dermatologists agree that AHAs are as effective as their manufacturers say they are. Many contend that over-the-counter products are really not strong enough to have any effect. Some dermatologists worry that the skin will eventually adjust to the AHA and that higher and higher concentrations may be required for any noticeable change. As it stands now, many people find that even low levels of AHAs can be irritating. In addition, some doctors express concern about potential hazards resulting from the long-term use of these new products. They point out that no one knows what, if any, ill affects could arise after several decades of use. What's even more alarming is that some skin salons offer AHA treatments using concentrations of up to 70 percent, which could cause damage. My advice is, proceed with caution. I don't believe that using the lower concentrations of AHAs (under 10 percent) will be harmful as long as you can tolerate it. If you develop any irritation, discontinue the product. Unless the label says otherwise, do not apply an AHA product near the eyes.

SALICYLIC ACID

Similar to AHAs, salicylic acid also sloughs away dead cells and promotes cell turnover (the production of new cells). Salicylic acid may be less irritating for some people, and some dermatologists believe that it is somewhat more effective. At least one study suggested that it promoted faster cell regeneration than AHAs.

ANTIOXIDANTS

Antioxidants are substances that can prevent damage caused by free radicals, unstable oxygen molecules that can destroy healthy cells. UV light in particular can wreak havoc on the skin by creating more of these troublesome free radicals. Antioxidant vitamins such as beta-carotene, E, and C and superoxide dismutase, an antioxidant enzyme that is produced by the body, are included in many skin care products. Although not everyone is convinced of the effectiveness of the external use of antioxidants, it seems plausible that they may help to prevent UV damage. In addition, some researchers believe that antioxidant creams may help to prevent skin cancer.

Chapter 8

A Guide to Commonly Prescribed Drugs

Growing older in the United States has become synonymous with taking pills. Consider the following:

- A study performed at Johns Hopkins University of patients in an ambulatory clinic who were over sixty showed that the typical patient was taking 6.1 drugs simultaneously—4.9 were prescription drugs and the rest were over-the-counter medications. About 25 percent of the patients reported experiencing unpleasant side effects from one or more drugs. About 25 percent of all patients in the study did not even know why the drug or drugs had been prescribed!
- Another study recently published in *The Journal of the American Medical Association* found that close to 25 percent of all Americans over sixty-five were given prescrip-

tions for medications that were either unsafe or ineffective for the elderly. In many cases, side effects resulting from drug interactions or inappropriate medication were dismissed by both patients and their physicians as the normal aches and pains of aging.

Ironically, despite the barrage of drugs, older Americans are none the better for it. In fact, many are worse off. Many of the drugs that are routinely prescribed for older people are not designed for an aging body and often interact badly with other medications. In addition, many of the problems commonly associated with the elderly, such as dizziness, confusion, and weakness, are often caused by the very medication that is supposed to make them healthy! In my opinion, many of the ailments that the elderly are commonly treated for could easily be managed through natural alternatives, such as herbal remedies, diet, and changes in lifestyle.

People of any age should wary of popping pills indiscriminately, but this is particularly true for people over fifty. As we age, our bodies react differently to drugs. An impaired digestive system can interfere with drug absorption. A slowing down of liver and kidney function can lead to problems with breaking down and eliminating a drug, which can cause a toxic buildup. Memory or vision problems or other physical ailments could be affected by medication. Therefore, it is critical for older people to be very wary of taking any medication without first asking specific questions, such as:

What is this medication for?
Can this medication interact with any other medication that I am taking?
Do I have any other medical problem that could be adversely affected by this medication?
Are you giving me the lowest possible dose?
Is this medication safe and effective for a person my age?
What are the side effects?
Do I discontinue the drug or reduce the dose if I experience any side effects?

Are there any alternatives to this medication?
Do I take this drug with food or on an empty stomach?

It is my hope that a healthy lifestyle can eliminate the need for drugs. However, I recognize that it is sometimes necessary to take medication, and the right medication at the right time can indeed be a lifesaver. As a pharmacist, however, I believe that no more than three drugs should be taken simultaneously to avoid interactions or side effects, and that includes over-the-counter medications. If you must take several drugs simultaneously, be sure that you are being closely monitored by your physician.

I have compiled a list of the top thirty drugs prescribed for older people, detailing their potential side effects. Although some of these side effects are rare, I feel it is important for you to know about them. If you do experience any difficulties with medicine, you should notify your doctor immediately. I also discuss possible drug interactions with foods or other drugs, and whenever possible, I recommend natural alternatives. However, if you are taking any prescription medications, do not discontinue your medication for any reason without first checking with your physician. Do not substitute these natural alternatives for your medication unless you are under the supervision of a physician or natural healer.

(Drugs are listed alphabetically by their generic names followed by their common trade names.)

SOURCE: *Physician's Desk Reference*, 1995.

Allopurinol (Zyloprim)

Facts. Prescribed for the treatment of gout.

Possible Side Effects. Skin rashes, hives, itching, fever, headaches, dizziness, drowsiness, nausea, vomiting, diarrhea, stomach cramps, loss of hair from head, chills, joint pains, swollen glands, kidney damage, inflammation of the liver, seizures.

Diet Tips. Watch your vitamin C intake—2 grams (2000 milligrams) of vitamin C can acidify the urine and possibly increase kidney stone formation when used with this drug. Follow a low-purine diet. (See p. 204.)

Caution: Allopurinol can increase the effectiveness of azathioprine and mercaptopurine. It can also thin the blood. When taken with ampicillin, it can cause a skin rash. If you experience drowsiness from this drug, beware of driving or operating heavy machinery.

Personal Advice. Try drinking 1 cup of cherry juice daily to control gout.

Alprazolam (Xanax)

Facts. Mild tranquilizer used to treat anxiety and nervousness.

Possible Side Effects. Drowsiness, light-headedness, headaches, dizziness, fatigue, blurred vision, dry mouth, confusion, hallucinations, depression, excitability, agitation, allergic rash or hives, nausea, vomiting, diarrhea.

Diet Tips. Avoid caffeine, alcohol, and tobacco. Take extra calcium and magnesium, tyrosine, and L-phenylalanine.

Caution: This drug can be addictive. It should not be discontinued abruptly if taken for more than 4 weeks. When taken with digoxin, it can produce toxicity. Smoking may reduce its effectiveness. Other drugs such as levodopa can reduce its effectiveness.

Personal Advice. Exercise is a great stress reliever. Take B vitamins with extra pantothenic acid. Herbs such as passionflower, valerian, hops, skullcap, and chamomile can help reduce tension.

Ambien (Zolpidem)

Facts. Sleep aid.

Possible Side Effects. Drowsiness, dizziness, headaches, nausea, vomiting, amnesia, drug dependency.

Diet Aids. A cup of warm milk or chamomile tea before bedtime can help. Avoid caffeinated beverages and alcohol.

Caution: Do not take other sleep-inducing drugs at the same time as ambien. Be careful of over-the-counter drugs when taking ambien.

Personal Advice. Try using melatonin, valerian, hops, passionflower, skullcap, and calcium and magnesium, which are all natural sleep aids.

Atenolol (Tenormin)

Facts. Used as a treatment for angina and high blood pressure.

Possible Side Effects. Lethargy, fatigue, cold hands and feet, slow heart rate, light-headedness, dizziness, insomnia, abnormal dreams, indigestion, nausea, vomiting, constipation, diarrhea, edema (retention of fluid), joint and muscle discomfort, mental depression, anxiety, chest pain, shortness of breath, decreased libido in both sexes, and impaired erection in men.

Diet Tips. Avoid too much salt. Do not drink alcoholic beverages.

Caution: Do not smoke when taking this drug. Avoid becoming overly heated or overly cold. Be careful when driving or operating heavy machinery. Avoid overexertion. Do not stop drug abruptly; a gradual decrease over 2 to 3 weeks is recommended. This drug can increase the effects of other high blood pressure medications. Monitor closely when taken with insulin. Several drugs can alter the effectiveness of this

296   Earl Mindell's Anti-Aging Bible

drug; check with your physician or pharmacist before taking any other medications.

Personal Advice. Garlic(fresh or supplements), an increase in potassium-rich foods, decrease in sodium, a calcium–magnesium supplement, and celery can help control blood pressure naturally.

Beclomethasone (Vanceril)

Facts: Used to treat asthma.

Possible Side Effects. Fungal infections, skin rashes, dry mouth, sore throat, allergic reactions.

Diet Tips. Check with your physician to make sure that food allergies are not aggravating your condition.

Caution: Do not smoke with this drug. Certain medications including epinephrine (commonly found in cold and allergy medications) can increase the effectiveness of this drug. Check with your physician or pharmacist before using any medications in conjunction with this drug.

Personal Advice. Ephedra tea (also called ma huang) may help with asthmatic symptoms. Use only as directed. If abused, this herb can cause serious side effects including fatal arrhythmias. If you have asthma, do not self-medicate. Consult with a physician or a skilled natural healer.

Captopril (Capoten)

Facts. Treatment for high blood pressure.

Possible Side Effects. Skin rash; swelling of face, hands, and feet; fever; loss of or altered taste; mouth and tongue sores; palpitations; decreased male libido.

Diet Tips. Watch your salt intake. Do not use salt substitutes with potassium or a potassium supplement with this drug unless recommended by your physician. Do not use with alcohol. Food sensitivity may occur with this drug.

Caution: Captopril and potassium could cause serious heart rhythm problems. Captopril can interact poorly with several drugs. Aspirin can decrease effectiveness of captopril. Check with your physician or pharmacist before taking other medications.

Personal Advice. I also recommend eating garlic, losing weight, and reducing your salt intake.

Cimetidine (Tagamet)

Facts. Used to treat peptic ulcers.

Possible Side Effects. Skin rashes, hives, fever, headaches, dizziness, weakness, blurred vision, fatigue, muscular pain, diarrhea, kidney damage, liver damage, agitation, confusion, delirium, hallucinations, slowed heart rate, abnormal bleeding or bruising, decreased libido, impotency, decreased male erection, male breast enlargement, female breast enlargement with milk production.

Diet Tips. Eat a low-protein diet (protein increases stomach acid production). Take a vitamin B_{12} supplement (sublingual or intranasal).

Caution: Citmetidine increases the effectiveness of blood thinners, which can cause internal bleeding. Citmetidine can increase the effectiveness of several other drugs, so check with your pharmacist or physician before taking any other medication. Do not smoke marijuana while using this drug.

Personal Advice. Most specialists feel that an antibiotic is the treatment of choice for this condition, although it is still underprescribed for ulcers. If you are taking cimetidine, ask about antibiotic therapy. In addition, try papayas (whole fruit or tablets), bananas, and a good digestive enzyme. Potato juice, aloe vera juice, and acidophilus capsules may also help relieve symptoms. Marshmallow herb is a time-honored treatment for ulcers.

Conjugated Estrogens (Premarin)

Facts. Estrogen replacement therapy.

Possible Side Effects. Bloating, swelling, and tenderness of the breasts; tan spots on face; skin rashes; hives; itching; headaches; nervous tension; irritability; migraine; depression; stroke.

Diet Tips. Eat foods such as tofu and rye, which are rich in phytoestrogens.

Caution: Be careful about taking estrogen with warfarin (an anticoagulant). Several drugs can adversely react with estrogen. Check with your physician or pharmacist before taking any other medication.

Personal Advice. For relief from menopausal symptoms, try using evening primrose oil, dong quai, vitex, and calcium and magnesium.

Diazepam (Valium)

Facts. Anti-anxiety, anti-alcohol withdrawal symptoms, antiseizure, muscle relaxer.

Possible Side Effects. Drowsiness, lethargy, unsteadiness, rash or hives, dizziness, fainting, blurred or double vision, sweating, nausea, liver damage, low platelet count, bone marrow depression, fever, sore throat, anger, rage, menstrual irregularities, male impotency, inhibition of orgasm in women.

Diet Tips. Restrict coffee, colas, and other caffeinated beverages. Do not use with alcohol.

Caution: Heavy smoking may reduce the effectiveness of this drug. Do not use with marijuana. Do not drive or attempt any hazardous activity while taking this drug. Be careful about overheating your body while taking this drug. Do not discontinue abruptly. Taper off dosage to prevent unpleasant withdrawal. Digoxin and phenytoin may decrease the effectiveness of this drug. Several other drugs including cimeditine and oral contraceptives may increase the drug's effectiveness. Check with your physician or pharmacist before using this drug with another medication.

Personal Advice. A B-complex vitamin, calcium and magnesium, valerian, hops, passionflower, and chamomile would greatly decrease the need for this drug.

Digoxin (Lanoxin, Lanoxicaps)

Facts. Heart stimulant used in congestive heart failure that helps to maintain normal heart rate and rhythm.

Possible Side Effects. Headaches; drowsiness; confusion; blurred or yellow-green vision; nausea; vomiting; diarrhea; allergic reactions, including skin rashes or hives; decreased libido; impotency; breast enlargement in males.

Diet Tips. Eat potassium-rich foods including potatoes, canteloupe, and bananas. Avoid caffeinated drinks. Don't smoke tobacco or marijuana.

Caution: Do not take diuretics (water pills) or quinine. Many drugs are synergistic (can increase the effectiveness) with digoxin, such as ibuprofen, captopril, and indomethacin. Check with your physician or pharmacist before taking any other medication, either prescription or over the counter.

Personal Advice. Herbs such as hawthorne berries and cayenne are cardiotonics. Vitamins and supplements including vitamin E, coenzyme Q_{10}, and L-carnitine, which can strengthen the heart muscle, help metabolize fats and dissolves blood clots.

Diltiazem (Cardizem)

Facts. Used to treat angina and high blood pressure.

Possible Side Effects. Fatigue, light-headedness, changes in heart rate and rhythm, palpitations, skin rashes, hives, itching, headaches, drowsiness, dizziness, nervousness, insomnia, depression, confusion, hallucinations, nausea, indigestion, constipation, male impotence.

Diet Tips. Avoid too much salt. Do not use with alcohol.
Caution: Do not smoke tobacco or marijuana when using this drug. When taken with beta-blockers or digitalis drugs, diltiazem can cause heart rhythm disorders. Cimeditine increases the diltiazem's effectiveness.

Personal Advice. Garlic, celery, calcium and magnesium, passionflower, valerian, a B-complex vitamin, coenzyme Q_{10}, hawthorn berries, vitex.

Dyazide (Hydrochlorothiazide and Triamterene)

Facts. A diuretic used to treat congestive heart failure.

Possible Side Effects. High potassium blood level, low sodium level, low blood pressure, dehydration, discolored urine, skin rash, itchiness, headaches, dizziness, unsteadiness, weakness, drowsiness, lethargy, dry mouth, nausea, vomiting, diarrhea, anaphylactic shock, confusion numbness, tingling of lips and face, slow heart rate, shortness of breath.

Diet Tips. Do not increase intake of potassium-rich foods or take potassium supplements while taking this drug. Avoid salt substitutes containing potassium. Do not use this drug if you are nursing. Drink alcohol with caution or not at all.

Caution: Avoid taking with captopril, indomethacin, and lithium. Amantadine and digoxin can increase the effectiveness of this drug. Withdraw from this drug slowly. If you are over sixty, take this drug for 2 to 3 weeks and then check with your physician to make sure it is working properly. Dehydration (loss of body fluid) can occur, which can lead to stroke, heart attack, and thrombophlebitis. Do not operate heavy machinery if dizziness or drowsiness occurs. This drug can cause sensitivity to sunlight.

Personal Advice. Weight loss, exercise, garlic, and calcium and magnesium can help reduce the need for this drug.

Enalapril Maleate (Vasotec)

Facts. Used to treat high blood pressure.

Possible Side Effects. Dizziness; light-headedness; fainting; skin rashes; fatigue; itching; headaches; nervousness; numbness; tingling; rapid heart rate and palpitations; digestive disorders; excessive sweating; muscle cramps; swelling of face, tongue, and vocal chords; abnormal bleeding; bruising.

Diet Tips. Do not use salt substitutes while taking this drug without first checking with your physician; they usually contain potassium, which can cause serious complications when taken with enalapril maleate. Salt intake should be adjusted by your physician. Alcohol consumption should be moderated.

Caution: Avoid potassium supplements; they can cause serious heart rhythm disturbances when taken with this drug. Enalapril maleate combined with certain drugs can also lead to dangerously high potassium levels. Do not take any medications without first checking with your physician or

pharmacist. **Do not overheat your body; blood pressure can drop precipitously, causing serious effects when using this drug.**

Personal Advice. Weight loss, salt restriction, garlic (fresh or supplements), calcium and magnesium, and celery can go a long way to reduce the need for this drug.

Fluoxetine Hydrochloride (Prozac)

Facts. Used to treat depression.

Possible Side Effects. Decreased appetite, weight loss, skin rash, hives, itching, headaches, dizziness, fatigue, difficulty concentrating, changed taste, nausea, vomiting, diarrhea, seizures, weakness, fever, joint pain, fluid retention, dry mouth, impaired erection or orgasm, suicidal tendencies.

Diet Tips. Do not use with alcohol.
Caution: Do not drive if this drug causes drowsiness. Prozac increases the effectiveness of digitalis drugs, coumadin (an anticoagulant), antidiabetic drugs, and other monoamine oxidase inhibitors, including meperidine hydrochloride and phenelzine sulfate.

Personal Advice. Tyrosine, taurine, L-phenylalanine, B-complex, and exercise can reduce the need for this drug.

Flurazepam Hydrochloride (Dalmane)

Facts. A short-term treatment for insomnia.

Possible Side Effects. Hangover upon rising, drowsiness, lethargy, unsteadiness, skin rash, hives, burning eyes, tongue swelling, dizziness, fainting, blurred vision, double vision, slurred speech, nausea, indigestion, nervousness, irritability, apprehension, euphoria, excitement, hallucinations, impaired white blood cell production, liver damage, sore throat, fever.

Diet Tips. Caffeine should be restricted within 4 hours of taking this drug. Do not use with alcohol.

Caution: This drug may be habit forming with long-term use. Smoking heavily will decrease the effectiveness of flurazepam hydrochloride. Do not use marijuana while taking this drug. If you are over sixty, use the smallest possible dose to avoid overdose. Don't drive or operate heavy machinery while taking this drug. Do not discontinue drug abruptly. Flurazepam hydrochloride can increase the effectiveness of digoxin and phenytoin; I would not advise taking these drugs together. Flurazepam hydrochloride can decrease the effectiveness of levodopa, cimetidine, birth control pills, and other drugs. Check with your pharmacist or physician before taking flurazepam hydrochloride with other drugs.

Personal Advice. A calcium and magnesium supplement, passionflower, hops, valerian, and exercise can greatly reduce the need for this drug.

Furosemide (Fumide, Lasix)

Facts. A diuretic used for congestive heart failure, high blood pressure with other medication. Increases calcium excretion.

Possible Side Effects. Skin rashes, hives, fever, headaches, blurred vision, ringing in the ears, numbness, tingling, fatigue, weakness, digestive complaints, jaundice, abnormal bleeding or bruising, impotence in men, can increase the likelihood of diabetes, gout, and drug-induced lupus.

Diet Tips. Diuretics can sap your body of important minerals including potassium. Eat a high-potassium diet including bananas, potatoes, cantaloupe, and plain yogurt. Decrease salt intake to prescribed amount. Watch all processed food for sodium content. Watch your drinking: alcohol and furosemide can cause blood pressure to drop too low.

Caution: Be careful of sun exposure: some people develop photosensitivity (sensitivity to sunlight). Beware of interactions with many other drugs, including digoxin and indomethacin. If you are over sixty, start with a very small dose until your response can be determined. Too high a dosage can lead to stroke, heart attack, or vein inflammation with a blood clot.

Personal Advice. To reduce your need for this drug take a calcium–magnesium or garlic supplement. Chew on celery stalks. Drink lots of water. Eat fresh dandelion leaves or take dandelion root capsules. Vitamin B$_6$ is also a natural diuretic.

Ibuprofen (Advil, Motrin, Rufen)

Facts. Treatment for moderate or severe pain, available over the counter in doses of 200 milligrams. Prescription strengths also available at 400, 600, and 800 milligrams per tablet or capsule.

Possible Side Effects. Fluid retention, discolored urine, skin rash, hives, itching, headache, dizziness, blurred vision, ringing in ears, depression, mouth sores, indigestion, nausea, vomiting, constipation, diarrhea, severe skin reactions, peptic ulcers, liver damage, kidney damage, menstruation irregularities, male breast enlargement and tenderness, mild anemia, suppressed bone marrow.

Diet Tips. Do not use with alcohol.
Caution: Drive with caution. Ibuprofen can increase the effectiveness of acetaminophen and anticoagulant medicines. Check with your physician or pharmacist before taking ibuprofen with other drugs.

Personal Advice. Try the amino acid D,L-phenylalanine and white willow bark for moderate pain control.

Lorazepam (Ativan)

Facts. Used to treat anxiety.

Possible Side Effects. Sedation, dizziness, weakness, unsteadiness, disorientation, depression, nausea, change in appetite, headaches, sleep disturbances, agitation, vision problems, rashes.

Diet Tips. Do not use with alcohol. Restrict caffeinated beverages.
Caution: Heavy smoking may reduce the effectiveness of this drug. Do not use with marijuana. Do not drive or attempt any hazardous activity while taking this drug. Be careful about overheating your body while taking this drug. Do not discontinue abruptly. Taper off dosage to prevent unpleasant withdrawal. Digoxin and phenytoin may decrease the effectiveness of this drug. Several other drugs including cimetidine and birth control pills may increase the drug's effectiveness. Check with your physician or pharmacist before using this drug with another medication.

Personal Advice. A B-complex vitamin, calcium and magnesium, valerian, hops, passionflower, and chamomile would greatly decrease the need for this drug.

Lovastatin (Mevacor)

Facts. Used to treat high cholesterol.

Possible Side Effects. Abnormal liver function, skin rashes and itching, headaches, dizziness, blurred vision, digestive disturbances, nausea, muscle pain, cataracts, bleeding ulcers.

Diet Tips. Eat a low-fat diet with no more than 20 percent of calories from fat. Avoid saturated fat.

Personal Advice. Vitamins E and C, garlic, psyllium, charcoal, yogurt, pectin, and oat bran can reduce the need for this drug.

Metoprolol (Toprol XL)

Facts. Used to control mild to moderate blood pressure.

Possible Side Effects. Lethargy, fatigue, cold hands and feet, slow heart rate, light-headedness, dizziness, insomnia, abnormal dreams, indigestion, nausea, vomiting, constipation, diarrhea, edema (retention of fluid), joint and muscle discomfort, mental depression, anxiety, chest pain, shortness of breath, decreased libido, impaired erection.

Diet Tips. Avoid too much salt. Do not use with alcohol.
Caution: Do not smoke when taking this drug. Avoid becoming overly heated or overly cold. Be careful when driving or operating heavy machinery. Avoid overexertion. Do not stop drug abruptly; a gradual decrease of 2 to 3 weeks is recommended. Metoprolol tartrate can increase the effects of other high blood pressure medications. Monitor closely when taken with insulin. Several drugs can either increase or reduce the effectiveness of this drug. Check with your physician or pharmacist before taking any other medication.

Personal Advice. Garlic (fresh or supplements), an increase in potassium-rich foods, decrease in sodium, a calcium–magnesium supplement, and celery can help control blood pressure naturally.

Naproxen (Naprosyn)

Facts. Pain reliever, anti-inflammatory.

Possible Side Effects. Fluid retention, prolonged bleeding time, skin rash, hives, itching, localized swelling, spontaneous bruising, headaches, dizziness, nausea, vomiting, abdominal pain, diarrhea, inhibited evacuation (one report), menstrual irregularities.

Diet Tips. Do not use with alcohol.

Caution: Naproxin can increase the effectiveness of acetaminophen and anticoagulants such as coumadin and can increase bleeding with aspirin and other drugs. Be sure to check with your pharmacist or physician if you are taking this drug with other medication.

Personal Advice. D,L-phenylalanine, white willow bark, quercetin, and bromelin are also good pain relievers and anti-inflammatories.

Nifedipine (Procardia)

Facts. Used to treat angina and mild to moderate high blood pressure.

Possible Side Effects. Low blood pressure, rapid heart rate, swelling of feet and ankles, flushing, sweating, skin rash, hives, itching, fever, headaches, dizziness, weakness, nervousness, blurred vision, palpitations, shortness of breath, wheezing, coughing, heartburn, nausea, abdominal cramps, diarrhea, tremors, muscle cramps, altered menstrual cycle, excessive menstrual flow.

Diet Tips. Avoid excess salt. Do not use with alcohol.
Caution: Do not smoke tobacco or marijuana. Do not overheat yourself. Do not stop taking this drug cold turkey; gradually taper drug off under a physician's supervision.

Personal Advice. Try using hawthorn berries, garlic, cayenne, calcium and magnesium, hops, valerian, and chamomile.

Piroxicam (Feldene)

Facts. Prescribed for mild to severe pain and inflammation.

Possible Side Effects. Fluid retention, prolonged bleeding time, skin rash, itching, bruising, headaches, dizziness, blurred vision, ringing in the ears, drowsiness, fatigue, difficulty concentrating, nausea, vomiting, abdominal pain, diarrhea, peptic ulcers, ulcerative colitis, mild anemia.

Diet Tips. Do not use with alcohol.
Caution: Piroxicam can increase the effectiveness of acetaminophen and anticoagulants. Do not drive when taking this drug. Check with your doctor or pharmacist before using piroxicam with other drugs.

Personal Advice. D,L-phenylalanine, white willow bark, fish oil, quercetin, and bromelin can be used instead of piroxicam.

Propanolol Hydrochloride (Inderal)

Facts. Used to treat angina and high blood pressure and to prevent migraine headaches.

Possible Side Effects. Lethargy, fatigue, cold hands and feet, slow heart rate, light-headedness, dizziness, insomnia, abnormal dreams, indigestion, nausea, vomiting, constipation, diarrhea, edema (retention of fluid), joint and muscle discomfort, mental depression, anxiety, chest pain, shortness of breath, decreased libido, impaired erection in men.

Diet Tips. Avoid too much salt. Do not use with alcohol.
Caution: Do not smoke when taking this drug. Avoid becoming overly heated or cold. Be careful when driving or operating heavy machinery. Avoid overexertion. Do not stop drug abruptly; a gradual decrease of 2 to 3 weeks is recommended. This drug can increase the effects of other high

blood pressure medications. Monitor closely when taken with insulin. Several drugs can alter the effectiveness of this drug; check with your physician or pharmacist before taking any other medications.

Personal Advice. Garlic (fresh or supplements), an increase in potassium-rich foods, decrease in sodium, a calcium–magnesium supplement, and celery can help control blood pressure naturally.

Ranitidine Hydrochloride (Zantac)

Facts. Used to treat ulcers.

Possible Side Effects. Skin rash, headaches, dizziness, feeling ill, nausea, drowsiness, constipation, diarrhea, confusion in elderly, hepatitis, bone marrow depression, weakness, sore throat, bruising, decreased libido, male impotency, breast enlargement in men.

Diet tips. Do not use with alcohol. Ranitidine hydrochloride can increase your blood alcohol concentration by 34 percent. Talk to your physician about a special diet. A high-protein diet can increase stomach acid secretions, which can worsen your condition.

Caution: Be cautious when using ranitidine hydrochloride with anticoagulant; it can increase the risk of bleeding. This drug can make you drowsy. Be careful when driving or operating heavy machinery.

Personal Advice. Most specialists feel that an antibiotic is the treatment of choice for this condition, although it is still underprescribed for ulcers. If you are taking ranitidine hydrochloride, ask about antibiotic therapy. In addition, try papayas (whole fruit or tablets), bananas, and a good digestive enzyme. Potato juice, aloe vera juice, and acidophilus capsules may also help relieve symptoms. Marshmallow herb is a time-honored treatment for ulcers.

Terfenadine (Seldane)

Facts. Antihistamine.

Possible Side Effects. Dry nose, mouth, and throat; skin rash; itching; headache; nervousness; fatigue; increased appetite; indigestion; nausea; vomiting; swollen breasts in women.

Diet Tips. None.
Caution: Do not use this drug with ketoconazole. Check with your physician or pharmacist before taking this drug with other medications.

Personal Advice. Try ephedra tea or ma huang. Use only the prescribed dose. If abused, this herb can cause serious side effects including fatal arrhythmias.

Theophylline (Theo-Dur)

Facts. Anti-asthmatic and bronchodilator

Possible Side Effects. Nervousness, insomnia, rapid heartbeat, increased urination, skin rashes, hives, headaches, dizziness, irritability, tremors, fatigue, weakness, loss of appetite, nausea, vomiting, abdominal pain, diarrhea, excessive thirst, flushing in the face.

Diet Tips. Do not have caffeine with this drug.
Caution: This drug can interact adversely with several drugs. For example, it decreases the effectiveness of lithium and phenytoin (which means you may require a higher dose) and increases the effectiveness of allopurinol and oral contraceptives (which means you may require a lesser dose). Check with your pharmacist or physician before using theophylline with any over-the-counter or prescription drug.

Triamcinolone Acetonide (Azmacort)

Facts. Used to treat bronchial asthma.

Possible Side Effects. Yeast infections of mouth and throat; irritations of mouth, tongue, and throat; skin rash; swelling of face; hoarseness; cough.

Diet Tips. Check to see if food allergies could be worsening your condition.

Caution: Albuterol, ephedrine hydrochloride, terubaline, and theophylline may increase the effectiveness of this drug.

Personal Advice. Try ephedra tea or ma huang. Use only the prescribed dose. If abused, this herb can cause serious side effects including fatal arrhythmias. Asthma should be treated by a physician or skilled healer.

Triazolam (Halcion)

Facts. Short-term treatment for insomnia.

Possible Side Effects. Drowsiness, dizziness, light-headedness, euphoria, tachycardia, fatigue, confusion, memory impairment, abdominal cramps, pain, depression, visual disturbances.

Diet Tips. Do not use with alcohol. Restrict caffeinated beverages.

Caution: Heavy smoking may reduce the effectiveness of this drug. Do not use with marijuana. Do not drive or attempt any hazardous activity while taking this drug. Be careful about overheating your body while taking this drug. This drug can be habit forming. Do not discontinue abruptly; taper off dosage to prevent unpleasant withdrawal. Digoxin and phenytoin may decrease the effectiveness of this drug. Several other drugs including cimetidine and oral contraceptives may

increase the drug's effectiveness. **Check with your physician or pharmacist before using this drug with another medication.**

Personal Advice. Melatonin, calcium and magnesium, hops, passionflower, and valerian are also good for insomnia.

Verapamil Hydrochloride (Calan)

Facts. Used to treat angina, high blood pressure, and heart rhythm irregularities.

Possible Side Effects. Low blood pressure, fluid retention, skin rash, hives, itching, aching joints, headaches, dizziness, fatigue, nausea, indigestion, constipation, menstrual irregularities, male breast enlargement and impotency.

Diet Tips. Avoid too much salt. Do not use with alcohol.
Caution: Do not smoke tobacco or marijuana when taking this drug. Verapamil can increase the effectiveness of carbamazepine and digoxin. When taken together with beta-blockers, this drug can affect heart rhythm. Cimetidine can increase the effectiveness of verapamil.

Personal Advice. Garlic (fresh or supplements), celery, calcium and magnesium, passionflower, hops, valerian, a B-complex vitamin, hawthorn berries, vitex, coenzyme Q_{10} are also excellent for lowering blood pressure.

Selected Bibliography

Acoustic Neuroma Association Notes, no. 36 (December 1990).

Adlercreutz, Herman. "Plasma Concentrations of Phyto-Oestrogens in Japanese Men." *The Lancet* 342 (November 13, 1993): 1209–1210.

———. "Lignans and Phytoestrogens: Possible Protective Role in Cancer." *Frontiers of Gastrointestinal Research* 14 (1988): 165–176.

Adlercreutz, H., E. Hamalainen, S. Gorbach, and B. Goldin. "Dietary Phyto-oestrogens and the Menopause in Japan. *Lancet* 339 (May 16, 1992): 1233.

"Aloe Update." *The Lawrence Review of Natural Products* 3 no. 21 (November 15, 1982).

Anderson, James W. "Dietary Fiber and Diabetes." *Journal of the American Dietetic Association* 87, no. 9 1189–1197 (September 1987).

———. *The HCF Guide Book.* Lexington, Ky: HCF Diabetes Foundation, 1987.

Armstrong, S. M., and J. R. Redman. "Melatonin: A Chronobiotic with Anti-Aging Properties." *Medical Hypotheses* 43 (1991): 300–309.

Aspirin as a Therapeutic Agent in Cardiovascular Disease. Dallas, Tex.: American Heart Association, 1993.

Balch, James F., and Phyllis A. Balch. *Prescription for Nutritional Healing.* Garden City, N.Y.: Avery Publishing Group, 1990.

Barbul, Adrian, et al. "Arginine Stimulates Lymphocyte Immune Response in Healthy Human Beings." *Surgery* 90, no. 1 (1981): 244–251.

Be Your Best: Nutrition After Fifty. Washington, D.C.: American Institute for Cancer Research, 1988.

"Beyond Deficiency: New Views on the Function and Health Effects of Vitamins." Howerde E. Sauberlich and Lawrence T. Muchlin, eds. *The New York Academy of Sciences* (February 9–12, 1992) (abstracts).

Bitterman, Wilhelm A., et al. "Environmental and Nutritional Factors Significantly Associated with Cancer of the Urinary Tract Among Different Ethnic Groups." *Urologic Clinics of North America* 18, no. 3 (August 1991).

Bland, Jeffrey. *Bioflavonoids: The Friends and Helpers of Vitamin C in Many Hard-to-Treat Ailments.* New Canaan, Conn.: Keats Publishing Inc., 1984.

Block, Gladys, Donald E. Henson, and Mark Levine, eds. "Ascorbic Acid: Biologic Functions and Relation to Cancer." Proceedings of the National Institutes of Health, Bethesda, Md., September 10–12, 1990. *American Journal of Clinical Nutrition* 54, no. 6 (suppl.) (December 1991).

"Blocking Skin Cancer Through Diet?" *Tufts University Diet and Nutrition Letter* 12, no. 5 (July 1994).

Blumenthal, Mark. "Echinacea Highlighted as Cold and Flu Remedy." *Herbalgram,* no. 29 (1993): 8–9.

"Borage Seed Oil and Evening Primrose Oil May Relieve Arthritis Pain and Swelling." *Environmental Nutrition* (March 1994).

Borum, Peggy R. "Carnitine." *Annual Review in Nutrition* 3 (1983): 233–259.

Bowman, Barbara. "Acetyl-Carnitine and Alzheimer's Disease." *Nutrition Reviews* 50, no. 5. 142–143.

Bradlow, H. Leon, and Jon Michnovicz. "A New Approach to the Prevention of Breast Cancer." *Proceedings of the Royal Society of Edinburgh* 95B (1989): 77–86.

Brody, Jane. "Folic Acid Emerges as a Nutritional Star." *New York Times,* March 1, 1994.

Bunce, George Edwin. "Nutritional Factors in Cataract." *Annual Review of Nutrition* 10 (1990): 223–254.

". . .But Study of Women Finds Iron May Contribute to Higher Coronary Disease Risk." *News from the American Heart Association,* (June 13, 1994).

Burtin, Ritva B., Carolyn Clifford, and Elaine Lanza. "NCI Dietary Guidelines: Rationale." *American Journal of Clinical Nutrition* 48 (1988): 888–895.

Butterworth, C. E., et al. "Folate Deficiency and Cervical Dysplasia." *Journal of the American Medical Association* 267, no. 4. 528–533 (January 22/29, 1992).

Cancer Facts and Figures—1993. Atlanta, Ga: American Cancer Society, 1993.

Caragay, Alegria B. "Cancer-Preventive Foods and Ingredients." *Food Technology* 46, no. 4 (April 1992): 65–68.

Castleman, Michael. "Red Pepper Is Hot!" *Medical Selfcare* (September/October 1989): 68–69.

Cerda, J. J., et al. "The Effects of Grapefruit Pectin on Patients at Risk for Coronary Heart Disease Without Altering Diet or Lifestyle." *Clinical Cardiology* 11, no. 9 (September 1988): 589–594.

Chen, K.J., and Chen, K. "Ischemic Stroke Treated with Ligusticum chuanxiong." *Chinese Medical Journal* 105, no. 10 (October 1992): 870–873.

Chinthalapally, Rao V., et al. "Inhibitory Effect of Caffeic Acid Esters on Azoxymethane-Induced Biochemical Changes and Aberrant Crypt Foci Formation in Rat Colon." *Cancer Research* 53 (September 15, 1993): 4182–4188.

"Chronic Stress is Directly Linked to Premature Aging of the Brain." *National Institute on Aging, Research Bulletin* (October 1991).

Cutler, Richard G. "Antioxidants and Aging." *American Journal of Clinical Nutrition* 53 (1991): 373S–379S.

Darlington, L. Gail. "Dietary Therapy for Arthritis." *Rheumatic Disease Clinics of North America* 17, no. 2 (May 1991): 273–285.

Darlington, L. G., and S. W. Ramsey. "Clinical Review: Review of Dietary Therapy for Rheumatoid Arthritis." *British Journal of Rheumatology* 32 (1993): 507–514.

Devi, P.U., et al. "In Vivo Inhibitory Effect of *Withania somnifera* (Ashwagandha) on a Transplantable Mouse Tumor, Sarcoma 180." *Indian Journal Experimental Biology* 30, no. 3 (March 1992): (169–172).

Diet and Cancer. Washington, D.C.: American Institute for Cancer Research, Information Series, 1992.

Diet, Nutrition, and Prostate Cancer. Washington, D.C.: American Institute for Cancer Research, Information Series, 1991.

Dizziness, Hope Through Research. U.S. Department of Health and Human Services, National Institutes of Health, September 1986.

"Do Monounsaturated Fats and Vitamin E Provide Double-Barreled Protection Against Coronary Ills?" *News from the American Heart Association* (April 11, 1994).

Dorgan, Joanne F., and Arthur Schatzkin. "Antioxidant Micronutrients in Cancer Prevention." *Hematology/Oncology Clinics of North America* 5, no. 1, 43–68.

Duke, James A. "An Herb a Day: Clubmoss, Alias Lycopodium Alias

Huperzia." *Business of Herbs* (January/February 1989).

Elegbede, J. A., et al. "Regression of Rat Primary Mammary Tumors Following Dietary d-Limonene." *Journal of the National Cancer Institute* 76, no.2 (February 1986): 323–325.

"Estrogen and Alzheimer's." *Harvard Women's Health Watch* 1, no. 11 (July 1994).

Evans, W. J. "Exercise, Nutrition and Aging." *Symposium: Nutrition and Exercise, Journal of Nutrition* 122: 796–801, 1992.

"Exercise and Arthritis: The Importance of a Regular Program." *University of California, Berkeley, Wellness Letter* (April 1994).

"Exercise in 90-Year-Olds Increases Muscle Strength and Mobility." *National Institute on Aging Research Bulletin* (September 3, 1990).

Fackelmann, K.A. "Chicken Cartilage Soothes Aching Joints." *Science News* (September 25, 1993): 198.

———. Do EMFs Pose Breast Cancer Risk?" *Science News* 45 (June 18, 1994): 145.

———. "Nutrients May Prevent Blinding Disease." *Science News Letter* 145 (September 12, 1994).

"Facts and Fiction About Memory Aging: A Quantitative Integration of Research Findings." *Journal of Gerontology* 48, no. 4 (1993): 157–171.

Facts on Prostate Cancer. Atlanta, Ga.: American Cancer Society, 1988.

Feldman, Henry A., et al. "Impotence and Its Medical and Psychosocial Correlates: Results of the Massachusetts Male Aging Study." *Journal of Urology* 151 (January 1994): 54–61.

Fiatarone, Maria, Evelyn F. O'Neill, and Nancy Doyle Ryan. "Exercise Training and Nutritional Supplementation for Physical Frailty in Very Elderly People." *New England Journal of Medicine* 330, no. 25. 1769–1775 (June 23, 1994).

"Flax Facts." *Journal of the National Cancer Institute* 83, no. 15 (September 7, 1991): 1050–1052.

"The Food Guide Pyramid." *Department of Agriculture, Home and Garden Bulletin,* no. 252 (August 1992).

Garland, Cedric F., Frank C. Garland, and Edward D. Gorham. "Can Colon Cancer Incidence and Death Rates Be Reduced with Calcium and Vitamin D?" *American Journal of Clinical Nutrition* 54 (1991): 193S–201S.

"Garlic Fights Nitrosamine Formation . . . as Do Tomatoes and Other Produce." *Science News* 145 (1991): 190.

"Ginger and Atractylodes as an Anti-inflammatory." *Herbalgram,* no. 29 (1993): 19.

Giovannucci, Edward, Eric B. Rimm, and G. Colditz. "A Prospective Study of Dietary Fat and Risk of Prostate Cancer." *Journal of the National Cancer Institute* 85, no. 19. 1571–1579 (October 16, 1993).

Graf, Ernst, and John W. Eaton. "Antioxidant Functions of Phytic Acid." *Free Radical Biology and Medicine* 8 (1990): 61–69.

Hackman, Robert M. "Palm Oil Carotene: An Exciting New Innovation in Nutrition Supplementation." *Whole Foods* (December 1993).

Heart and Stroke Facts. Dallas, Tex.: American Heart Association.

Heimburger, D.C., et al. "Improvement in Bronchial Squamous Metaplasia in Smokers Treated with Folate and Vitamin B_{12}: Report of a Preliminary Randomized, Double-Blind Intervention Trial." *Journal of the American Medical Association* 259, no. 10 (March 11, 1988): 1525–1530.

"Herbs and Spices May be Barrier Against Cancer, Heart Disease." *Environmental Nutrition* 16, no. 6 (June 1993).

al-Hindawi, M. K., S.H. al-Khafaji, and M.H. Abdul-Nabi. "Antigranuloma Activity of Iraqi Withania Somnifera." *Journal of Ethnopharmacology* 37, no. 2 (September 1992): 113–116.

Hobbs, Christopher, and Steven Foster. "Hawthorne: A Literature Review." *Herbalgram*, no. 22, (Spring 1990): 19–33.

Hocman, Gabriel. "Prevention of Cancer: Vegetables and Plants." *Comparative Biochemistry and Physiology* 93B, no. 2 (1989): 201–212.

Hodge, Marie. "Immunity Breakthrough: The 6000-Year-Old Rx." *Longevity* (January 1993).

Horwitt, Max K. "Therapeutic Uses of Vitamin E." *Resident and Staff Physician* (December 1982): 38–46.

Horwitz, Crystal, and Alexander R.P. Walker. "Lignans—Additional Benefits from Fiber?" *Nutrition and Cancer* 6, no. 2 (1984): 73–76.

How Men Stay Young. Emmaus, Pennsylvania: Rodale Press, 1991.

"Improved Physician/Patient Communication Can Minimize Some Drug Side Effects." *National Institute on Aging Research Bulletin*, (January 30, 1989).

"In Vino Veritas—and Something for Your Heart." *Heartstyle* 4, no. 3 (summer 1994).

Jaakkola, K., et al. "Treatment with Antioxidants and Other Nutrients in Combination with Chemotherapy and Irradiation in Patients with Small-Cell Lung Cancer." *Anticancer Research* 12 (1992): 599–606.

Jain, Adesh K., et al. "Can Garlic Reduce Levels of Serum Lipids? A Controlled Clinical Study." *American Journal of Medicine* 94 (June 1993): 632–635.

Johnson, Kathleen, and Evan W. Kligman. "Preventive Nutrition: An 'Optimal' Diet for Older Adults." *Geriatrics* 47, no. 10 (1992): 56–60.

Johnston, Carol S., Claudia Meyer, and J.C. Srilakshmi. Vitamin C Elevates Red Blood Cell Glutathione in Healthy Adults." *American Journal of Clinical Nutrition* 58 (1993): 103–105.

Joosten, Etienne, et al. "Metabolic Evidence That Deficiencies of Vitamin B_{12} (Cobalamin), Folate, and Vitamin B_6 Occur Commonly in Elderly People." *American Journal of Clinical Nutrition* 58 (1993): 468–476.

Kamikawa, Todashi, et al., "Effects of Coenzyme Q_{10} on Exercise Tolerance in Chronic Stable Angina Pectoris." *American Journal of Cardiology* 56 (1985): 247–251.

Khachaturian, Zaven S. "Calcium and the Aging Brain: Upsetting a Delicate Balance?" *Geriatrics* 46, no. 6, 78–79, 83 (1991).

Khan, A. et al. "Insulin Potentiating Factor and Chromium Content of Selected Foods and Spices." *Biologic Trace Element Research* 24, no. 3 (March 1990): 183–188.

Kravitz, Howard M., Hector C. Sabelli, and Jan Fawcett. "Dietary Supplements of Phenylalanine and Other Amino Acid Precursors of Brain Neuroamines in the Treatment of Depressive Disorders." *Journal of the AOA* 84, no. 1 119–123 suppl. (September 1984).

Kune, Gabriel, Susan Bannerman, and Barry Field. "Diet, Alcohol, Smoking, Serum ß-carotene and Vitamin A in Male Non-melanocytic Skin Cancer Patients and Controls." *Nutrition and Cancer* 18, no. 3 (1992): 237–244.

Lee, H. P., L. Gourley, and S.W. Duffy. "Dietary Effects on Breast-Cancer Risk in Singapore." *Lancet* 337 (May 18, 1991): 1197–1200.

Leighton, Terrance, Charles Ginther, and Larry Fluss. "The Distribution of Quercetin and Quercetin Glycosides in Vegetable Components of the Human Diet." Paper presented at the Royal Society of Chemistry Conference, September 1992.

Lipkin, Richard. "Wine's Chemical Secrets." *Science News* 144, (October 23, 1993): 264–265.

"Long-Distance Runners Double 'Dilating' Capacity of Their Coronary Arteries, Researchers Find." *News from the American Heart Association,* (April 12, 1993).

Mabey, Richards, ed. *The New Age Herbalist*. New York: Collier Books, 1988.

"Magnesium Lowers Blood Pressure in Some Diabetic Hypertensives." *News from the American Heart Association*, (September 13, 1990).

"Major Study Reports 'Huge' Variance in Heart Rates Among Nations." *News from the American Heart Association*, (July 11, 1994).

McCaleb, Rob. "Astralagus." *Herb Research Foundation* (July 30, 1990).

————. "Bilberry: Microcirculation Enhancer." *Herb Research Foundation* (April 29, 1992).

McKeown-Eyssen, Gail E., and Elizabeth Bright-See. "Dietary Factors in Colon Cancer: International Relationships." *Nutrition and Cancer* 6, no. 3 (1984).

McMurdo, Marion E. T. and Lucy Rennie. "A Controlled Trial of Exercise by Residents of Old People's Homes." *Age and Ageing* 22 (1993): 11–15.

Meydani, M., et al. "Protective Effect of Vitamin E on Exercise-Induced Oxidative Damage in Young and Older Adults." *American Journal of Physiology* 264 (*Regulatory Integrative Comparitive Physiology* 33) (1993): R992–998.

Michnovicz, Jon J., and H. Leon Bradlow. "Induction of Estradiol Metabolism by Dietary Indole 3-Carbinol in Humans." *Journal of the National Cancer Institute* 82, no. 11. 947–949 (June 6, 1990).

"Mining for Minerals—Zinc is Worth Its Weight in Gold." *Environmental Nutrition* 17, no. 9 (September 1994).

"Mining for Toxic Minerals Hidden in Our Diets." *Environmental Nutrition* 15, no. 3 (March 1992).

Moriguchi, Satori, et al. "Functional Changes in Human Lymphocytes and Monocytes After in Vitro Incubation with Arginine." *Nutrition Research* 7 (1987): 719–728.

National Institute on Aging, Research Bulletin, (February 20, 1990).

National Institute on Aging, Research Bulletin, (April 1991).

National Institute on Aging, Research Bulletin, (July 1991).

National Institute on Aging, Research Bulletin, (October 1991).

National Institute on Aging, Research Bulletin, (August 1992).

National Institute on Aging, Research Bulletin, (November 1992).

Negri, Eva, Carlo La Vecchia, and Silvia Francheschi. "Vegetable and Fruit Consumption and Cancer Risk." *International Journal of Cancer* 48 (1994): 350–354.

Nelson, Miriam E., Elizabeth C. Fisher, and Avraham F. Dilmanian. "A 1-Year Walking Program and Increased Dietary Calcium in

Postmenopausal Women: Effects on Bone." *American Journal of Clinical Nutrition* 53 (1991): 1304–1311.

Newsome, D. A., et al. "Oral Zinc in Macular Degeneration." *Archives of Ophthalmology* 106, no. 2 (February 1988): 192–198.

"Niacin: Double-Edged Sword for Lowering Cholesterol." *Tufts University Diet & Nutrition Letter* 12 no. 6 (August 1994).

Nielson, Forrest H. "Studies on the Relationship Between Boron and Magnesium Which Possibly Affects the Formation and Maintenance of Bones." *Magnesium Trace Elements* 9 (1990): 61–19.

———. "Ultratrace Minerals Mythical Elixirs or Nutrients of Concern?" *Biologic Association of Medicine of Puerto Rico* 83 (1981): 131–133.

"NIH Consensus Development Conference: The Treatment of Sleep Disorders in Older People." *National Institute on Aging Research Bulletin* (September 3, 1990).

1995 Heart and Stroke Facts Statistics. Dallas, Tex.: American Heart Association.

Nixon, Daniel W., Myron Winick, and Michelle Maher. "Metabolic Efficiency, Energy Intake, and Cancer." *Cancer Prevention* 1, no. 3 (1991).

"No Need for Kidney Stone Sufferers to Curb Calcium." *Environmental Nutrition* (September 1993).

"Noise and Hearing Loss, Consensus Statement." *NIH Consensus Development Conference* 8, no. 1 (January 22–24, 1990).

Odens, Max. "Prolongation of the Life Span in Rats." *Journal of the American Geriatrics Society* 21, no. 10 (1973): 450–451.

"On the Link Between Diet and Gout." *Tufts University Diet & Nutrition Letter* 10, no. 9 (November 1, 1992).

Packer, Lester. "Protective Role of Vitamin E in Biologic Systems." *American Journal of Clinical Nutrition* 53 (1991): 1050S–1055S.

Panush, Richard S. "Does Food Cause or Cure Arthritis?" *Rheumatic Disease Clinics of North America* 17, no. 2 (May 1991): 259–271.

Penn, N.D., et al. "The Effect of Dietary Supplementation with Vitamins A, C, and E on Cell-Mediated Immune Function in Elderly Long-Stay Patients: A Randomized Controlled Trial." *Age and Ageing* 20 (1991): 169–174.

Perchellet, J.P., et al. "Antitumor-Promoting Activities of Tannic Acid, Ellagic Acid, and Several Gallic Acid Derivatives in Mouse Skin." *Basic Life Sciences* 59 (1992): 783–801.

Peto, R., et al. "Can Dietary Beta-Carotene Materially Reduce Human Cancer Rates?" *Nature* 290 (March 1981): 201–207.

Press, Raymond I., Jack Geller, and Gary Evans. "The Effect of Chromium Picolinate on Serum Cholesterol and Apolipoprotein Fractions in Human Subjects." *The Western Journal of Medicine* 152, no. 1 (January 1990): 41–45.

"Preventing Wintertime Bone Loss: Effect of Vitamin D Supplementation in Healthy Postmenopausal Women." *Nutrition Reviews* 50, no. 2 (February 1992): 52–54.

"Preventive Nutrition: Disease-Specific Dietary Interventions for Older Adults." *Geriatrics* 47, no. 11 (November 1992): 39–49.

"Prostate Cancer and Red Meat." *University of California, Berkeley, Wellness Letter* (February 1994).

Pryor, William A. "Can Vitamin E Protect Humans Against the Pathological Effects of Ozone in Smog? *American Journal of Clinical Nutrition* 53 (1991): 702–722.

"Pumping Immunity." *Nutrition Action Healthletter* (April 1993).

Raloff, Janet. "Hearty Vitamins: Sparing Arteries with Megadose Supplements." *Science News* 142 (1991): 78.

Regan, T. J. "Alcohol and the Cardiovascular System." *Journal of the American Medical Association* 264, no. 3 (1990): 377–381.

"Reviving Your Taste Buds When Taste and Smell Wane." *Enviromental Nutrition* (February 1993).

Risch, Harvey A., et al. "Dietary Factors and the Incidence of Cancer of the Stomach." *American Journal of Epidemiology* 122, no. 6 (1985).

Robertson, James McD., Allan P. Donner, and John R. Trevithick. "A Possible Role for Vitamins C and and E in Cataract Prevention." *American Journal of Clinical Nutrition* 53 (1991): 346S–351S.

Roe, Daphne, A. "Overview of Effects of Aging on Nutrition." *Clinics in Geriatric Medicine* 6, no. 2 (May 1990): 319–334.

Roebothan, Barbara Vera, and Ranja Kuma Chandra. "Relationship between Nutritional Status and Immune Function of Elderly People." *Age and Ageing* 23 (1994): 49–53.

Rose, David P. "Diet, Hormones and Cancer." *Annual Review of Public Health* 14 (1993): 1–17.

———. "Dietary Fiber, Phytoestrogens, and Breast Cancer." *Nutrition* 8, no. 1 (January/February 1992): 47–51.

Rosenberg, Irwin H., and Joshua W. Miller. "Nutritional Factors in Physical and Cognitive Functions of Elderly People." *American Journal of Clnical Nutrition* 55, (1992): 1237S–1243S.

Rusting, Ricki L. "Why Do We Age?" *Scientific American* 267, 1 (December 1992): 131–141.

Sandyk, Reuven. "Possible Role of Pineal Melatonin in the Mechanisms of Aging." *International Journal of Neuroscience*. 52 (1990): 85–92.

Schardt, David. "Alzheimer's in the Family." *Nutrition Action Healthletter* (June 1994).

Schmidt, Karlheinz. "Antioxidant Vitamins and ß-Carotene: Effects on Immunocompetence." *American Journal of Clinical Nutrition* 53 (1991): 383S–385S.

"Seedy Remedy for Rheumatoid Arthritis?" *Science News* 144 (November 6, 1993): 302.

Selkoe, Dennis J. "Aging Brain, Aging Mind: Structural and Chemical Changes." *Scientific American* 267, no. 3 (September 1992).

Sharma, Om P., et al. "Soy of Dietary Source Plays a Preventive Role Against the Pathogenesis of Prostatitis." *Journal Steroid Biochemical Molecular Biology* 43, no. 65 (1992): 557–564.

Shephard, Roy J. "Exercise and Aging: Extending Independence in Older Adults." *Geriatrics* 48, no 5. 61–64 (May 1993).

Siani, Alfonso, et al. "Increasing the Dietary Potassium Intake Reduces the Need for Antihypertensive Medication." *Annals of Internal Medicine* 115 (1991): 753–759.

Simopoulos, Artermis P. "Omega-3 Fatty Acids in Health and Disease and in Growth and Development." *American Journal of Clinical Nutrition* 54 (1991): 438–463.

Smigel, Kara. "Vitamin E Moves on Stage in Cancer Prevention Studies." *Journal of the National Cancer Institute* 84, no. 13 (July 1, 1992).

Snyder, Jessica. "Solving the Alzheimer's Jigsaw." *Longevity (January 1992)*.

Soni, K.B., A. Rajan, and R. Kuttan. "Reversal of Aflatoxin Induced Liver Damage by Turmeric and Curcumin." *Cancer Letter* 66, no. 2 (September 30, 1992): 115–121.

"Staying Physically Active May Help to Stave Off Blood Vessel Ills, Two New Studies Suggest." 33rd Annual Conference on Cardiovascular Disease Epidemiology and Prevention. *News from the American Heart Association* 18 (Abstract 17).

Stern, Yaakov, et al. "Influence of Education and Occupation on the Incidence of Alzheimer's Disease." *Journal of the American Medical Association* 271, no. 13 (April 6, 1994).

Tanaka, T., et al. "Inhibition of 4-Nitroquinoline-1-oxide-Induced Rat Tongue Carcinogenesis by the Naturally Occurring Plant Phenolics Caffeic, Ellagic, Chlorogenic and Ferrulic Acids." *Carcinogenesis* 14, no. 7 (July 1993): 1321–1325.

Teas, Jane. "The Consumption of Seaweed as a Protective Factor in the Etiology of Breast Cancer." *Medical Hypotheses* 7 (1981): 601–613.

Teel, R.W., and A. Castonguay. "Antimutagenic Effects of Polyphenolic Compounds." *Cancer Letter* 66, no. 2 (September 30, 1992): 107–113.

"A Test to Take (and Not to Take) for Colon Cancer." *University of California, Berkeley, Wellness Letter* 9, no. 12 (September 1993).

Thun, Michael J., et al. "Risk Factors for Fatal Colon Cancer in a Large Prospective Study." *Journal of the National Cancer Institute* 84, no. 19. 149–1500(October 7, 1992).

"Triglycerides Finally Unmasked as 'Bad Actor' in Coronary Artery Disease Drama, Researchers Say." *News from the American Heart Association,* (July 1994).

Troll, Walter, and Ann R. Kennedy, eds. "Workshop Report from the Division of Cancer Etiology, National Cancer Institute, National Institutes of Health. Protease Inhibitors as Cancer Chemopreventive Agents." *Cancer Research* 49 (January 15, 1989): 499–502.

Tucker, Don M., et al. "Nutrition Status and Brain Function in Aging." *American Journal of Clinical Nutrition* 52 (1990): 93–102.

"23-Year Study of Middle-Aged Men in Hawaii Confirms: Physical Activity Will Lower Risk of Heart Disease." *News from the American Heart Association,* (June 13, 1994).

U.S. *Department of Agriculture, Food and Nutrition, Research Briefs* Washington, D.C. (January–March 1993).

U.S. *Department of Agriculture, Food and Nutrition, Research Briefs* (July–September 1993).

U.S. Department of Agriculture, Human Nutrition Research Center on Aging at Tufts University, Research Program Description.

U.S. *Department of Agriculture, Research Briefs* (April–June 1993).

Varma, Shambhu D. "Scientific Basis for Medical Therapy of Cataracts by Antioxidants." *American Journal of Clinical Nutrition* 53 (1991): 335–345S.

"Vitamin B_6 and Immune Function in the Elderly and HIV-Seropositive Subjects." *Nutrition Reviews* 50, no. 5 (May 1992): 145–147.

"Vitamin E May Guard Against Artery Blockage by LDL." *Heartstyle* (Fall 1993).

"Vitamin E Supplementation Enhances Immune Response in the Elderly." *Nutrition Reviews* 50, no. 3 (March 1992): 85–87.

Walsh, Nicolas E., et al. "Anagesic Effectiveness of D-Phenylalanine in Chronic Pain Patients." *Archives of Physical Medicine Rehabilitation* 67 (July 1986): 436–439.

Wei-Hua, Lu, Jiang Shou, and Xi-Can Tang. "Improving Effect of Huperzine A on Discrimination Performance in Aged Rats and Adult Rats with Experimental Cognitive Impairment." *Acta Pharmacologica Sinica* 1 (January 1988): 11–15.

Wuethrich, B. "Higher Risk of Alzheimer's Linked to Gene." *Science News,* 144 (August 14, 1993).

You, W.C., et al. "Allium Vegetables and the Reduced Risk of Stomach Cancer." *Journal of the National Cancer Institute* 81, no. 2 (1989): 162–164.

Ziegler, Regina G. "Vegetables, Fruits, and Carotenoids and the Risk of Cancer." *American Journal of Clinical Nutrition* 53 (1991): 251S–259S.

Znaiden, Alex. "The Science Behind Successful New Skin Care Products." *Avanstar Communications* (January 1994).

Index

or—.

SMALL ROCKS RISING

western literature series

SUSAN LANG

SMALL ROCKS RISING

UNIVERSITY OF NEVADA PRESS ▲▲ RENO & LAS VEGAS

WESTERN LITERATURE SERIES

University of Nevada Press,

Reno, Nevada 89557 USA

Copyright © 2002 by Susan Lang

All rights reserved

Manufactured in the

United States of America

Design by Carrie House

Library of Congress

Cataloging-in-Publication Data

Lang, Susan, 1941–

Small rocks rising / Susan Lang.

p. cm. — (Western literature series)

ISBN 0-87417-504-6 (pbk. : alk. paper)

1. California, Southern—Fiction.

2. Women landowners—Fiction.

3. Women pioneers—Fiction.

I. Title. II. Series.

PS3612.A555 S63 2002

813'.6–dc21   2001008688

The paper used in this book meets

the requirements of American National

Standard for Information Sciences—

Permanence of Paper for Printed Library

Materials, ANSI Z39.48–1984. Binding

materials were selected for strength

and durability.

FIRST PRINTING

11 10 09 08 07 06 05 04 03 02

5 4 3 2 1

In memory of the women of Pipes Canyon

We are but thoughts in the mind of rock

ACKNOWLEDGMENTS

My profound gratitude to all the friends and colleagues who supported and/or critiqued this and other endeavors, most especially Ron Carlson, T. M. McNally, John Nichols, Marge Piercy, Ira Wood, Carol Rawlings, Carol Houck Smith, John Shannon, and my editor, Trudy McMurrin.

I am indebted also to the southwestern desert mountains that inspired this work of fiction, though readers should be aware that many aspects of the actual geography have been reconfigured to meet the dramatic needs of this novel, and that much of the landscape of this work is now fictional, as are the characters who live out their stories within these pages.

SMALL ROCKS RISING

W hen Ruth arrived on the truck loaded with her supplies, she headed straight for the first of four pinyons that enclosed her cabin site. While Matt guided John Olsen's backing of the flatbed, she boosted herself up the trunk of the pine and inched her way out onto a wide lower limb, until she could wrap her hand around a rusted tin can hanging from the branch above. Ruth had been picturing that moment since the day she signed the form and paid the fees for her homestead, March 15, 1929, nearly three weeks before. At that moment, she had made up her mind to erase all sign of the place's history as a stopover for cowboys who couldn't tolerate a few drops of pine pitch on their shirts. Can-Tree Springs, indeed: not a fit name for her land.

Ruth yanked on the can, but it remained stubborn. After twisting the tin several times to loosen the baling wire, she jerked down again. Both wire and can came off in her hand. After she had removed the three other cans, Ruth patted the rough bark beside her. She would free the other trees once the men left. With a finger she caught one of the clear drips of pitch that covered the sides of the can—trying the turpentine taste on her tongue. The rest of the sticky drip she smeared on the back of a hand, its scent merging with her own, then she dropped to the ground to help the men unload her belongings.

Matt and John had already begun piling building materials in front of the furthest pinyon, beside an odd-shaped boulder that reached to just above Ruth's waist.

"Wait," she called out to Matt, who was ready to throw more planks onto the pile. "Not there. Don't put any more there. How about over by that scrub oak?"

"What's the matter with here?" Matt leaned the planks against the boulder and swiped his forehead with the back of a hand. Sunlight turned his hair the color of fresh-churned butter. "Seems here would be handier for you." His pale blue eyes settled on her as John Olsen came up beside him lugging a huge sack of cement.

"I'd just have to move it all again," she said. "That's why." Ruth picked up a fallen twig. "Look. I'll show you," she said, pacing out the area as she drew an approximate rectangle in the dirt. "Here's where my cabin will be, between the pinyons, where the ground's nice and flat. You can see you're putting all that inside my cabin."

"If you draw your rectangle the other way, we won't be," Matt said. "Just turn your house around." With one foot he began to redraw the floor plan.

"No," Ruth said. "I want to walk right out into morning sun. My front door has to face east."

"Ya, Rute," John Olsen said, hunkering beside the stone. He rubbed at the white stubble on his jaw. "But what you do about the boulder?"

Ruth walked over and squatted beside the old Swede, who

smelled of goat and infrequent baths. Baths would not come easy here in this canyon, she realized. She ran a palm across the cold exterior of the rock. It appeared strangely alive. The smooth saddle of its back, the way it rested on a rounded belly made it seem like some kind of mineral beast. "I guess I'll have to move it, then," she said.

Both men laughed. Matt patted her shoulder. "Ruth," he said, "you may be the most capable woman I ever met. Honest. But not even John and I together could move that boulder."

Ruth felt her face flush. For once Matt's big smile didn't turn her to goo. "Just put the building materials over there, Matt Baxter," she said. "I'll move this rock. You wait and see." She marched toward the truck to escape the men's looks of amusement. John Olsen rose and began shifting the pile.

With three of them, it didn't take long to finish the unloading. While Matt and John set up her tent and carried in her cot and chest of drawers, Ruth gathered wood and built a fire in the circle of rocks that cowboys in the past had constructed. Then she picked up a bucket and walked across the wash to the patch of green that surrounded her spring. She knelt among the wiry sprigs of succulent grass, some more than a foot high, and dunked her bucket into the shallow pool of water—careful to avoid skater bugs and the gray beetle floating upside down near the water's edge. Behind the spring, the exposed roots of a cottonwood dropped a tangled skirt down the bank. When her bucket was full, she dipped a cupped hand into the water and brought it to her mouth. No water had ever tasted so sweet. Her very own, fresh from the earth. Her earth.

Later, the three of them sat in canvas camp chairs and christened her new homestead with cups of cowboy coffee. Containing her eagerness for the men to leave, Ruth sat savoring the smell of coffee and campfire smoke. She listened to the drone of passing flies and admired the sunlight puddling on Matt's soft curls. Caught up as she was in details close to her, she almost didn't notice, just over Matt's head, a man descending the bluff across the wash, dropping so smoothly he appeared almost to float down the rocks. She was too surprised to say a word, but her face spoke for her: John Olsen followed her eyes over to the stony base of Rocky Mountain.

"It just Jim, Rute. Indian Jim," John said, pulling pipe makings from his pocket.

"But I thought you and Kate were my nearest neighbors," Ruth said, "What is he doing . . ."

"Ya, Rute. Jim stay on the mountain sometime. In summer. He set svedges at the mine. Good worker, Jim is. Smart too." Olsen tamped the tobacco in his pipe.

Ruth got up and walked to the campfire, where she wrestled the enamel pot off to the side of the rocks. Using a stick to tip the hot pot handle, Ruth poured coffee into her cup while the man made his way toward the camp. She wondered what she would have done if Matt and John hadn't been there. What could she have done? She decided to take up Matt's offer and borrow his rifle until the one she had ordered came in at Matt's General Store. Not that she'd ever shot a rifle.

The man was dark-skinned, with definitive, rugged features. Abundant black hair hung loose halfway to his waist, except where it was bound by a red bandana around his forehead. Ruth had seen Indians before in El Paso, Mexican Indians who came across the border for supplies or business. She had never spoken to one, but had always been curious because of the rumors about her mother, Cally. No one in the family would speak of it directly—not even her mother—but Ruth had overheard enough hushed snatches of stories those years she lived with her aunt, whispers about the "half-breed bastard" her grandfather had brought home to raise. And once when Ruth was very young, she remembered a time on the streets in El Paso when a well-dressed woman spat at her mother's feet and hissed the word *squaw*.

Matt nodded when John Olsen made the introductions, did not rise or offer his hand. Ruth was surprised to see suspicion and discomfort in his face. She could tell the Indian noticed it too: not that the expression on Jim's face did more than harden around the eyes as he looked at Matt. She made a point of walk-

4

ing over to offer her hand, though Matt's disapproval lent stiffness to her action.

"There's hot coffee," she said, resuming her seat. "The cups are in the box there. Feel free."

"Thanks," Jim said, his face softening into the suggestion of a smile. "I do." Ruth stifled a laugh of surprise.

"Have they told you," Jim said as he tipped the coffeepot to pour, "about the inscripted rocks up there on the mountain?"

"Inscripted rocks?" Ruth asked, confused as much by the Indian's manner and clear speech as by what he said. He was more than simply smart. "What kind of inscriptions?" A picture formed in her head of cowboys attacking the rocks with pen and ink.

"Figures people long ago made on rocks. Your people call them petroglyphs. I'll show them to you sometime if you want. It means this place was important once. Possibly a major hunting area. My own people had a strange name for it. Something like 'place where rocks reside.' Something like that but not quite. Maybe more like 'small rocks rising.' Some things just don't translate," he said.

From her two years at Sarah Higgins Academy, Ruth recognized the educated nature of his speech—curious in such a man. But underlying that was some kind of Indian inflection that moved his voice smoothly over words, blunting the sharp edges of sound the way flowing water rounds off sharp rocks. She looked at Matt, who was studying the man with a wary interest.

"So before the cowboys came here with their tin cans, there were Indians," Ruth said.

"That's true everywhere, isn't it?" Jim sat on a small flat rock next to the fire. "Good coffee," he said, swirling the liquid in his cup so that light from its surface scattered patterns on the pinyon branches overhead.

"You come down to house, Jim? Could use help." Olsen tapped out finished tobacco onto the ground and rubbed it into the dirt with one foot. "Go up for a load in the morning. Stay tree or four day." He returned the pipe to his shirt pocket.

"Thought I might. I'll catch a ride down with you, John. Spotted your truck from near the top."

"Why don't I leave that rifle with you, Ruth?" Matt said, his eyes on the Indian. "Come on. I'll instruct you." He got up and walked to her chair, reached out a hand.

Ruth allowed him her hand and followed him back to the truck. Matt seemed distracted as he gave her a lesson on loading the .22. When he showed her where the safety was located, he seemed unaware of how close his arm came to her breast. "I want to make sure you're safe," he told her, once the rifle was loaded. "I'll be back in a week. No telling who might wander by meanwhile. Here," he said, "I'll show you how to shoot it."

Picking up one of the cans Ruth had discarded from the pine, Matt placed it on top of a rock near the bank of the wash. As she aimed the rifle, he came up behind and reached both arms around her, snuggling the rifle into the crotch of her shoulder. "Now keep the rifle firm here. Line up those two sights on that can," he said, leaning in closer. She could barely breathe with the warm outline of his body fitted tight against her.

Ruth felt him suck in his breath. She closed one eye and lined up the sights so the can sat square in front of the two posts, fighting all the while to concentrate against the pounding in her body. "Now," Matt whispered, "pull the trigger." A great rush of blood swept to Ruth's head as she snapped back the lever.

The shot ricocheted from the cliff across the wash. The can flew off the rock.

"Good shot." The Indian's voice came from behind them. Matt stepped back, and Ruth turned to find Jim and John Olsen heading toward the truck.

"It wasn't hard," Ruth said, keeping all trace of surprise from her voice. She would not be flustered, though she couldn't help but be impressed with herself. So that's all there was to it; it pleased her to have so easily broken through one of the mysteries of the male world. She sashayed back toward her camp, taking the rifle with her.

Setting the rifle and box of shells inside her tent, she went back out to say her good-byes. Matt reached out the truck win-

6

dow as John started the engine. "See you next week," he said. "I'll bring up those supplies from the store. Maybe your twenty-two will be in by then." He gave her arm a quick squeeze when she came up beside him. "Be sure to keep that rifle handy."

"I'll be all right," Ruth said. She climbed on the running board and poked her head in the window. "Thanks, John. For your help. Your truck too. And tell Kate thanks for the food."

"We neighbor now, Rute. Maybe you crazy, but neighbor." Shaking his head, John put the truck in gear. "Up here . . . all by yourself. Think you can move that boulder."

"I will move that rock," she assured him, though the truth was she'd forgotten all about her promise until he reminded her.

"Maybe John can loan you some dynamite," Matt said, laughing.

"Ya. We don't use the dynamite. We svedge the onyx." As the truck began to move, Ruth jumped from the running board and stood to one side while they backed onto the rut road. She gave a wave to Jim, who sat on the wooden flatbed, his back leaning against the cab. The Indian nodded, held her eyes as the truck pulled out and bumped on down the rough road.

Ruth watched the truck disappear around the far bend of Rocky Mountain, waited until the drone of motor grew faint. Grateful as she had been for the men's help, she had felt the canyon would not be fully hers until they were gone. When the engine sound faded into rushes of air playing in the pinyons, she lay flat on ground warm with March afternoon sun, nothing but a cotton shirt between her back and the place she had come to claim. Rough pebbles pressed into her skin beneath the cloth. Thin clouds spilled over the tops of the pine tree she had freed, its branches no longer encrusted with rusty tin cans. From somewhere an oriole strung a song through the air. She took in deep breaths of wildflower and pine and let the place seep into her, wanting the canyon to inhabit her as fully as she meant to inhabit it.

When her senses were saturated, she burst to her feet, stretched her arms above her head. "Mine. Oh, it's mine. Really all mine!" she yelled, then listened as her words bounced back from the bluff across the wash. Of course, the place wasn't quite hers yet. She still had to prove up on her homestead—to construct herself a structure out of the heap of building materials. And to move that damnable rock. She was required to stay three years in this place to make it hers. What sweet torture—living here three whole years! Crazed with joy, Ruth cackled out into the quiet canyon, and the rock cliff across the wash returned the sound of her laughter.

When the echoes died, she walked over to the rock and studied it. As ridiculous as it seemed, there was something willful about that rock. As if it would move—or not move—all of its own accord. She climbed up on the saddleback of the stone, curved her legs around its cool sides. "Giddyup," she said, almost expecting to ride the boulder like a small pony out of the range of her cabin site. The boulder didn't budge. She knew it didn't want to move anywhere. She knew also that this place could never be hers until she had moved this rock from her chosen spot. She had traveled far to find this place, so many things had come together to bring her here—those months spent in nurse training that enabled her to come west, all the small details dovetailing to bring her to this canyon. She couldn't let one rock stop her now.

Matt said she'd been lucky to get the building materials, thought it miraculous the way they'd come available the day after she filed her claim. The sixty-five dollars needed was exactly what she had left after paying the filing fees. She suspected it was destiny at work—though she hated to think the death of the Henleys' child and their sudden departure had come about in order to present her with the odd assortment of materials she needed.

Can-Tree Springs in Rattlesnake Canyon had been the last of the sites Matt had taken her to see, and even then he seemed reluctant. Not even he had thought a woman would be interested in homesteading such an isolated claim so many miles away from Juniper Valley—or he didn't want her to be. But the place did have water, Matt admitted. Ruth hadn't known herself just what she was looking for, but she knew the minute she found it.

They had followed an old mining road that wound around the base of Rocky Mountain and into the long wash that led up Rattlesnake Canyon, Matt's Model A bucking the rough road all the way up. In the first hour they surprised three deer and stopped to kill a rattler. Hawks and buzzards circled overhead. When they started out, Ruth had a qualm or two about the isolation, but the farther they drove the more at home she felt. The very wildness of the canyon excited her.

Some four miles up, the road cut through a long thicket of willows, and a small stream rose aboveground on one side. A few minutes later they arrived at a stone house tucked back on a flattened knoll. Goats galloped up and down the mountain, poked heads out from behind willows in the wash. "The Swedes' place," Matt said as he stopped in the road and set the hand brake. They would be her closest neighbors if she took the homestead, Matt told her, a mere four miles down canyon from her. The "Swedes" turned out to be John Olsen, his wife, Kate, and several men who slept in tents beside the stone house and hacked out a living mining onyx up the North Fork.

Olsen strode down from the knoll to greet them, large and muscular, wearing a silver badge on each of his suspenders: one badge read "Fire Marshal," the other, "Fish and Game Warden." Then Kate, who must have weighed nearly three hundred pounds, lumbered out the door, her round face beaming as she shouted, "Velcome, Velcome." Ruth didn't know who was the more impressive.

Kate took Ruth out to see her new garden. In the dark rich soil around the willows, Kate said vegetables grew several times normal size, which seemed appropriate for the woman. She insisted they stay for "someting Svedish," which turned out to be a delicious pastry baked on her woodstove and served with what Kate called "cowboy coffee." Ruth felt dubious about the coffee, grounds poured into boiling water, simmered briefly, then pulled off the fire to settle. She forced herself to taste what had come to look like chocolate mud. That one taste had convinced her, and not a day had gone by since that Ruth hadn't brewed some for herself.

Over coffee, John Olsen had given Matt directions. About two miles up, he said, the canyon split at the base of Rocky Mountain. The fork to the right went up past the old Rose Mine and ended at Onyx Peak. The left went to Can-Tree Springs by way of an old cattle trail that had only recently become a rut road. The very names of places seemed to give character to this canyon, and it took considerable effort on Ruth's part not to run for the car as soon as she'd taken the last swallow from her cup. She burned to see what lay ahead.

The Olsens assumed that Matt and Ruth were a couple, having seen Ruth before behind the counter at Matt's store. When Ruth explained that she had only been helping out and nursing Matt's tubercular wife, now recovered, and that she would be homesteading alone—if she decided on the place—the Olsens disapproved. "Ya, not good for woman without man. Too far. Find other place, Rute," John told her. It was the same old story, though Ruth liked the Olsens well enough to forgive them.

Once Ruth saw Can-Tree Springs, nobody else's opinion mattered anyway. She knew at once that it was a match. Standing under the pinyons, she had looked across the wash, where three huge cottonwood trees huddled above the spring, the wind flickering sunlight through their leaves. Already an early showing of purple monkey flower and desert gold carpeted the mountainsides and banks above the wash. The scene reminded her of a poem she'd read at Sarah Higgins, about a poet who once saw a crowd of daffodils and who ever after, back at his dwelling in the city, would close his eyes and remember them. But Ruth knew she would never be content somewhere else remembering this place. She intended to stay right here and live her life with these pinyons and wildflowers. "Glory Springs," she had said in a hushed voice to Matt, not wanting to break the spell. "I'll name it Glory Springs." It deserved better than to be named after tin cans.

And she had done it. Renamed it and claimed it. Now she had work to do. Ruth slid down from the rock and began storing food supplies and large pots under the writing table in the tent. She arranged the cooking utensils in wooden crates stacked as shelves by the fire ring. Then she climbed the pinyons after the remaining cans, which took up more of the afternoon than she had imagined. The other pines were harder to scale, the cans more difficult to reach. Some she had to bat off with a thick stick, leaving the baling wire dangling. When she dropped down from the last branch, Ruth was as covered with pitch as some of the cans she'd removed. Bark had scraped her arms in several places. She lifted the lid of the water cooler and dipped out a ladle of water, looking back at the stack of lumber and building materials. Someday soon she would have to make sense of them. Meanwhile, she felt more like the yellow butterfly that fluttered up over her two paneless window frames, then dipped down to land on a stalk of apricot globemallow.

Ruth continued on to the high bank of the wash, where bluebells grew knee deep. A cottontail rabbit sat in absolute stillness in a clearing near the spring. Beside her, lupine stalks reached nearly to her shoulder, the blossoms busy with honeybees who seemed to be enjoying the fragrance as much as she was. The lupines reminded Ruth of Texas bluebonnets, except these were lavender and somehow more elegant. And they were hers. How far this place felt from her life in El Paso, from the feud between her mother and aunt that Ruth thought she would never escape. Certainly far from that ridiculous finishing school her late father's family had exiled her to. It was a finishing school, all right—meant to finish off her spirit. But here she was shed of all that.

The sun was about an hour from the horizon. She still had time to get her bedding spread on the cot inside the tent, to revive the campfire and heat the goat stew Kate had sent up for supper. For a moment more Ruth stood basking in her new freedom, then brought her mind back—a person couldn't afford to let it wander for long out in the wild. She picked up the enamel bucket and walked down the path to the spring; she would need more water for the cowboy coffee her taste buds were craving.

Ruth had not counted on the nights being so dark and wild, so full of strange sounds that made the canvas walls around her seem flimsy. For a long while that first night, she tossed on her cot and listened to crickets and coyotes. She tried not to think of Matt—he was someone else's husband—but when she closed her eyes she would remember the way he had of looking up at her from across the room as they sat reading by lamplight long after May had gone to sleep. Yet she doubted Matt would ever act on what had passed unspoken between them; he seemed far above any other man she had known, so gentle and caring with a wife who was infirm. It might be shameful to think it, but Ruth thought he deserved more from a wife. And Matt was certainly mountains above that fool Karl in El Paso. She had been blinded by curly hair and a motorcycle. If it hadn't been for Cally, Ruth would have been undone that time. Her nurse training hadn't given her any help in that regard, and for once she was grateful for her mother's strange skill with herbs.

Tossing in the wake of memory and the turmoil of strange surroundings, Ruth wondered if she would ever sleep again. After some time, she got back up and lit a candle.

She sat at the tiny wooden table and opened the journal she'd thought herself too tired to write in earlier. Though the white canvas did its best to reflect the glow of the flame, the light was still so dim she couldn't be sure ink actually flowed from the pen, so she wrote on faith. She had felt alone her whole life, she wrote, but always with people around her. This was the first time she had ever been as alone outside as she was inside. It felt right. She dipped her pen and went on to recount the events of her first day, trying to find words for the beauty of the place and her feelings for it.

A scream, eerily high-pitched and not quite human, cut through the quiet tent. Ruth jerked to her feet. The sound was like nothing she had ever heard. Then she remembered what the Olsens told her about the night cries of mountain lions. She considered the rifle leaning next to the table, but put down the pen and picked up two pots from a box. Unlatching the flap of the tent, Ruth stood by the doorway and banged the pots together. When the mountain quieted, she went in and tied up the canvas flap as tightly as she could. She lit a second candle, though she only had four to last the week.

Ruth resumed her pen and journal, but sat without writing a word, watching the wavering shadows cast by candlelight. A tiny insect smaller than a ladybug landed on the blank page and began moving smoothly across the white space. She studied the attractive black-and-white patterns etched on its shell as if they were letters she had yet to learn. When it flew off, she put down the pen and closed her journal.

Unknotting the straps, Ruth stepped outside the tent door. She forced herself to remain in the alien darkness, refusing to entertain the images leaping up from her imagination, the cougars and bears crouched behind black patches of scrub oak and juniper. Instead, she looked up at the ink sky with its stars close enough to touch. She imagined the light dripping down on her like rain, bathing her and washing away her fear until she became part of the mystery she felt around her. How then could she be afraid?

F or the next three days Ruth cleared stubborn, thorny shrubs from the ground that was to be her cabin floor. The days were long and hard. She would set to work early, after a breakfast of oatmeal and coffee, not quitting until the long shadows of late afternoon stretched out across the canyon. Sometimes it took hours to remove one bush, especially the cat's-claw, whose barbed branches fought her inch by inch and whose roots went so deep they seemed attached to the center of the earth. Cholla cacti were even more dangerous; the spiny sections reached out to embed themselves in her clothing and boots when she came near, each spine carrying stinging venom in its tip. It was no wonder the plant was referred to as jumping cactus. Ruth was grateful that only two small cholla occupied her ground and that their roots were shallow compared to those of the cat's-claw. Before long, her sun-darkened arms bore deep scratches as proof of her victories.

She began to notice, as she dug around shrubs to loosen their roots, that what she sometimes assumed were pieces of flat rock were not stone at all, but shards of broken pottery, most of them crude and earthy-red, a bit like the unpainted terra-cotta she'd seen in border shops in El Paso. Many had been blackened by fire. A few, and these intrigued her, had indications of stripes or swirls. She became adept at spotting the unnatural shape of these objects and, whenever she came across one in her digging, would brush off the dirt packed around it and place it in a tin on the flat rock that served as a secondary table by the campfire.

It was midmorning on the fourth day when Ruth felt ready to tackle the boulder. She pulled out a plank from her building supplies to give her leverage, thinking if she could just nudge the rock's rounded bottom and make it roll over by the pinyons where the ground began its downward slope, it would be out of her way. After scraping away enough loose topsoil so she could jam the end of the board under the edge of the rock, Ruth walked around to the other end and lifted the plank. She found she couldn't raise the board above her waist, so she got to her knees and put her back and shoulder underneath, straining upward until she thought her leg bones would crumble. She rested and lifted again. And again. Time after time, Ruth repeated the process. With each lift, either the board or her flesh gave more than the stone. After dozens of tries, her only achievement was to emboss red welts on her shoulders.

Her next idea was to rest the middle of the plank on a smaller rock carried over from the campfire, then to jump up and down on the raised end. About the fourth try, Ruth thought she had it, thought she felt the boulder budge. She jumped once more as high as she could and came down hard. The plank snapped in two. After several jumps so did the second board she used. The next plank she chose carefully for strength and resilience and, indeed, it took her nearly a dozen jumps before it, too, snapped. The stone stood its ground.

Leaning the shovel against the recalcitrant rock, Ruth eased her rear onto the stone's curved surface, ignoring the muscles that protested each movement. She ran a dry tongue over her cracked lips and thought about walking the few yards to the water bucket but could not bring herself to take even the first step. She pushed back her hair and undid the top button of her blouse, fanning air into the sweat that poured between her breasts. Afternoon sun burnt fiercely through the cotton of her shirt, though it was barely April. Ruth swiped at tears welling against her will. She wasn't going to give in to them. Bodysore, every cell cried out to admit defeat, to give in to the hard cold creature, and turn her house around. But to be humbled by a mere stone was more than her spirit could bear. She'd overcome bigger obstacles just to get out of Texas. Besides, such capitulation was just what Cally and her aunt Myrtle would expect to happen. That Ruth would come crawling back someday was the first thing she could remember the two of them ever agreeing on.

Ruth lurched to her feet and staggered to the tin water cooler beside the pinyon. Dropping the ladle into the cool liquid, she gulped down two full dippers, then dipped again and poured the water over her forehead, letting it drip down inside her shirt. She stood assessing the pile of building materials that had once seemed such a blessing. The mystery of how to turn such things into a place to live overwhelmed her. The sheer labor of it. Ruth shook her head in wonderment. How had she ever expected to construct a house when she couldn't even manage to clear the land to put it on? Yet inexperience had never stopped her in the past—else she would never have come west in the first place, never hitched rides back to El Paso from Sarah Higgins. And what a stir that caused. The thought still amused her.

Ruth dropped the ladle back into the cooler. No use beating herself against that rock anymore today. The sun was already about halfway to the horizon. Tomorrow, once she dug out the rest of the cat's-claw root, she'd find some way to move the boulder. After the way Matt had laughed, she had to. Too tired to walk as far as the tent for a pillow, Ruth sank down into the shade of the pinyon. She could not remember a bed more welcoming than the simple ground at that moment. She closed her eyes and relished the soft afternoon breeze brushing the hairs on her arms.

The smell of smoke startled her awake. The sun was down and its light nearly faded. Ruth jerked to her elbows at the sight of flames leaping above her campfire. Confusion paralyzed her. Was she dreaming? That fire had been dead out since morning; she was sure of it. Another smell penetrated, coffee and something very like flour baking. Then she saw the figure silhouetted against the tent—where her rifle was stashed, she realized, lunging to her feet.

"Sorry to scare you," the Indian said. "I thought about waking you, but didn't have the heart." He turned and walked toward the campfire. "I knew the smells would wake you sooner or later. Coffee?"

Ruth tried to clear what felt like drips of pine pitch from her head. She hurried to her tent door. The rifle lay in plain sight on her cot. She promised silently that she would never allow herself to be so unprotected again. What if . . . she shuddered to think. He'd had plenty of opportunity. He must not have meant her harm.

Jim held out a steaming cup as she came up to the fire. "You must like to surprise people," she said. "I keep thinking I'm alone in the canyon. That's why I chose this place. But what is it I smell?"

Squatting on the other side of the campfire, Jim used a stick in the handle to lift the lid from Ruth's cast-iron Dutch oven. The glow of coals seeped out from around the edges of the pot. Inside, the bottom was covered with lightly browned biscuits. The smell made her weak in the knees; she'd had nothing since oatmeal at breakfast.

"We finished the swedging early. Kate sent you up some cheese. She likes to feed people. There," he said, "on the rock beside you. Biscuits go good with it."

Not knowing what to say or feel—whether to be mad at the intrusion, impressed by the man's culinary skills, or just plain grateful for the food—Ruth unwrapped the bundle. The cheese was curdy and white with a pungent aroma. "Goat," Jim said. "Nothing better."

She gave him no argument, and indeed Ruth would never forget the taste of those hot biscuits smeared with goat cheese and washed down with fresh cowboy coffee. She didn't miss in the least the Hereford corned beef and beans she'd planned.

Sitting on the ground in front of the fire, they ate without speaking, while stars seeped out and the cricket chorus deepened. A lemon slice of moon accentuated the night sky. When the biscuits were gone, Ruth got to her feet and moved around the campfire, tipping the pot with the stick to fill her coffee cup. "Thanks," she said. "Those were great biscuits."

Jim leaned over to hold his cup under the spout, his dark hair falling across his bare arm like an extension of night. "You looked hungry enough to eat rocks if I'd warmed them up," he said, looking over past the tent into the dark. "You've made progress around here."

"Some." Ruth settled the coffeepot back on the rocks and removed the stick from the handle. "What's this swedging you do?"

"It breaks loose the onyx deposits. I climb cliffs and hammer pegs into the cracks—sometimes I drill a little to get them in. Then soak the wood so it swells up and breaks the rock apart."

It sounded like a tall tale to Ruth, this breaking of rock with wood and water, hardly possible—yet she felt a surge of something like hope.

As if he read her mind, Jim said, "It wouldn't work with your hunk of granite, though. Not the same. Too hard. And you need flaw lines."

"So that's what that thing out there is, then, granite?" she said, looking into the dark where she could feel it looming, mocking her. Set in its ways.

Jim nodded. Though she could see only his outline against the fire, she sensed a suppressed smile. "That's what it's made of anyway," he said.

Granite rock-flesh, Ruth thought, lying back to look at the

stars, her head pillowed on her hands. The man was educated. She wondered where he'd gone to school to speak so properly, why he'd come back home to hammer pegs into rocks and walk miles up this rugged canyon to bring a strange woman cheese. Someday she might ask him. It seemed a parallel to the one facing her overhead.

Her appetite satisfied, drowsiness came over her, modified somewhat by the effects of the earlier water and the coffee. Her usual practice—until she decided where to dig an outhouse—was to wander out and find a spot a few yards away from her campsite. But she didn't usually have to hide herself from anyone. She became aware, too, of how unwashed she was—only a couple of splash baths in four days. Already, she fit right in with the customs of other canyon inhabitants, could probably give John Olsen competition. She was grateful the campfire smells were so strong around her.

Beside her, Jim stretched his arms upward, then got to his feet. "Miles to go," he said.

"Will you show me sometime how to cook biscuits like that?" Ruth gathered enough energy to force her sore muscles back to a sit.

"Nothing to it. Just coals in a hole beside the fire. Biscuit dough in a greased pot. Coals on top. But keep your nose on it. Smell will tell you when to check." He began walking away from the campfire.

"How can you see where you're going? It's four miles."

Jim stopped and turned back toward her. "I'm an Indian, remember? We can see in the dark."

"What about cougars and bears? They eat Indians, too, I've heard." She wondered whether to offer him a candle to carry.

"I always carry a tiny bow and arrow," he said. "Right here in my knapsack behind this." He pulled out a carbide miner's lamp. Poking a thin twig into the campfire, Jim lit the lamp, pointing it first at her face, then onto the ground in front of him. For a few seconds she could hear his retreating footsteps soft in the wash sand, finally evaporating into cricket song.

"Smart-aleck Indian," Ruth said, rising to pee. Afterward, she shoveled dirt over what was left of the coals and stumbled into the tent. Tomorrow she would treat herself to a bath, and though it would only be a sit bath in a #8 corrugated tin, she fell asleep imagining herself lying back in a full-sized porcelain tub, submerged to her neck in hot bubbly water.

In the morning, while she prepared oatmeal and coffee, Ruth averted her eyes from the rock, banishing even its image from her mind. She would not allow it to weigh on her. When her dishes had been set to dry in the sun, she went over to appraise the situation, circling the stone in hope of inspiration, of some notion occurring to make its removal possible. Bending to inspect the stone's shape for clues, she ran her palm over a rough ridge that traveled along the sorrel side down to the circular bottom. "You think this is your spot, don't you?" Ruth said to the rock. "But it's mine now." She waited quietly, as if the stone would answer her. "Look," she explained, "I know you've been here a long time. Maybe you like this place. But it's my turn. I live here now." Ruth pushed against the side of the rock. "Move over and make room for me."

Ruth stood, shaking her head. She couldn't help smiling at how silly she must look, talking to a rock. As a matter of fact, she felt pretty silly and was glad Matt wasn't here to witness it. Brother! Would he ever laugh about this one: when she didn't have the strength of a man to move the boulder, she acted like a woman and tried to persuade it to move. "Never mind," she said to him out loud. "So you and John together couldn't move it, huh? Well, just you wait, Matt Baxter."

Despite her resolve, Ruth hadn't come up with a plan to make good her promise. She didn't want to damage any more planks either, so she set to work clearing brush until an idea could come to her. She started on the thick knot of cat's-claw root that persisted above the surface, rising into the area planned for her concrete foundation. Yesterday she'd managed to hack away most of the bush with her shovel, but the blade would not penetrate much beneath the loose layer of topsoil. Now she jammed her boot down on the rim of the shovel blade, cutting an inch at a time into the packed subsoil. Metal sparked in protest against buried chunks of mineral. Again and again, Ruth forced the blade against the ground, removing a mere tipful at a time. Gradually, she made a shallow recess around the fibrous knot. When the ground became completely impossible, Ruth chopped at the root with the shovel, slightly below the surface of the soil. Just before severing it, she stopped and walked to the water cooler.

Ruth drank, surveying the root stump. She didn't trust it, wasn't at all sure the remnant wouldn't someday raise its snakelike head again and break through the concrete she intended to cover it with. She might just end up with a cat's-claw bush in the middle of her living space. As she drained the last of the water from the ladle, an idea struck her as soundly as her shovel had hit the small stones. Of course.

A bucket of water hauled from the spring filled the recess. Ruth waited while the thirsty ground drank in the liquid. After she had emptied yet another bucket and let it soak in, Ruth picked up the shovel. With a bit of coaxing from her foot, the blade slid nicely into the softened soil. She couldn't help but feel smug as she loosened the earth around the root, then reached in and plucked it out as easily as a carrot from a garden. With only the pinyons audience to her triumph, Ruth flung the rope of root toward the wash, where it looped over a silver sage and hung defeated. Now she was ready for the rock.

Digging through the pile of building materials, Ruth found two coils of rope. One rope felt soft and flexible, the other thick and hard to bend. She chose the flexible rope. As she had hoped, it fit nicely into the grooves of the ridge across the rock. She looped twice for strength, and secured it around her waist. If she could just get the rock tipped on its belly—even a smidgeon— that would be a start. Then she could rock the boulder back and forth, inch by inch, hour by hour over toward the pinyons. She merely needed to move it a few feet. It didn't matter how long it took; she had the time. The trick was to get the momentum started.

Ruth braced herself and walked forward until the rope pulled tight. She took another step and pulled, straining her weight forward while the rope cut deeply into her waist. She stepped back and started over, tugging as the rope carved into her belly and cut back her breath. Still the stone stayed immobile. She loosened the knot and rolled the rope down over her hips, then forced her body to advance until the rope between herself and the boulder stretched taut as the string on a guitar. She leaned her body into space, only her tie to the rock keeping her from pitching forward. Relaxing the tension on the rope, she tightened it again and began rocking, front and back, back and front, again and again, hoping to entice mobility from the stone.

She might as well have been asking the mountain to move. After numerous pulls that did more to dislocate her hips than to move the boulder, Ruth untied herself and sat cross-legged under the pinyon. She just didn't have the strength to drag the rock forward. If only rocks had roots, like the cat's-claw, she could loosen it with water. But there was no use imagining such things, she chided herself; even her silliness in talking to the rock was more useful than that—for all the good it had done her. Yet the image of the root hung over the sage stayed with her, and when she rose to get a drink of water, the notion came to enlist the help of the pinyon.

Looping the second coil of rope around the tree, Ruth wrapped one end around her waist. It took several tries to knot the thick strands tight enough to hold. Then she retied herself also to the softer rope wound around the rock and walked toward the pine. When the rope between herself and the rock became tense, Ruth picked up the end of the rope she had winched around the tree, winding the strand around her wrist. She began to pull herself—and she hoped the rock—toward the pinyon. Hand over hand, she fought for each frustration of an inch, straining her body closer to the pinyon.

With the pinyon's strength, Ruth was certain the rock would roll and, with ropes pulling her waist in both directions, she did feel something begin to budge ever so slightly. Motivated, she pulled even harder, every muscle straining, winding the rope over her wrist until it twisted her hand halfway back around— painful, almost beyond standing. But this time she was sure something was beginning to give. Triumph rippled through her, swelled, then surged, as she felt a great release on the rope and pictured the boulder rolling over with her motion.

Ruth found herself propelled toward the tree, her legs moving rapidly to keep her body from smacking the ground. She felt the rope whip from her waist as she ran headlong for the tree. Only the arms she held out in front of her kept her from smashing face first into the rough bark of the trunk.

When she recovered, Ruth looked back at the rock. The rope was no longer attached; its unknotted end lay halfway to the tree. The stone appeared precisely as before. So sure Ruth had been of its movement that she dropped to her knees and inspected the dirt close to the rock's belly for tracks, expecting some kind of indication that it had actually moved as she pulled. She saw none. Still, that didn't stop her from several times repeating the winching process—after she had soaked the rope and tied tight triple knots—before giving up for the day, bruised, but refusing to be daunted.

Exhausted as she was, Ruth forced herself toward the spring with the bucket. Once she'd replenished the water cooler and filled the coffeepot, she took off her blouse and let air pour over her sweaty body. She made four more trips to halfway fill the tin tub, then another bucket to heat on the campfire and warm her bath above the chill temperature of her spring. While the water heated, she sliced up a can of corned beef and opened a can of beans, managing to eat half of each cold from the can. The sun was just sliding behind the far ridge of Rocky Mountain as Ruth stepped into the tepid tub, wincing as water insulted the scratches on her calves, then her thighs when she bent her knees and sat. Despite the stinging when she soaped, the bath revived her. Ruth was surprised at how much of what she'd assumed was dirt did not wash off. Her olive skin had been considerably darkened by sun. She allowed her dry skin to soak up the cooling fluid until she heard the sizzle from her coffeepot that told her the water was readying to boil. When she stood to leave the tub, the water was a murky gray-black.

Ruth climbed onto the rock and dried herself with the towel

she'd set there. She had placed the tub beside the troublesome boulder for the practical purpose of keeping her wet feet and body from the sand. But she couldn't help enjoying the fact that she sat on top of the rock. She felt safe and in charge, using it to her own ends. That fact seemed to shift their relationship. Once her feet were dried, Ruth lifted the tub by its handle and dumped the water onto the ground beside the rock. Naked in the balmy twilight, she walked toward the campfire to prepare the rest of her evening meal.

The next morning, Ruth was dragged out of dreams by the harsh scolds of jays—as if they had peered into her sleeping activities. She shut her eyes and tried to return to the soft lips and insistent arms of the faceless man who had been about to enter her. But he had evaporated and taken everything with him but her longing. Left unrequited with such a burning, Ruth put her hand to herself. She knew she should not, but could not stop, the faces and bodies of men raging through her like a river on rampage: Karl, Matt, Ramon—her first, even the Indian, all swirling into one huge swell that cast her finally onto a shore of shame and release.

Such feelings were not normal for a woman, she knew. At Aunt Myrtle's teas, Ruth had heard whispers about wives "doing their duty," listened to talk of their boredom while the men "went about their business." So what were these feelings in her? It frightened her that in such moments she did not even attach her passion to any particular man. She had been told men felt such things. Was she more like a man in this way? But what man would long after other men? Some things might better remain unexamined.

The mountaintops were barely flushed with dawn when Ruth stepped from her tent. The sight of the pink ridges, the sound of an oriole singing in the morning, weakened her resolve to get an early start on the rock, and when she walked into the wash and found a deer with its fawn drinking at the spring, that resolve evaporated completely, the scene filling her with an unexplained joy. On a whim, she packed a knapsack with a hunk of the canned meat and the last of the half-burned biscuits she had made the night before—next time she would do better—and spent the first tender hours of the day exploring the lower ridges of Rocky Mountain. As she looked down on the bright green cottonwoods and cluster of pinyons that marked her spot so clearly, she reminded herself that this was the freedom she had come here to find. She resolved that once she managed to get her cabin built, she would spend as much time as she wanted meandering the landscape. Today, she would content herself with merely the early hours, examining the stands of bluebells and splashes of apricot mallow as the sun's low heat wafted a potpourri of fragrances. She hoped to come upon the Indian inscriptions in her wanderings; the nature of such a thing intrigued her. Several times she thought she spotted odd markings on boulders. Each time, closer inspection found the marks to be merely natural marbling of colors. Like most mysteries, the writing was not to be easily discovered.

Though hungry as she descended the narrow draw that led down into the wash, Ruth wanted first to quench her thirst in cool spring water. A startled cottontail perched at the basin took off through the tall grass. She cupped her hands and drank, cupped again and poured cool water over her face and neck. The thick grass invited and she leaned back against the shady bank beside the spring. As she sank into the soft, damp sediment, from somewhere in the loamy dirt behind her back came the muffled but unmistakable sound of a rattler.

In an explosion of motion, Ruth leapt upward, landing several feet from the basin, unsure whether the current that knifed up her spine was from fear or a rattler's strike. Hers was physical terror of the most basic kind, registering in her body before it ever reached her brain. That terrible buzzing continued while she felt beneath the back of her shirt, fingers searching for any trace of wound. And though her knees remained spongy as spring grass and her brain rang with anxiety, she could find no openings or marring of her skin.

Inspecting the noisy bank, Ruth at first saw nothing more than several layers of gray clay formation. Then she discerned a small hollowed opening between the roots; inside, a segmented tail whirred. The reptile hugged into the clay bank appeared quite small—but she'd heard that even baby rattlers were deadly. Ruth looked around carefully for siblings, her eyes combing the innocent grass for danger.

She retrieved the .22 from her tent and backtracked to the spring. Aiming the rifle carefully, Ruth shot several times into the opening. The rattler quieted, as did her heartbeat. She felt instead a peculiar swelling in her chest, and with it flowed through her a certainty that nothing could stop her. She could take care of herself—even here in this wild place. If anything got in her way, she would remove it—even if she had to kill to do so. With disdain, she remembered the day May had screamed and jumped up on the porch when some harmless bull snake slithered across the desert in front of their house. Matt had come running outside to protect her. Well, Ruth wished he were here now to witness the way she had taken care of a real danger.

Not wanting to touch the snake, but not wishing it to rot above her spring, Ruth used the end of a stick to pry the mangled body from the bank, turning her head when the mutilated cord of body hung on the stick in front of her. Without looking, she flung it toward the wash.

Back at the camp she inspected the rock. Stars of sunlight reflected back from mica embedded in the stone's reddish back. A forest of green lichen covered one side. As alive and willful as the stone seemed, it was not possible to simply kill it and fling it into the wash. Granite, the Indian said, impossibly hard beneath her hand. She hadn't the strength to pull its weight, she admitted, as she squatted and waddled around to the stone's other side. Something about that rounded bottom seemed a clue for its removal. There had to be a way to roll that rock. Ruth picked up her knapsack and sat in the shade of the pinyon, continuing to watch her nemesis as she constructed a makeshift sandwich of her drying corned meat and crusty biscuits. When she finished, she leaned back against the tree and closed her eyes. She pictured the rectangle of her house turned the other way, the front door facing the rocky side of the mountain. A nice enough view, but not the view she wanted. For a moment, she considered building her house around the rock—it could be done. But to have its presence as a constant reminder of her defeat did not sit well. And behind the image of the boulder in her house, she could hear the sound of Matt's laughter.

She conjured up instead a scene of triumph, Matt walking into her camp to find the boulder over between the pines. She would ignore the look of incredulity on his face as she offered him a cup of campfire coffee, casually, as if nothing at all were remarkable. Then, in the midst of her imagined victory, it occurred to her that this was the sixth day she had been here. Matt would arrive tomorrow. How stupid she had been to spend the morning on the mountain.

All at once, Ruth stood and strode to the stone. She positioned herself flat on her back, perpendicular to the rock, legs bent, feet pressed against the granite. She would roll this rock as surely as she had killed the snake, as surely as she had left El Paso behind her.

Ruth began straightening her legs, straining all their strength against the stone. As her legs straightened, her body slid away. She repositioned herself, and tried again. And again, only her torso moved. After two more attempts, she rose and retrieved the rope, looping it around the pinyon. To keep her body in place, she lay down on the side of the rock opposite the tree and wound the rope ends tight around her wrists.

Keeping the rope stretched between herself and the pinyon, Ruth slowly forced her legs to straighten. As she did, her back arched upward until only her shoulders and head touched the ground, then simply her head. She curled and pushed again, with the same result.

"Damn. Damn. Damn." Ruth lay back and kicked the rock until her soles hurt. Then she sat up, took off her boots, and rubbed her feet, still cursing and holding back all but a few tears, which she quickly wiped away. "You're going to move, damn you," she informed the hunk of granite in front of her. "I don't know just how yet, but you're going to move. Even if I have to take a hammer and remove you from this place chip by chip."

Her early start the next morning did Ruth little good, except for giving her time to concoct stories for Matt about how she would soon have the rock out of the way, running through imagined scenarios as she worked. She began with the ropes again, but after very few tries went back to using planks for leverage, selecting only the most sturdy boards. She stopped often to listen, thinking she heard the sound of a motor. Each time a plank broke, she dropped it over the edge of the wash, so the evidence of her wasted efforts would be well out of sight when Matt arrived. By late afternoon, she was both relieved and disappointed when he had not showed. Surprised, though. She had counted on his word that he'd be back in a week. Her food was running low. At least she had a day or two of coffee left, maybe more. When she sat down with her next-to-last can of pork and beans for supper, Ruth felt a strange tightness in her throat that made it hard to swallow her food. Matt knew she would need supplies. She had thought he'd be eager to see her.

Gradually, the mixture of coffee and campfire smoke began to lull her. She was making too much of it, she decided. He must be tied up somehow—maybe at his store, maybe May's condition had worsened again. Surely he would be here tomorrow. She should be glad she still had time to find a way to move the rock before he arrived. Getting to her feet, she used most of the lard to put together a fairly decent pan of biscuits, of which she used half to make bean sandwiches and saved the rest. For a long time she sipped coffee and listened to the ringing night while the waxing half-moon rose over the ridge beside her. Coyotes began to yip and howl. They sounded nearby, probably across the wash. For a moment she considered going for the rifle positioned against the stone. Instead, she stood, lifted her chin, and joined in the cacophony.

Ruth started on the rock soon after dawn. It had occurred to her sometime during the night that the broken pieces of plank might make stronger levers than the full-sized boards, since they were shorter and harder to break, so the first thing she did was retrieve the planks least damaged from the wash and even up their ends with a saw. Then, with her shovel, Ruth scraped more dirt from under the edge of the stone so the sheared end of the wood fit snugly under its bottom.

She searched the wash, where flash floods had piled countless rocks of various shapes and sizes, seeking the perfect fulcrum— not wanting a rock so small it wouldn't give enough movement, but neither a large one that would leave the free end of the board pointing straight for the sky, so she couldn't get her boot down to apply sufficient weight. This day's effort, she knew, was her last chance. She had run out of ideas to compensate for her lack of muscular strength. But her resolve was strong.

Balancing both feet on the intact end of the short board, Ruth jumped up and down, bouncing until the moving board flung her off. She climbed back on and resumed the springing motion. Several times she repeated the action, the only result being that the rock gradually smoothed and sanded down the end of the plank placed under it.

The climbing sun beat down through her shirt. After a quick drink to wet her dry mouth, Ruth decided the rock would only roll if more force were applied—and quickly. After fitting another short plank under the boulder, Ruth climbed the saddleback of the rock itself and jumped onto the lever. The first time, she sprang forward from the board and had to run to stay up. Still, the method was promising—and the only idea she had left. She tried again. And again. And again. Each time she became more adept at staying on the plank when she landed. When the board at last began to splinter, she replaced it with the one sturdy piece she had left, then leapt on it from the rock with a vengeance.

Five times more Ruth climbed the boulder and jumped onto the board. Each time, her weight hit the wood without affecting the stone. When she finally squatted to check the end of the plank, she found it too worn to be of any use. The sun now directly overhead, she stared down into the shadow pooled beneath her knees, then at the boulder, which appeared to have no shadow at all but remained solid and immovable in its entirety.

"Damn you goddamned piece of granite," Ruth shouted, pushing at the rock. She stood and kicked at it with the sole of her boot, first one foot, then the other. "You goddamned thing, you." She wouldn't give in to the burning behind her eyes, she just wouldn't.

Ruth stomped to the tin water cooler and gulped down two full dippers of water. Lifting a third to her lips, she found her throat so constricted she couldn't swallow. All she wanted to do was smash the rock to smithereens. In a fit of rage she flung the dipper at the boulder, the ladle clanging against the surface, to spill her drink onto the dry ground.

For a moment Ruth stood impotent. What a useless act—the waste of precious water she had to haul from clear across the wash. She stared at the small splotch of dark on the dirt, feeling tears again about to overpower her. She imagined her tears pouring out over the ground like the water from her tub, flowing in a river toward the rock, carrying the massive mineral away. The thought of soft wet earth left behind the tear river made her smile. It would be earth easily dug.

Ruth began hauling water buckets from the spring, dumping them onto the ground beside the boulder. She chose the spot where she had emptied her tub days before, hoping some of that dampness had been retained beneath the harsh soil. After the first few trips across the wash, Ruth removed her shirt and worked bare-chested as she had seen men do down on the desert. After all, it seemed certain by now that Matt wasn't coming—not that she cared much anymore. Bucket after bucket she poured onto packed earth that drank it in as quickly as she could drain her container, wetting, then digging into layer after layer of softened soil. When her back and breasts began to burn, she wet her shirt and kept it on during the long hours it took to loosen, then dig down into what had been hard ground. Her digging also turned up a number of the odd pottery shards. Intent as she was on her project, Ruth did her best to toss as many of these as she could toward the rock by the campfire. About the time the hole beside the boulder was waist high, her shovel brought up an odd, triangular-shaped object. Not a shard, but also not natural. She spat on it, swiped it across her pantleg, and examined it. A small thrill ran through her. An arrowhead. She stuck it in her pants pocket and persevered in her shoveling, dousing and digging, until the hole grew a few inches deeper. The sun had dropped behind the mountain and spread a thick twilight across the canyon when she climbed out of the pit she had created.

Standing with her legs apart at the edge of the hole, Ruth reached in with her shovel and chipped at the ledge of dirt that kept the boulder from rolling into the depression. She moved to the other side and repeated the action until the rock hung over the edge of the hole more than a foot. Ruth counted on the same weight that had made the boulder immovable to work in her favor now. Once she had placed another long plank from her pile under the far side of the stone, she again pried the rock toward the opening, lifting the end on her back. This time she felt definite movement. But not enough to push it in.

Straining to see in the dim light, Ruth stretched as far as she could without tumbling into the cavity and hacked away a few inches more of the dirt with her shovel, then walked back around. To maximize leverage, she shoved a rock under the middle of the plank as fulcrum again and went to the raised end. She closed her eyes, pictured the stone in the grave she had dug for it, then jumped as hard as she could onto the end. The plank snapped, flinging her onto the ground just as the boulder rolled over the edge and thudded into its final resting place.

For the briefest of moments, Ruth felt a twinge of sympathy for the rock she had unseated. Then she struggled to her feet, shouting in triumph. She peered down at the fallen boulder. Strange as it seemed, she could still imagine it escaping from her trap. Exhausted or not, she wasn't taking any chances. Piling wood high on her campfire, she struck a match to it, then by firelight, threw shovelsful of dirt into the space around and over the boulder. Afterward, she spread the extra dirt around her site. Finally, it was done; she had won. The boulder was out of her way, buried forever under what would be the foundation of her cabin.

With due ceremony, Ruth set the unusable pieces of plank on the campfire, along with a couple of pine logs. She peeled off her sweaty pants and shirt and, wearing nothing but boots, danced in her victory, cackling and hooting in the flickering red firelight as she stamped down the dirt to pack it. This was her night to send wild screams echoing off the mountainsides. She almost expected to hear creatures out in the dark bang pans to shut her up.

But no one was around to shut her up. She could dance and shout naked around her fire if she felt like it. And she felt like it. This was the freedom she had dreamed of. No one came to constrain her. Not her aunt with admonitions of impropriety, not her mother with dark and bitter eyes. No one at all. Ruth had conquered the boulder. Whatever else life chose to hand her, she was ready.

The next morning Ruth woke before the sun was up, her belly rumbling. She had finished off half of the last can of beans after she buried the stone and had just enough coffee for one more pot. She'd saved a biscuit, too, though it seemed near hard enough to break teeth on.

It was now her tenth day. Or was it the ninth day; she was no longer sure. All she knew was Matt had promised he'd be back with supplies for her in a week, and it had been longer than that. Her check would have arrived at his store days ago. She was tired of finding excuses for him—didn't care if May had had a relapse. Ruth was sick of always being on alert, several times a day mistaking wind in the pines for Matt's Model A. He hadn't even arrived to witness her triumph over the rock. She was sick of beans, too; hungry as she was, she couldn't bring herself to eat them. One thing was sure—she wasn't going to wait around for him until she starved to death. It was time to do something on her own. Get herself something to eat and walk down to the Swedes'. Ruth picked up the rifle—she could thank Matt for that at least—and headed up the wash past the spring.

She hadn't gone far before she spotted the cottontail, pink ears pointed skyward, as it basked in new sun beside a clump of sage. Ruth took aim with the rifle, bringing the sights together in front of the rabbit's head; she gripped the trigger with her index finger. The rabbit hopped a few inches closer to the bush, then stopped, hunched back its ears. Ruth resighted. The cottontail appeared sweet and innocent, not at all menacing like the rattler she had shot. Certainly a far cry from the spit-roasted rabbit she had been served at the Paxtons' cookout. She was almost ready to drop the barrel and walk back to camp when her stomach groaned again. She thought about the half can of beans drying in the cooler, a thick skin forming around the edges. Damn you, Matt, she thought, and pulled back the trigger.

The rabbit flopped onto one side, kicking its hind legs wildly in the air as Ruth ran toward it, blood splattering onto the sand as the creature propelled itself across the clearing, emitting a fine high-pitched squeal. She pushed the rifle barrel against the rabbit's head to still it and pulled the trigger once more. The cottontail's body jerked once, then went limp.

For a moment when Ruth first took hold of the soft, warm carcass, its fur sticky with oozing blood, she was willing to re-sign herself to a life of pork and beans. But the deed was done. It would be wrong to waste this rabbit's death and leave it to rot in the sun as she had the snake, whose odor now hung heavy in the warming air. The problem was how to turn the creature into a meal she could actually eat—she'd not so much as plucked a chicken before, though she'd seen it done often enough. And fur, like feathers, had to come off.

At camp, with the end of the soft rope, Ruth tied the rabbit's hind feet, then looped the rope over a pine branch. Using her butcher knife, she cut the fur from around the bound feet, and pulled, peeling off the skin like pajamas from a small child, exposing the shape of naked muscle. An ugly purple wound gaped in the right shoulder. By this time Ruth's stomach was more queasy than hungry. She had lost all desire to eat the raw and bloody meat hung in front of her by furry feet. But she couldn't just quit, though she wanted to more than ever. Taking up the knife again, Ruth slit open the balloon of belly. The sweet smell of intestines made her own stomach churn. Swallowing back her nausea, she reached in quickly and yanked out the colored coils of intestine, dropping them onto the ground, reached in again to pluck the heart and pink sponge of lungs from the chest cavity. The last thing she removed was a line of little round pellets, wrapped in a membrane tube like a row of chocolate balls.

The knife would not slice through the delicate ankle bones. She grabbed hold and snapped them, then cut through the muscle and ligaments to free the dressed carcass. Carrying the feet and guts down to the wash, Ruth buried them in a shallow grave of sand. That done, she poured water from her bucket over the rabbit and wrapped it in a wetted burlap bag. The rest of the water she used to rinse the blood splotches from her own hands and arms, thinking of the trip she would soon make to the Swedes'. Perhaps she would take them the rabbit.

Her body filthier than a few splashes of water could take care of, Ruth began hauling buckets from the spring to fill her tub, which she placed next to the spot where she had buried the rock. When her coffeepot was on the fire, Ruth stepped into the unwarmed tub, goose bumps popping out over her skin as she willed herself down into the chill water. She got on her knees and ducked her hair into the water, lathered and rinsed it before attacking the rest of her body with the fat bar of Ladies Joy, finally using a pine needle to clean the dirt from under nails so ragged they had caught on her hair as she washed it.

Yet all the while Ruth had a nagging feeling that something was amiss. Her eyes scanned the bluffs on the other side of the wash and the brush around her camp. No graceful Indian man was gliding down the cliffs or appearing out of nowhere. The .22 was near enough, propped against the tent. There had been no boulder to lean it on—as there would be none to climb on to dry without plastering her feet with sand. Then she realized it was the rock that she missed. Somehow its absence loomed as large as its presence once had. She was just marveling over that absurdity when she heard the first hint of an engine in the distance.

Ruth sat in the gray-black water, listening for a moment before dismissing the sound as another false hope. She poured cold water over her hair from the smaller bucket she had placed beside the tub, then stood to clean-rinse the rest of her body. Still the sound persisted. She was rinsing the last of the soap from her arms when Matt's Model A appeared down by the bend. He gave three hoarse blasts of horn.

Ruth bounded from the tub to the tent, grabbing up her towel as she went. More horn blaring disrupted the canyon. She ran back out to dump the tub. By the time Matt pulled into her camp, she had a clean blouse and slacks over her undried body and stepped out of the tent to greet him, her hair still wet and anarchic, though she managed to finger-comb and fluff it as she walked.

Matt's lanky form unfolded from the car. He smiled and shook his head when she stopped in front of him. For a moment she thought he might hug her. "Ruth," he said, pulling at one earlobe as he did when he was trying to find words, "you look beautiful, like . . . well, like some kind of wild woman. So . . . untamed. I'd guess your skin is near dark as that Indian's. Honest."

Ruth reached up to straighten the collar of her blouse. "I was getting ready to walk down to the Swedes," she said, "if you hadn't come." The sound of her voice speaking in normal words and sentences after all these days surprised her, seemed to settle her back into a civility she had almost forgotten. "I'm out of food—nearly coffee too."

"Not anymore, you're not." Matt reached into the rear of the Model A. Three big boxes of groceries were jammed into the space behind the seat. He extracted a five-pound can of coffee and held it out. Ruth hugged the can to her while he picked up one of the boxes. "I got a good deal on the gun, too. You'll see," he said as they walked toward the campfire, where the water in the pot was splashing and hissing onto the flames. Ruth poured in the last of her coffee and pulled the pot to the edge.

Matt placed the box on the flat rock near the fire ring and looked around at the ground she had cleared. "Well, I'll be," he said. "How did you ever . . ." He walked out to the middle of the clearing. "But what did you do with it?" He stood surveying the campsite, then looked back at her. "Boulders don't just disappear," he said.

He stopped, broke into a sudden smile. "I know what happened. John must have brought his men up here to help," he said, laughing. How yellow and pointy his teeth were, sort of ratlike, she thought, so out of place in an otherwise handsome face. Funny she'd never noticed it before.

"I said I'd move that rock by myself, Matt Baxter. And that's what I did," Ruth said, facing him. "Nobody helped me."

"But it's not even here. Someone had to haul it off."

"It's buried. I buried it. Directly under where you stand."

He cocked his head to one side. "Buried it?"

"It was simple. I dug a big hole and pushed it in. Getting rid of that rock was sure easier than digging out all those cholla and cat's-claw bushes," she lied. "It didn't take strength but brains — a mule has brute strength. Seems to me any fool would have thought of it."

The half-smile seemed frozen on Matt's face. He looked quite dumbfounded. Ruth gave a quick toss of her damp hair, acutely aware of the sun on her skin, the smells of pine and lupine, of her heart pumping blood through her toughened body. It was if some power radiated up from the ground into her bare feet, bringing with it a desire to howl out loud. The invincibility that had visited her the night before roared back in full force. She threw back her head and laughed.

"My hat's off to you, Ruth," Matt finally said. "I never dreamed you would actually do it." He looked down at the loosened earth. "I still find it hard to believe." Ruth was certain he would stop to ask John Olsen on the way down, just to make sure.

She turned toward the campfire. "I'm having coffee," she said. "Want some?" Not waiting for an answer, she poured hot frothy liquid into two tin cups. Her noisy stomach reminded her she had forgotten its earlier request. "I could use some food too."

"You have plenty to choose from now. Two more boxes in the car." Matt walked over to pick up his cup from the rock. "And I brought that jug of . . . well, you know, what you said you wanted for cooking. It's good, too—from my brother's vineyard."

"Thanks," Ruth said, taking the jug from the box and pulling the cork. She brought the crock up under her nose. "It sure smells good." Matt had no trouble supplying folks with whatever they wanted, she had learned working at his store. What law there was out here looked the other way.

She threw kindling and two logs onto the coals. Cup in hand, she dropped into the camp chair beside Matt. "I thought I might fry up the rabbit I've got in the cooler first," she said casually, all her squeamishness set aside by the opportunity to further impress Matt with her homesteading skills. "Shot and skinned it just this morning." Yet when she looked over to find him regarding her intently, the expression on his face was not one of admiration, but discomfort, with a hint of caution. What kind of a woman are you, anyway, he seemed to be wondering. She supposed he would be more comfortable if she brought out her knitting, like his wife might do—except that Ruth had never owned a knitting needle, wouldn't know what to do with one. Didn't care to know.

"How's May?" she asked then; she had almost forgotten Matt had a wife.

"Holding her own," Matt said, his eyes turning back to the area Ruth had cleared, "thanks to all the care you gave her. She does get tired out easily, though. I've had to take over most of the cooking again." He looked back at Ruth. "That kind of thing," he said, nodding toward Ruth's future foundation, "would likely kill her. Didn't seem to do you any harm, though."

"It wasn't easy," Ruth said, "but not so hard either."

They sat facing each other in the shade of the pinyons. For a few minutes Matt caught her up on happenings in Juniper Valley. After talk fell off, Matt raised his cup. "A toast. Here's to you, Ruth," he said. "The wild woman of Rattlesnake Canyon. You'd be a challenge for any man."

"I'm not sure I want to drink to that." Ruth pulled back the cup she had raised. "At least not to being a challenge. Who wants to be that?" She tried to smooth down the hair that had dried so impossibly disheveled. "There are better things for a woman to be for a man."

Matt looked at her and swallowed, yet didn't pull his eyes from hers. His face reddened slightly. "Well, then," he said, "let's drink to the wild woman."

They clanked tin cups. When they finished their coffees, Matt rose and carried over the rest of the groceries. Ruth put the rabbit to fry on the campfire. She stacked the supplies while Matt wrapped new burlap around the wire mesh of the cooler. It warmed her to glance over and see the sun in his hair, to have him fixing for her the way he always did for May, to have his eyes keep coming back to her. She wondered what it would be like if he were hers, her man and not May's. Not a husband, really—she couldn't picture herself as a wife, back under someone's control—but her man. She was ready for the arms and lips—and the rest of it. Desire for the faceless man of her dream flooded her body.

It wasn't that she'd been with many men. There had been only one before Karl—Ramon, the son of one of Aunt Myrtle's kitchen workers. It happened shortly before she had been sent to Sarah Higgins. All summer, Ruth had found herself setting her reading aside to stand at the window and watch how the muscles of the young man's back gleamed as he raked leaves from the huge lawn or pulled weeds from the flower beds. She wasn't sure he was aware of her until that day he came to the door to ask for water. His look asked for much more. Ever since she could remember, she had known the word for what was going on all around her. Those early years with Cally had been informative. Now was her chance to experience it for herself. And she wasn't disappointed. Afterward she understood that she wasn't cut out to be like other women—in it for the man's sake, married, or being paid to supply him, then blamed for doing it, like the prostitutes that Aunt Myrtle's women's group wanted to eradicate. Ruth had as much right to that pleasure for herself as any man; Cally had taught her that much. A few weeks later, when they sent Ruth to Sarah Higgins, she wondered if they hadn't found out somehow. Why else would her late father's family suddenly offer to pay her way to an Eastern boarding school? Clearly they were all trying to save her from becoming her mother's daughter. Well, they needn't have worried; Ruth wasn't about to take that route either.

The rabbit turned out to be tasty but tough and hard to chew. Ruth was hungry enough by this time to tear the meat from the bones with her teeth, but forced herself to use a fork and knife, for Matt's sake. She gave each of them a meaty hind leg. Hers was gone in short order, before Matt's was half finished. She looked up, after being intent on extracting every last piece of flesh from the bone, to see Matt regarding her with a bemused glance.

"Don't know that I've ever had wild rabbit before," he said. "Interesting taste." He straightened up from the plate in his lap and put his silverware on top of his food.

"You don't like it?"

"Of course I do, honest, but it does take some getting used to. Same with venison. Excellent once you acquire the taste." He stood, set his tin plate on the rock beside her and began walking toward the Model A. "You haven't seen your new twenty-two yet," he said. "I'll go get it." When his back was turned, Ruth reached for the rabbit leg he had barely touched. She bit off a mouthful, then put the rest down quickly.

When Matt returned, he carried a shinier version of the rifle he had loaned her. "It looks a lot like yours," she said.

"A newer model." He sat beside her, leaned the .22 against her chair. "This and the groceries took up most of your check. Here's what's left." He held out a few dollar bills.

Ruth slipped them into her slacks pocket. "It was good of you to bring supplies, this rifle, all the way up here. You must have closed up the store to do it?"

"Today's Sunday," he said, shaking his head. He looked at her intently. "I would have closed it if I had to, though. I've missed you, Ruth. I was glad to have a reason to come see you."

"I'd been wondering if you'd changed your mind."

"I couldn't get away any sooner. Had to make a trip into San Bernardino for May's medicine and supplies for the store—I picked up the gun while I was there. Then May was feeling poorly again. I couldn't leave her alone."

"I suppose not. I was about to walk down to the Swedes' and hitch a ride to town to get what I needed."

"Don't ever think I'll let you down, Ruth. I don't want you to think that. Promise me." He reached over and took her hand.

Ruth looked away, struggled to speak through wings fluttering inside her. "Who am I to count on you?" she said. "Why should you do for me? You have a wife to look after."

"Thanks to you she's still alive. But that's not . . . You know why, Ruth." He let go of her hand and waited until she looked up at him. "You must know how I feel about you." He glanced down, then back up to catch her eyes directly. "Some things are best left unsaid . . . as long as it's understood."

"What if understanding isn't enough? What if more is required?"

"What would that be, Ruth? What would you require?"

"I don't know," she said, getting up. "But what use to talk about it?" She took hold of the rifle. "Did you bring more bullets?"

Matt rose and stood beside her, laid a hand on her shoulder. "What would you require, Ruth?"

She felt the pressure of his fingers through the cloth of her shirt, heard his breath coming deep and irregular. "Sometimes in the dead of night, while May's asleep beside me . . . I know it's wrong to tell you this. But . . ." His hand closed around her shoulder, his voice becoming a hoarse whisper. "I remember the way you look at me . . . the way you walk across the room . . . it's been so long since . . ."

The very smell of the man's sweat drew her toward him. Ruth felt herself propelled toward those pale desert-sky eyes. Only the ground under her feet held her back. That and the sound of footsteps crunching up the sandy wash behind them.

Even before Ruth turned, she knew, so the sound of the Indian's voice did not surprise her, nor did the look of displeasure that swept over Matt's face. What did surprise her was the lift she felt at Jim's appearance, despite considerable irritation at the interruption.

"Can't see how you missed me waving you down as you drove by. I was right out there by the garden," he said to Matt. "Kate wanted to send Ruth these early squash and tomatoes. Some goat jerky too. We expected you to stop. It's customary. Check in next time you come up." Jim held a lumpy flour sack out toward Ruth. "I went ahead and brought them up myself. That way I can still catch a ride back down when you go." He turned to inspect the spot where the boulder once sat. "You must have been persuasive," he said, glancing back at Ruth.

"You might say that. There's some rabbit left in the pan, Jim," Ruth told him. "Coffee over there too. Help yourself. Can't offer you any biscuits, though. I'd already used up all the flour . . . that is, until Matt brought me a whole new supply." She looked up at Matt, whose eyes were fixed on the Indian.

"You tried your hand at it, then?" Jim said as he walked to the campfire. "Must have had enough for two or three batches when I left."

"So you have had company," Matt said quietly to her, still staring at Jim with what could only be termed hatred. "And the rock . . ."

"I told you. I moved it myself," Ruth whispered, taken aback by the intensity of Matt's response. "Kate sent Jim up with fresh goat cheese nearly a week ago." Ruth touched his arm lightly. "How about more coffee?"

Matt looked back at her, his eyes still iced with anger, as if trying to decide whether to believe her. Then he took in a breath and nodded. "I think it's best I head back now," he said, starting toward the cooler. "I'll get my tools together." Ruth watched his retreating back. She swallowed her disappointment. It wasn't only what had been lost at the interruption, all that had not happened, but what was yet to be lost. She wasn't ready for either of them to leave—the first company she'd seen in days—and could have spent a good deal of time drinking coffee and talking around the campfire. But the company didn't mix, and while she could have enjoyed either of them alone, it would never work with the two of them.

"Shot this yourself?" Jim called from the campfire. He picked up a foreleg and took a bite. "Not bad," he said. Ruth carried the vegetable sack to the rock table and began removing squash and tomatoes, placing them in her favorite ceramic bowl, yellow with tiny blue flowers. Except for the potatoes Matt had just brought, these were the first fresh vegetables she'd seen in a long while.

"You might simmer these last two pieces in a bit of the wine you have in that jug there and see what happens," Jim said, as he cleaned the last of the meat from the leg bone with his teeth.

"Now that's something to look forward to," she said, imagining the two dry hunks of rabbit transformed into succulent morsels. She could even picture squash and potatoes in the sauce beside them. "You always have such good ideas for food."

"You probably would have thought of that one yourself," he said, his eyes crinkling slightly at the corners. Ruth wanted to show him the pot shards in the tin but noticed that Matt kept glancing over as he stashed tools behind the front seat of the car. She placed the bowl of vegetables in the burlap cooler, then went to the tent to retrieve Matt's rifle. When she returned he was standing near the tent flap.

"I'm ready," he said to the Indian.

"Thanks again for loaning me your twenty-two," Ruth said. She stepped out to hand Matt his gun.

"Don't mention it. It's best to be safe. Now you have one of your own. You never know just who's going to show up—even out here. Could be someone who means you harm," Matt said as the three of them walked toward his Model A.

"There's a dance at the Olsens' next Saturday, Ruth," Jim said. "They said to tell you. Just about everyone from Juniper Valley will come for Kate's pastries alone—the Hudsons, Talmadges.

Shorty with his fiddle. John said he'd bring the truck up to get you." Jim opened the passenger door. "You come too, Matt. Bring your wife," he said.

Matt remained looking at her. He appeared to be over his anger. "Looks like I'll be back next week, then," he said, giving her hand a quick squeeze in full view of Jim. He climbed behind the wheel. "No need for John to get you, with guests coming and all. I'll be up for you myself."

Ruth waved as they drove off, staring after them as if that might bring the men back. She sighed as the Model A grew smaller, finally disappearing around the far bend, and the solitude of the canyon wrapped quiet arms around her. The thought of the coming dance comforted her, the food, music, conversation. How she loved to dance. She had danced a lot those months after she left the finishing school, when she'd cut her hair and considered herself a flapper. She pictured herself dancing, whirling around with a variety of faceless men. The idea of dancing close up with Matt made her skin tingle. And she wondered what it would be like to put her arms around Indian Jim, to feel the hard muscle of his shoulder beneath her fingers, the strands of his long hair brushing the skin on the back of her hand. Her breath caught at the prospect.

Shaking off her fantasies Ruth revived the small fire and set about making a sauce of wine and water, stirring to dissolve the crust at the bottom of the frying pan and adding the last of the rabbit with squash and potatoes, and a tomato for good measure. While it simmered, she prepared the best biscuits she had yet made. At dusk, she savored the pungent stew, washing it down with a cup of wine. The flavors helped to quiet, though not quite satisfy, her hunger.

The next stage of house building gave Ruth a clearer idea of the realities she faced. While clearing her land, she had merely been readying to build. Now that she was starting on the actual structure, she became more aware of how much she did not know about constructing a house—which was nearly everything. Whatever had made her so sure she could undertake this project, she wondered again as she inspected the dirt surface for her foundation. She had been instructed to make the ground as level as possible beneath the concrete and to outline the rectangle of its shape with long strips of wood that would serve as a form for her cement. John Olsen's warning that a proper foundation was of crucial importance served to emphasize her ignorance and to underscore the importance of somehow overcoming that ignorance. This was not to be an undertaking she could brazen her way through, as she had most other endeavors. Unsure of herself, she worked with great care.

Ruth continued to uncover pottery shards as she shoveled and raked to level the soil. She found a few more the day she dug a hole for her outhouse behind a scrub oak. Though she saw no more arrowheads, she did unearth a large shard that was particularly attractive, one side lightened with a kind of glaze, its surface depicting a fragment of intricate design. She ran a finger over the dark swirling lines as she carried the piece over to put with the others, conscious that someone long ago had taken care to make it lovely in much the same way that someone more recently had covered her yellow ceramic bowl with small blue flowers. Finding the arrowhead had confirmed Ruth's notion that the pottery belonged to the Indians that Jim said once occupied her land. Now, as she spread the shards out on the rock to inspect them, she wished she knew more about the people who made and used them here. Another fragment appeared blackened by fire. A hole fashioned through its lip caused her to wonder if it hadn't once hung at the same fire she used for her own cooking: the fire ring she assumed had been constructed by cowboys might be of even earlier date. She sat on the rock and tried to imagine these people who had dropped arrowheads and broken vessels here, what they must have been like. The best she could do was to people her spot with versions of Jim.

About midweek the temperature cooled slightly, and a few puffy clouds came to drift aimlessly overhead. Ruth felt herself slip into their languorous mood. She had, after all, already dug the hole for her privy and completed the wooden outline for the foundation. She had even experimented with test batches of cement, which convinced her she must speak again with John Olsen before she attempted to prepare and pour the concrete. She would talk to him at the dance, an event that itself occupied a great deal of her attention as she worked dreamily at sawing and hammering the last of the usable broken planks into a seating arrangement over her outhouse hole, her mind filled with visions of herself in men's arms, with snippets of fantasized conversation. Even a few nicks with the saw and a fairly bruised index finger resulting from her divided attention were not enough to bring her back. When Ruth was not imagining herself at the Olsens' party or picturing a female Jim squatting beside a cooking pot, her eyes searched the lower parts of Rocky Mountain while she pondered the whereabouts of the hidden inscriptions.

The day before the dance, she hung her party dress to straighten on the rope strung for skinning the rabbit, which had now become her clothesline. The dress was the same one she had worn in the fall to the dance at the Hudsons', but that did not much concern her. She had purchased it when she stopped in Los Angeles before she came to the desert, and it looked good enough on her to do for many dances. Besides, she had no choice, since she did not sew. Scarlet was the best color for her, too, set off her skin and hair, and she liked the way the bodice lowered at the neck to show just enough bosom to be interesting. And she had enough bosom to be interesting, she thought smugly as she stood before the small mirror in her tent the afternoon of the dance, turning sideways to admire herself in profile.

Matt's response confirmed her view, and, though she still felt some distance when he arrived to fetch her, it was clear he couldn't keep his eyes off her. Ruth knew from the mirror that her excitement had given a flush to her cheeks, overruling even her tanned skin, and she couldn't help but be aware of how she must appear in his eyes as they drove down canyon toward the Swedes', making small talk and speculating about the evening's highlights.

Goats ran crisscross between the line of parked cars as Matt pulled up in front of the Olsens'. In the wash beside the car, several horses stood grazing, hobbled or drop-reined. A brown billy leapt onto the front fender as Matt pulled on the brake. He squeezed the horn twice and the goat slid to the ground. "We better join the crowd. May's been waiting to see you." Matt placed a hand over hers. "You'll save a dance for me, won't you, Ruth?"

"More than one, if you like," Ruth said, taking hold of the door handle with her free hand. They looked at each other and smiled long enough for her body to remember what had happened between them last weekend. Then she pulled the lever and pushed the door open.

She knew it would be some time before the dancing started. First would come food and conversation. Then a few folks would pack up and leave, but most—whole families—would stay to bed down late after the music stopped. At least that was the way it had been at the two dances Ruth had gone to in Juniper Valley. People lived spread out, traveled a long way to each dance; some, like the cowboys, came on horseback.

May waved and several other women seated next to the stone house turned to nod as Ruth approached. Otherwise she would have been tempted to join the men who stood around talking and laughing, especially the cowboys from the Heart Bar. And she did want to have a close look at the concrete slab out where the dancing would take place.

May put aside her knitting and held out her hand. "It's so good to see you again, Ruth. I've missed your company," she said as Ruth came near. "I'm sorry I couldn't come all the way to get you." May managed a weak smile. "But I'm afraid just riding this far has tired me greatly." Though the woman's face was sallow and drawn and her brown hair lacked luster, the tubercular flush of her cheeks presented a false appearance of health.

"Just look at you," May said. "You look like you've been living in the wilderness for years, like you were born here. How dark you've become." Ruth followed May's eyes down to where their hands joined, one creamy white, the other bronze in contrast.

"How are you feeling?" Ruth asked. "Matt tells me you're doing well. Are you still taking walks?"

"Some days. I feel stronger again now that I have dear little Lily to come in and help me. She's been assisting Matt in the store too. You remember Lily Rose, don't you, Ruth?" May turned to place her hand on the young woman beside her.

Ruth nodded, wondering why Matt hadn't mentioned it. "Hello, Lily. Hello, Mrs. Rose," she said to the girl and the mother who appeared to be a faded version of the younger beauty. How could anyone not remember Lily Rose? The Angel of the Valley, they called her. And no wonder, Ruth thought, as Lily smiled sweetly up at her, giving her head a little toss that shook the golden ringlets framing her face. With her light blue eyes, she could be a sister to Matt, except for those full, white teeth. Ruth knew Lily was close to her own age, maybe nineteen to Ruth's new twenty-one, but her innocence made her seem younger than Ruth had ever been. The only thing Ruth had in common with her was the name, Ruth's middle name being Lilith, another form of Lily.

"Rute. Rute." Ruth turned in time to be clasped in Kate's bone-crushing hug. She thrust Ruth out at arm's length and held her there. "You werk too hard. I told Jim. Need the strudel to fatten you up." She let go of Ruth long enough to squeeze her upper arm. "Need meat on your bone," she said, pulling Ruth into another hug. "It good to see you."

Ruth couldn't help but smile. Kate's affection was so genuine and direct. "I'm glad to see you too, Kate. Thanks for all the cheese and vegetables you sent me. The jerky, too. Those seeds I planted haven't begun to sprout, and I've already tired of canned meat and beans. Luckily, Jim showed me how to make biscuits. Someday maybe I'll make them as good as he does."

"Ya," Kate said. "I have tomato for you take home. Now you sit. John and Jim bring over the goat pretty soon." Over behind the tents Ruth could see the two men shoveling out coals from a large pit. Jim worked without a shirt, the last of the afternoon sun sliding over his muscles as he moved. He made work appear so graceful. She wondered what she must have looked like clearing her land, had anyone seen her—awkward and inexperienced as she shoveled and pulled brush.

After forcing herself briefly to make small talk with Martha Hudson and Charlotte Paxton, whom she barely knew, Ruth disobeyed Kate's orders by following her into the stone house to see what was to be done. She could bear no more of the conversations around her about sewing and other domestic affairs. Even the talk of recipes—what good were they to her own campfire cooking? She would rather corner some of the cowboys gathered in a tight knot within the main collection of men. Besides finding the talk more interesting, she might even pick up some campfire cooking ideas she could use. Ruth wound her way through a group of boys tossing a wooden ball—all but one of the girls had remained sitting prettily beside their mothers—and walked through the open door of the house.

Kate allowed Ruth to carry out two of the many dishes kept warming on the huge woodstove for the "smorgasbord," as Kate called the potluck. When the women saw Ruth bringing out casseroles to set among the cold salads and fruit on the long table, others headed in to get their own concoctions. By the time everything had been put out alongside the pit-roasted goat, Ruth was witness to the most impressive spread she had ever laid eyes on. The goat, Kate's pastries, and fresh vegetables moved the repast far beyond anything she'd seen at other dance gatherings in the valley.

A few of the men, Matt among them, pulled up chairs and ate with the women, though many—all of the miners—stood holding their plates and talking as they ate. The cowboys squatted in a circle, as if they were hunkered around a campfire. Ruth kept her eye out for Jim, wanting to brag to him about her latest batch of biscuits and the rabbit-wine stew, but he had managed to slip away with a plateful of food and sat on a rock out of range of the gathering.

She settled into the chair Matt had pulled up for her in the small circle that consisted of himself and May and the two Rose women. Ravenous, Ruth had heaped her plate high at the table, the plate's circumference seeming inadequate for her appetite and the many dishes before her. Remembering Kate's admonition, Ruth had added two pastries on top of the rest. After trying to move aside her dessert to eat the main dishes, Ruth had finally decided to eat the strudels first and get them out of her way. About midway through her first, she looked up to see Matt staring down at the mountain of food in front of her. As was Mrs. Rose.

Ruth paused, teeth sunk into the delicious pastry, and glanced at the other plates in the group. The women had more space on their plates, it seemed, than food. For a moment, Ruth felt heat creep up the back of her neck, but she shook it off and bit down further, refusing to drop her eyes from Matt's. She chewed, instead, with relish, though the strudel's flavor had gone dry in her mouth. She bit down again and took an even larger mouthful, flicking her tongue out to get every last speck of filling that clung to her lips.

"Aren't Kate's strudels wonderful?" she said.

"I wouldn't know," Mrs. Rose said. "I haven't had time to complete the rest of my meal. But the casseroles are certainly delicious. I don't care much for the goat meat, though."

"Where are you going to put all that food, Ruth? That's a man-sized plateful," May said. "I couldn't eat all that in a month of Sundays."

"Mother's casserole is the best, don't you think?" Lily Rose said in a honeyed voice. "She makes the best cream sauce in Juniper Valley." Her blue eyes looked up for approval. Ruth noticed how dark and full her lashes were. Was there no flaw in this woman—besides a syrupy manner that Ruth could not abide? Everyone else, including Matt, seemed to adore her.

"Which dish is yours, Mrs. Rose?" Ruth asked, but before she got an answer a commotion started among the cowboys. Ruth looked over to see two of the men—she couldn't tell who— wrestling and punching as they rolled in the dirt by the tents. Other cowboys cheered the two on as John Olsen marched toward them.

"It's probably that Johnny Lee again, from Mound Springs," Lily Rose said to her mother, while Matt hurried toward the crowd of gathering men. "He's always stirring up trouble." And sure enough, when John reached in and extracted one of the cowboys, it was Johnny Lee. John shoved him away, landing the slender cowboy on his rear. The other, someone with orange hair whom Ruth didn't recognize, was struggling to sit up, his face smeared with blood.

"Whiskey," Mrs. Rose said. "That's what started it. Tippling. Always starts trouble."

"It's not simply the drink," May said. "Matt drinks whiskey, or did when it was legal; it never made him fight."

Mrs. Rose shot May a look that Ruth would have flinched at. "I've had whiskey before," Ruth said, in May's defense. "It never made me want to fight either."

Now the three women looked at her. All but May dropped their eyes. "I tried it once," May said, "but it tasted like turpentine. Only a man could drink it."

Ruth clamped her lips shut. As a matter of fact she was quite fond of whiskey. It was often available at her mother's. She hadn't indulged for some time until the last dance, when she granted Johnny Lee's request that she join him in "a little snort." Now she sat quietly while she finished her food. The women's small talk only served to make her feel more removed. Maybe later she would have a chance to greet Jim, though he was no longer anywhere in sight.

When her plate was empty, Ruth carried her own and May's into the house. Several women were already helping Kate with the cleanup, so Ruth walked back out to inspect the cement slab, where chairs had been set along the outside edges. When she squatted to judge the texture of the concrete, she spotted the Indian on a branch in the cottonwood overhanging the tents. Seeing her look up, he jumped down and came over to squat beside her.

"Poured your slab yet?" he asked.

Ruth shook her head, ran a hand over the level surface of concrete. "First I want to be sure I know what I'm doing. John said a foundation's important to get right. I mixed up a few test batches of cement with sand and water in a coffee can. It was fun to smooth it over a section of rock—sort of like frosting a cake," she said, ducking her head away from a kid that trotted up from behind and began nibbling at her hair. "Only I couldn't get it right. Once it slopped over the edge like thick soup and ran down the sides. Another time it piled up like whipped cream. None of it turned out anything like this, so nice and clean on top."

"Takes practice, like anything else, to get right," Jim said. "There's a lot to learn about such things."

"I suppose. It's true enough with biscuits, anyway. My first couple batches were pretty black. But I wish you could have seen the last batch. I might even give you competition someday." Ruth straightened and pushed the goat away. She looked down at the slab. "The problem with the cement is I only get one chance before it hardens into something I have to live with under my feet forever."

Jim nodded. "I've never seen you in a dress," he said, rising to stand beside her.

"It's the only one I have," she said. "My dancing dress. See?" She gave a little whirl to show how the skirt twirled out, then stopped, feeling silly before him.

Jim smiled. "Well," he said looking away, "the dancing should start soon."

"Shall I save a dance for you?"

His smile was dark. "Someday I'll dance with you," he said. "Not here." Jim said no more as the two of them watched John Olsen striding toward them.

"You want goat, Rute?" Olsen asked. "Take nanny home for milk?"

"What would I do with a goat, John? I've never milked one." Ruth said.

"Ya, we teach you. I bring one up."

"What I do want is to know more about making concrete for my slab," she said, describing her experiments and the questions they raised about the rest of the process. "I'm not even sure just where I can mix it," she ended by saying, "except maybe in my bathtub."

"Too big job for you," Olsen said, shaking his head. "I come up with Jim, maybe bring Ingmar and Olaf. We get done in a day."

"A woman can make concrete too, John—this one can, anyway. I simply want you to instruct me on a few things—the amounts to mix, how much sand and water, how thick it . . ."

"John doesn't mean the job's too big for a woman," Jim said. "It's a big job for any one person—with numerous and simultaneous steps."

"Well, tell me about the mixture anyway, so I can start fixing it in my mind," Ruth said, unconvinced. "And what things need doing all at once? Can't they happen one step at a time?"

"You a strange woman. Stubborn," John Olsen said, but he explained the process anyway, helping her to see how the type of sand she chose to mix with the cement, as well as the amount, had made such a difference in her experiments. The coarser wash sand was the kind she should use, he said, the small pebbles being what gave the concrete its strength. The more of them the better. As he went on to describe the way to mix and how to trowel and tamp, she began to understand how it might be difficult for one person to do, especially one who had never even seen it done before. She listened carefully and tried to memorize the details, but decided that if John were to offer his services again, she would certainly accept—though she would insist on being part of the crew. But she was not about to ask him.

By the time John and Jim began throwing wood on the roasting pit for the bonfire, several other men had straggled over to join the discussion: Matt first, then a few men from the valley and some of the cowboys, who each tugged down the front of his hat at her. When Larry Hudson began telling Matt what he needed ordered at the store, the orange-haired cowboy who had fought with Johnny Lee turned to her. "I hear tell you're camped out at Can-Tree, ma'am," he said. The cowboy's ears stood out under his hat brim, like opened car doors. His rancid breath nearly made her turn her face away. Something in his voice made her fidget. She had to force herself to stay and be civil when her body wanted to flee. He was not like Johnny Lee and the others with their easy friendliness.

"You hear wrong," Ruth said. "I'm not camped. And the place used to be Can-Tree Springs. It's now Glory Springs, my homestead."

"A watering hole's no place to homestead, ma'am. The cattle have rightful claim. Maybe you haven't heard of the law of the West. This here's open range." He pulled down his hat brim so it hid his eyes and slouched off toward the horses, two other cowboys close behind. She thought she heard him mumble something about a cattle drive.

Ruth turned back to Matt, a jumble of worries tumbling through her. "Is it true," she asked, "what he said?"

"What who said?" Matt asked, pulling away from his conversation.

"That cowboy over there. He said my water belongs to the cattle. That it's open range. Called it the law of the West."

"Beats me," Matt said. "You have papers on the land. Seems to me the law's on your side."

"Having the law on your side doesn't mean much when a herd of cattle want to get to your water hole," said Larry Hudson. "You got a fence? That might help."

Ruth shook her head. "I don't want a fence. I don't like fences."

"Don't worry, Ruth," Matt said, laying a hand on her shoulder. "That cowboy was just trying to start trouble. Don't let him ruin your evening."

Ruth nodded. Matt was right. Shorty and Zeke were already warming up fiddles at the head of the slab. The sun had dropped behind the mountain and a huge orange moon was rising on the other side of the sky. Ruth put the worry from her mind and let her spirits lift with the moon. She had come here for dance and fun. The round moon's promise made her feel heady, as if she'd had a shot of whiskey. She became strangely elated, as if before her were endless possibilities, an entire smorgasbord of men, and she wanted nothing more than to heap her plate high with tastes, selecting from whom among them she would take a large helping, from whom take the merest nibble: the dance to come, a sampling platter.

She sat out not one dance the entire evening. The music so excited her blood that, had she not been asked, she would have gladly danced without a partner. But there was no chance of that. For every tune she had three or four offers. Only Lily Rose was as popular, and Lily chose to sit out the faster melodies, the ones that Ruth loved best. Ruth preferred Johnny Lee for those, since he was the most skillful at swinging and twirling her around. She danced several slow tunes with Matt, though she noticed he danced with Lily a great deal, too, when he wasn't sitting at May's side or conversing with other men.

Toward the end of the evening, Ruth looked over to see Lily and her mother leading May toward the tent provided for women's cots. She finished the polka with Corky Warren, another one of the Mound Spring cowboys, and was immediately caught up by Johnny Lee again, who whirled her till she was so dizzy she could hardly stand. As they came to a laughing, staggering halt, Matt tapped Johnny's shoulder. "This one's mine," he said, sliding an arm around Ruth's waist. The sweet aroma of fresh whiskey wafted over her when he spoke. He pulled her close, and they began moving to the music. Neither spoke as she felt that familiar heat grow between them, drawing her body tight to his. She felt exposed by the bright moon overhead and the bonfire's light, so she closed her eyes to shut out anyone staring at them.

"Has May retired for the evening?" Ruth asked when the song finished and the musicians stopped for a drink.

"I'm afraid she was exhausted. Lily took her to the women's tent," Matt said as they walked to the circle of empty chairs. "She said to tell you she was saving you the cot next to her."

"Not for Lily?"

"Lily's on her other side. The Rose girl's been such a comfort to her."

"A help to you, too, May tells me," Ruth said, studying Matt's expression.

"She learns fast. Knows the inventory and prices almost as well as I do already." He looked over toward the tents. "The two of them get on well."

"May looks . . . well, a bit weaker than when I left."

"She's tired from the trip. I didn't think she'd be coming along with me." He looked back at Ruth. "You seem to be having yourself a good time tonight. You've certainly had enough partners."

"I am," she said as John Olsen came up in front of them. The fiddles were starting up again.

"How 'bout dance with old man, Rute?" Olsen asked.

Ruth got to her feet and took his arm. "What old man, John?"

The two dances following her dance with John were fast, and Ruth let herself be carried off by Johnny Lee. She was aware of Matt watching her, and he came to her side when the music slowed for the last dance of the night. His arm circled and brought her so close against him she could feel a hard knot against her skirt. She swallowed and met his eyes. For a few more beats they pretended to dance, then stopped. Everywhere around them was in motion.

"I'll walk you to the women's tent," he said.

They continued past the chairs, reaching the darkness between the tents just as the music ended. The moment they were out of sight, he pulled her to him and kissed her so hard she felt her lip split against his teeth. Then his tongue burst into her mouth and his pelvis probed hers, his hands gripping her buttocks. "Ruth," he rasped. "Ruth."

At the sound of approaching footsteps, he wrenched himself away. Ruth took a step backward to steady herself, watching him disappear around the far corner of the tent just as Martha Hudson's full form came into view on the other side. Ruth smoothed her skirt and moved aside to let the woman go into the tent ahead of her.

Overhead, cottonwood leaves rustled, though Ruth could feel no breeze. She looked up to see no one, but remembered the Indian perched there earlier. The thought sobered her. But why should it bother her, why should she care? What should bother her, she realized, was where she was headed with Matt. The fact that there was only one place she wanted it to head was not a good sign. She should feel guilty going in to sleep beside the man's wife, she told herself as she followed Mrs. Hudson down the middle aisle and sat on the empty cot. But her body was too full of longing to have room for guilt or worry. She slid beneath the blanket and tried to keep from tossing. Surrounded by the women's soft purring and May's quick, shallow breaths, Ruth remembered the hands of the woman's husband kneading her buttocks, felt again the hardness he pushed against her. Quietly, she put her hand to herself, imagining the rest. Even in this simulated scene, she could feel the Indian's eyes looking down on her from the cottonwood. She would not raise her own to meet them.

*S*hortly before dawn, a cough hacked its way into Ruth's dream, appearing as voices of little green jays fussing in her pinyons. When the noise became more insistent, she awoke. Once her eyes became used to the near dark, she could make out a figure sitting up in the cot next to her. "Are you ill again, May?" Ruth asked, raising to her elbow.

"I'll be fine. The cough always comes this time of the morning," May whispered.

"Since when?"

"Always."

"Not when I left."

"Yes, even then, though not so much."

"You never said. Matt never told me." Ruth reached over to feel the woman's forehead. "You're feverish." She couldn't remember May feeling quite this hot, even at the beginning of her care.

"I'll be all right as soon as the sun comes up, really." She coughed quietly into her handkerchief. "Go back to sleep."

Ruth lay back down and closed her eyes, but it was impossible to sleep. Each hack hammered another nail into her guilt.

When the tent began to lighten, Ruth left to fetch May some water. A rooster crowed as she walked to the well. By the time she lowered the bucket, brought it up, and found a cup, the nannies were demanding to be milked. Morning in the Swedes' yard—the men sleeping in the open on bedrolls, the emptied chairs, and scattered belongings—retained none of the magic of the night before. Ruth had the feeling she'd awoken from a long dream, or from a drunk—perhaps an intoxication with moon. Last night she'd been in Matt's arms; now she was back to nursing his wife. Ruth sighed and entered the tent.

Grateful, May drained the cup at once. "You must keep your liquids up," Ruth reminded her, operating from the textbook ingrained in her during the months of training. How quickly she'd fallen back into her role as nurse. But why should she? She was no longer under hire. She'd be better off if . . . Ruth pushed the hateful thought from her mind. "I'll see if Kate can't fix you some broth, too," she said. Stepping out of the tent in time to see the sun slide over the top of the mountain, Ruth stopped for a moment to watch it lift up from the ridge.

The risen sun did not stop May's cough, nor did the water, nor the chicken broth Kate made, and it was still early when Matt packed up to take her home, along with the Rose women who'd ridden up with them. In the atmosphere of concern surrounding May, Matt had not once met Ruth's eyes. He was now the concerned husband, failing even to acknowledge the care Ruth had given his wife before the others were up. Even the precious Lily Rose had slept on until her mother shook her. Matt's response left a bad taste in Ruth's mouth, transforming her guilt to resentment, mitigated only slightly by the anguished look Matt finally gave her as the departing group situated themselves in his Model A.

Ruth wondered, as the Model A pulled away, why May's relapse should cause Matt to disregard her so completely. That disregard seemed more wrong than had their furtive coming together by the tent, though she was certain others wouldn't see it that way. But how wrong could it be for Matt to want someone who could give him what his wife had no inclination for? And was it wrong of Ruth to take from him what May no longer had any desire for? Here Ruth knew her thinking was too much like her mother's, though Cally would have more plans for Matt than simply bedding him.

Where she had gone wrong, Ruth realized, was in counting on Matt. This was where her thinking differed from her mother's. Cally, in Ruth's opinion, depended on her lovers for far too many things. Early on, Ruth had learned to count only on herself. Cally had left Ruth to her own devices, and that was fine with Ruth. She had come to prefer it—which was why life became so difficult after she was made to stay with her aunt Myrtle, a woman who ruled her own home with an iron will. Not that Cally hadn't tried to control Ruth in subtle ways, too, hadn't wanted to limit Ruth's horizons to the world Cally made for herself after Thomas left. It was a world Ruth found disturbingly flimsy, that dependence on the goodwill of men, on the herbal sorcery that Cally used for healing practices, the midwifery, and on whatever was going on at the so-called rest home she managed. None of these things had much substance, as far as Ruth was concerned, and were not enough to base a life upon.

Ruth walked down the path through the willows toward the garden, where Kate had gone to gather vegetables. John had agreed to drive Ruth home when he finished helping the Hudsons start their Model T, since Jim had already left for the mountaintop. So far no progress had been made with the broken crank. Mrs. Hudson sat fanning herself in the passenger's seat, while her two children chased goats up and down the wash. Everyone else had driven off.

Kate had a bowl already filled with radishes by the time Ruth opened the garden gate, and was bent down searching under the large zucchini leaves for fruit. "Squash too small," she said, bringing out two zucchini somewhat bigger than cigars, "Like sausage. Few days be bigger."

"I'm happy with these, Kate. It will be midsummer before any of mine are ready." She helped Kate to her feet, then the two of them walked back to the house to see if John was ready to take her home.

It turned out the Hudsons' car had to be towed down to the valley. Rather than wait for John to drive her home when he returned, Ruth elected to risk her one pair of dress shoes and walk. Everything at the Swedes' served to remind her of the disturbing incident with Matt. She had been away from her place too long.

As she had anticipated, the further she walked up the rut road home, the less concern she felt about what had happened. The event at the Swedes', even the dance itself, became less real than the canyon around her: its dusty smells, the jays' sharp squawks in the pinyons, the shapes of ridges in front of her lightened each step. She could not let herself be deterred from what was important by her feelings for a man. And Ruth wasn't sure just what Matt did mean to her, other than being an attractive man she wanted, a man married to someone else.

She thought about the rough way he had grabbed at her, like an animal pouncing. At the time, she had been caught up in the excitement of surprise. But the way it had happened bothered her now. It held no tenderness. With Karl, there had been tenderness. Even her encounter with Ramon, whom she did not know at all, was sweeter, she thought, remembering the way he had touched her face, her body. The differences in men puzzled her.

Ruth had only a dim memory of her father—not surprising, since Thomas had left before she was three. She'd reconstructed her image of him from photos she found in Aunt Myrtle's attic. In one of the photos, her father stands close beside Myrtle. Behind them is a trellis with white tea roses, and Thomas's hair appears almost as light as the flowers. The photo must have been taken while he was still engaged to her aunt, before eloping with Cally, who was only sixteen at the time. What sweet revenge that must have been for the outcast half sister that Ruth's grandfather brought home to raise.

The marriage, of course, was doomed. At least Myrtle had that satisfaction. She loved telling Ruth how horrified Thomas's family was when they met the strange girl, how they did everything in their power to end the union. The Eastern family had barely approved of his engagement to Myrtle in the first place — considering Thomas's fascination with the Wild West a whim he would soon tire of. In the end, it was Cally who tired of him. At least that was her story. That he ended up dead three years later in New England, Cally cited as evidence of her continued power over him. To do the right thing, the family granted a small allowance for the child of the union, which Cally said was meant to keep herself and it out of their sight. Now that Ruth had emancipated herself from both Cally and Myrtle, with a career in nursing, the family sent the money directly to her, care of the Baxters, who they thought still employed her.

Ruth didn't know how long she could count on this guilt money — but she hoped the honorable intent of his family would last long enough to support her until she proved up her homestead; it would be nicer yet if in the future she came into a small inheritance as a severance settlement. Otherwise she'd be forced to find employment somewhere, and the nearest hospital was seventy-five miles away, in San Bernardino. Of course, tubercular patients other than May had come to recover in Juniper Valley. But caring for others was not the life Ruth wished to live — doing someone's bidding for her pay; even worse, it would keep her from her canyon. No, she would find a way to remain in her canyon — and without help from the likes of Matt.

Lost in these reflections, Ruth rounded the far bend at Glory Springs and walked up the wash to her campsite. It wasn't until she climbed the high bank of the wash and entered her camp that she saw the shaggy black rear protruding from her tent, cans and scraps of sacks strewn behind it. Her supplies! And her rifle under her mattress in the tent.

Without thinking, Ruth ran toward the tent, shouting to get the bear out of her groceries. When the animal began to move, Ruth changed course and ran to the shelves next to the fire ring. Her hand was on the cast-iron pot by the time the animal backed out of the tent and turned its head to look at her, white powder caked around its mouth and dusted over its face. The bear rose up on hind legs, front paws kneading the air, while a light wind riffled the glossy fur of its belly. Ruth let go of the pot, straightened, bared her teeth, and growled as loud as she could, her fingers shaped into claws raised above her head to shake at the bear.

For a long moment, both creatures stirred air with their forepaws. Ruth became aware of her pounding heart and of the size of the animal towering more than a foot above her. The .22 in the tent would not do much good even if it were accessible. The bear's power and beauty, its magnificent presence, and its absolute belonging to the wild awed Ruth almost to inaction, tempted her to give up trying to claim this canyon and just give it back to the bear. Then her senses took hold and she grabbed up the pot and flung it at the bear.

The creature was on all fours, turning to run when the heavy pot glanced off its shoulder. Ruth kept growling and shouting as she bolted into the tent for the rifle, and though the animal was no longer in sight when she came out, she aimed the .22 toward the bluff, where she knew the sound would echo, and fired off several rounds.

She had only glanced at the mess inside her tent when she went in for the gun, but once she was sure the bear was gone for good, she took a deep breath and stepped inside to face the damage to her supplies. The top strap that latched the tent had been torn off, though the bottom strap had simply come untied when the animal forced the flap back. The sight inside made her heartsick. Canned goods were scattered everywhere, on the chest of drawers, on and under her cot, as if the bear had tossed them in all directions. On inspection, she found that, other than a few dents, the cans were intact. Her dry goods were a different story. A light film of flour coated everything, and she imagined the bear had shaken the sack in its teeth. One five-pound sack was completely gone, even the cloth chewed to a pasty rag. The other sack had teeth and claw holes, as if the bear had just started on it, but most of the flour remained. The sugar had been ripped open, the paper sack licked clean, and the box that held her groceries shredded.

No use getting teary over it. She would have to cut back on her biscuits for the next month, that's all—and she didn't really use much sugar anyway, Ruth told herself as she did her best to sweep and wipe up the chaos created by the animal. She reminded herself that she was lucky not to have lost all of her flour, and that the bear hadn't touched the cooler. Yet the destruction deepened the despondency she'd experienced at the Swedes' and underscored the extent of her isolation. That evening she had no appetite for food. To chase off the blue devils, Ruth filled her cup twice with wine as she sat by the crackling campfire, determined not to brood. Afterward, in her journal, she did not whine but pressed her resolutions hard into the paper. She would build this house and make her life here. She would not be deterred. She would not seek the presence of Matt or any other man in her life. How frivolous she had been at the dance; she had forgotten herself. It reminded her of how silly she had once been about Karl back in El Paso, infatuated with his German accent and foreign ways, not once thinking ahead about what might happen to her. Even Cally had never warned her of the consequences until it was too late—then had told her of the use of vinegar and herb. But such things were behind her now.

What to do about these longings that sometimes drove her without her knowing, Ruth did not know. What she did do seemed only to increase her desire and was a poor substitute for connection with another's flesh. Yet she didn't want the dangers that came with such connections. The new prevention devices she'd heard about were too difficult to get, so she was left with only Cally's herbal remedy. The emotional attachment troubled her even more. The safest answer she could find was not to become attached, the way men sometimes did. But that was hard to do. She had to fight aspects of her nature that worked against it, she wrote, pressing down so hard the pen etched into the paper. She would not let even her own nature deter her. The silly girl who whirled at the dance would be banished from her.

Ruth blinked her eyes dry and put the cork in the inkwell. She must sleep, for she had work to do at dawn. In all the confusion of the morning after the dance, no further mention had been made of concrete for the slab, so she would complete the project by herself—no matter what the men had told her. Besides, other than begging for help, what choice had she? She now relished the idea of such a large project; the hard work and preoccupation would be good for her. She understood that choosing another woman's husband to help stave off attachment had not been a good idea, and lay back on her cot going through the steps John Olsen had outlined, forcing her mind away from other images—Matt's rough embrace, Indian Jim in the cottonwood. She wondered, though, why Jim had left so soon, allowing herself the thought since he was a friend and not in the same category as other men.

The next morning, Ruth woke to find her curse had come upon her, that aptly named scourge that was the burden of a woman's body to endure. She had been outraged to learn about this injustice—the inescapable condition of her fate; it was explained to her one day after she had buried all her bloodied undergarments in Aunt Myrtle's backyard and been caught filching more out of her cousin's drawer. She had thought herself the victim of some shameful and deadly disease and, even when her aunt had told her differently, could not bring herself to believe it for some time. Then, when she did believe, she could not accept the idea that such an awful event would continue to plague her through all the years of her life. Even now, residue from that early fury revisited her as she fastened the belt and pad that would be her imprisonment for the next three or four days and rinsed the blood from her sheet in the short stream trickling from her spring to vanish into the wash sand.

Once she had dispensed with this inconvenient delay, Ruth set about constructing the large board for mixing that John Olsen had said she would need. It turned out to look something like a huge breadboard, which she made from plywood rimmed with strips of thin wood and placed near her foundation to be. Rather than constructing a bottomless box for measuring sand, as Olsen had suggested, Ruth decided to use her bucket and count the number of trips she made. The whole project began to seem more and more like cooking up a recipe, and while some cooks measured carefully and used the perfect utensils, others managed to throw ingredients together with common sense and have better results for it. The latter method suited Ruth best.

For the next two days, she worked to create a layer of sand about three inches high, as John had prescribed, selecting for the most part sand with large pebbles, carefully cleaning out debris as she spread it out on the mixing board. The buckets of sand were considerably heavier to move than buckets of water, but the wheelbarrow simply buried its wheels deep in the sand of the wash, so she continued hauling the sand in buckets. She was most grateful on the second day, when puffy white clouds parked flat bottoms overhead, blocking the sun's heat while she worked. When she sat in the tub at the end of the day, the air carried a most delicious smell of rain somewhere in the distance.

The following day, Ruth used most of one sack of cement to cover the sand, distributing it as evenly as she could manage with her shovel and rake. But when the breeze came up just after lunch, cement went everywhere, in her hair, on the ground around the board, in the air. It took hours for her to turn the powder over into the sand, and she was again glad for the clouds that gathered overhead. John had said to blend the cement in evenly with the sand and pebbles so no pockets or streaks of sand or cement or pebbles remained, much the same way flour and baking powder and salt and lard mixed in a batch of biscuit dough. And what a giant batch she was fixing to bake for her cabin floor, she thought, as she turned the mixture over and dragged it back again and again, moving from side to side of the mixing board. The more she worked, the more confident she became of her success. She thought about how surprised the men would be with her accomplishment. By the end of the day she had the mixture ready for water.

Ruth sat by her campfire with coffee and canned stew as darkness deepened, planning out the timing and tools she would need the next day, while sheet lightning from a storm far off on the desert continually lit the ridges down canyon, lulling her to near sleep. She fell onto her cot tired as she had ever been, but with a strong sense of satisfaction. Tomorrow she would complete the foundation for her cabin.

After coffee and oatmeal the next morning, Ruth moved her #8 tub beside the mixing board and began hauling water to fill it, appreciating the lighter weight of the water buckets. She was grateful for the cloud puffs forming overhead, piling into a mountainous vapor above Rocky Mountain. A husky breeze cooled her further. With the tub filled to the brim, nine buckets' worth—she'd gotten into the habit with the sand of counting each bucket—she was just deciding where to begin pouring liquid onto the mixture when she heard the first sound of cattle.

At first she didn't believe her ears. The bawling came from somewhere near the bend, so she walked to the bank of the wash to look. There were definitely cattle in her wash, only a few, but more coming along behind. And the whole of them headed directly for her spring.

Ruth used a broom to shoo the first few, but not before their big hooves trampled the small plot where her seeds were about to sprout. The chicken wire over the plot meant nothing to the cattle, who simply walked right over it, dragging the wire askew with their hooves. And the cattle she had chased away didn't go more than a few yards, then remained to watch her as they pulled off huge mouthfuls of her bushes and grass and dropped large, stinky plops around her spring. Branded on the animal closest to her she could make out a heart with a line through the middle. More cattle bawls and mewling sounded from near the bend.

Ruth marched back across the wash to her tent to retrieve her rifle, knowing the nasty animals would be at her water before she could get back. Well, it might just be the last drink the stupid bovines ever had, she thought, snatching up both boxes of shells from her table. She strode back toward the spring, where one cow—steer, bull, how could she know—was about to drink. Ruth shouted and ran at the animal, who moved back a few feet and continued to chew as it viewed her.

She put the rifle to her shoulder and took aim. The beast was a large target at such close range, giving concrete meaning to the term *bull's eye*. And she figured a bullet between its eyes would indeed be a good start. But when she pulled the trigger, nothing happened. She remembered the safety, released it, and took aim again.

"I wouldn't do that if I was you, ma'am. You might spook 'em," a familiar voice to her right said. Ruth looked over to see the cowboy who had fought with Johnny Lee, the one who had been so rude to her. His hat was hanging behind him, and she got a good look at his stringy orange hair. It reminded her of the strands of orange fungus that wrapped themselves around rabbitbrush to strangle its life.

"And why not? These cattle are on my property. They're ruining my spring and garden." She kept the rifle to her shoulder, aimed at the cow, as she watched the man.

"The cattle always stop here to water. I told you that before." The cowboy set his hat on his head and pulled it down in front. He turned his face so she couldn't see his eyes.

"Are these your cattle, then? If they are, you better get them off my land before I shoot every last one of them." Just the sound of his ugly voice had filled Ruth with a bloody rage.

"With a twenty-two, ma'am? You'd only wound them. I couldn't let you do that. People like you don't belong in this place." He dusted his chaps and spat a stream of tobacco halfway to her feet, while his big buckskin stamped its hooves and raised its black tail to loose a stream of nuggets.

As Ruth turned to face him, she caught sight of the rifle strapped to his saddle; his hand lay ready to undo the knot. The idea of it pushed her over the edge, and words exploded from her. "Maybe I should just shoot you instead, then," she said. "Since you have no respect for me or my property." She kept the .22 to her shoulder, though she did not aim it at him.

The man looked at her now, his eyes as dead cold with hatred as her own must have been hot with anger. Neither moved nor spoke. Ruth knew her action had not been entirely sensible, and she waited to see what he would do next. But she stood her ground, holding fast to her rage for strength. Now was not the time to think straight.

It was the cowboy who finally pulled his eyes away, looking back over his shoulder at an approaching rider. In the gusty wind now whipping around them, Ruth hadn't distinguished the horse sounds from the trampling of the cattle. The second cowboy rode up beside the first and tipped his hat in greeting. "Name's Bobby Key, ma'am. I see you've already met Charlie Stine here."

"I can't say he introduced himself. I'm Ruth Farley and your cattle are trampling my homestead." Altogether there now totaled about twenty head.

"Not much of a homestead, from what I can see. Ain't no place to put one, neither," Stine said, glancing over at Ruth's tent on the knoll as he unscrewed the top of a whiskey flask.

"Aw, the cattle don't hurt nothin'," Bobby Key said. "They only want a drink a water, then they'll move on. They's just a few strays we're running back up the *cienaga seca* to the Heart Bar. Took the others up the North Fork."

"That spring is the water I drink from, mister." Ruth picked up a rock and tossed it at the cow that was munching its way through the grass to the pool. "The cattle don't need to drink here. You must have just come past the Swedes', where there's a stream a mile long."

"We've stopped at Can Tree long as I been herding cattle. Your tent there's in our camp," Charlie Stine said. "You haven't the right to stop us."

"I've filed papers on this land. Glory Springs is mine. That gives me the right." She hefted the rifle back against her shoulder.

"Not on a water hole it don't," said Stine.

"Don't be that way, ma'am. It'll just start trouble," Bobby Key said, watching her hand on the .22.

"It's you that's starting trouble. And I'll not run from it." Though she was outnumbered, outgunned, and certainly outexperienced, Ruth knew if she gave so much as an inch, she would lose everything she had worked for.

The cowboys looked at each other and Ruth could see some sort of unspoken conversation going on between them, one she couldn't read. "Anyway, John Olsen will settle this when he gets here. He and his men should be showing up anytime now," she said, surprised at the lie so readily springing to her lips like a gift from some great god of words, "to help me prepare concrete and lay the foundation. I've got the sand and cement all mixed on the knoll there, waiting for them. You're both welcome to stay and help—though I'll still not let your cattle into my spring." Ruth set the butt of her rifle on the ground, holding on to the barrel. She managed a smile. Much of the tension in her had dissolved, as though her saying the words, or the cowboys' belief in them, had made them real. After all, they could have been real, she thought, fully embracing the miracle wrought by language. "Is that a motor in the distance I hear?" she asked, turning to walk up the wash toward her knoll, not looking back. She imagined the cowboys' resigned glances at one another. By the time she set her rifle in the tent and walked back to the wash bank, the men were gathering the cattle to herd on. Before he spurred his horse, Charlie Stine gave a long last look over his shoulder to let her know she hadn't seen the last of him.

Ruth stood watching until the men and their cattle were out of sight up the ravine that led to the *cienaga seca*. Then she picked up a shovel and went down into the wash to tend to the cow and horse plops, flinging them as far from her spring as she could. Flies scattered in protest. Ruth smoothed out the huge tracks in the soil that held her seeds, squinting to keep sand from blowing into her eyes, and resecured the chicken wire to keep out rabbits. She didn't like the look of the sky overhead. The protective white puffs had turned dark and unfriendly during her encounter with the cattlemen and gobbled up the last of afternoon sun.

As she climbed the wash bank next to her camp, a gust of sandy wind peppered her face. Ruth squinted toward her mixing board and found she had another problem. Already the mixture had been altered, as wind lifted the cement from the sand and pebbles, powdering the ground around the board. Now that the gusts were fiercer, the sand was being whipped up too.

Ruth pulled out tarps from the building supplies to cover the mixing board, using a line of pot-size stones to hold down the edges and corners. It took her several attempts to secure the sides, with the wind ripping the canvas from her hands. A few drops of rain splashed her face as she dragged the unused bags of cement to the tent. Thunder followed a spear of lightning across the canyon, rumbled off the rocks on the bluff. More drops fell, the biggest she'd ever seen, like whole teacups of water dumped on her head. She dashed to her rock table, scooping up the oatmeal sack and coffee, and ducked into the tent. A towel drying on a bush went sailing off as she latched the bottom strap on her tent flap. Then the sky burst open, and Ruth thought the whole world would wash away.

Rain lapped inside the flap, which untied and danced wildly in the wind. Streams of water poured down from around the center pole as Ruth vainly tried to catch and tie the door strap, which kept escaping from her grasp. When wind began swaying and shaking the tent, she let go the flap and ran to the tent pole, holding it tight while rain coursed down her arms. Thunderclaps crashed on top of each other, magnified by the rocky bluffs across the wash. Wind tossed her, too, from side to side, so she dropped to her knees and held fast the loosening pole with all the weight of her body. She might have succeeded in keeping the tent upright if the canvas had not torn loose on one side from the baling wire that fastened its bottom to the ground. Then the pole gave way, the bottom half snapping up to whack Ruth on the side of the head.

In the dizzy jumble that followed, furniture toppled and rolled, her cot, bureau, table, and she with them, barely registering a slam in the face with canvas, the earlier blow to her head having knocked the sharp edge off of consciousness. She wriggled into a space between the tipped bed and table, where there were blankets and water wasn't pouring over her. She had no idea where the door might be and no desire to go out into the tempest if she had known. She struggled the free edge of a blanket around her shoulders and snuggled into that small pocket of warmth in the shambles made of her home. Lightning illuminated the darkened canvas cocoon, and thunder cracked close around her. Already she could hear water flooding in the wash. At least she'd managed to save the mix for her concrete, or most of it, she thought, as she sank down and let the turbulent darkness take her.

The next thing that penetrated her consciousness was light and bird chirps. Ruth opened her eyes to find the canvas strip beneath the tipped table lit with filtered sunlight. Her head was clear, though it throbbed on one side. She smiled, appreciating the birds' celebration of sun.

She sat up between the askew pieces of furniture. The interior was totally chaotic. She felt her clothing, which was only slightly damp, then the side of her head, with its sore and swollen knot. Gingerly, she half rose and, keeping her body bent, made her way around spilled cans, past the tent pole, to the chest of drawers. She pushed the bureau off its front side to reveal the tent door faced to the ground. It took her several minutes to push the furniture back to what had been the floor of the tent so she could free the front and sidewall to extract herself.

Ruth stood upright in the bright sun. Not a cloud in the sky. Beneath her feet, in the soaked ground and tracks of rivulets, lay what was left of yesterday's sky. Then she turned to look at the sight she had been avoiding. It was much worse than she had imagined.

One tarp was nowhere around. Later she would find it down the wash, caught on a cat's-claw. The other lay beyond the campfire. Her concrete mixture had been ruined; most of it had washed onto the ground and flooded with water before cutting a narrow pathway under the wooden strip around her foundation, etching straight across her would-be floor and out under the strip on other side, continuing on over the bank of the wash—except where it had pooled over the area above the buried rock, sinking in the dirt around it. The entire surface she had smoothed to pour the cement onto was webbed with rivulets that had washed away most of the looser soil. But the sight she most dreaded had also appeared. In the middle of the gray sink around the rock, she could see a clear patch of what could only be the rounded top of the boulder. Though the rock had not risen from its grave as she had feared, it had surfaced by lowering the earth that had embedded it.

Initially, Ruth's amazement at the spectacle of power she had witnessed was as strong as her dismay at the damage to her work. She couldn't help but be awed by forces she had no control over, that sometimes seemed to be working directly against her. An odd idea crossed her mind: that she would not be able to make her place here unless these potent forces let her do so. She did not, like the bear, belong unconditionally to the wild. How, she wondered, did that mesh with the sense of destiny she felt in finding the place? It seemed to her more and more that this place had a spirit and will of its own, one stronger than that of a person or animal, and that the spirit was somehow bound up with the boulder she had buried.

Ruth shook off these strange thoughts; they would not help her build her cabin, were not a sensible way to look at things, no more helpful than the tears she fought back at the thought of the work needed to make repair. She wondered, thinking of those poems gushing with daffodils and the beauty of nature, if that poet had ever spent any real time living in the nature he gushed about. If he had, she decided, he would have written differently of it. If he had come to know the other side of the pretty flowers, as she had, he would have shown at least as much respect as he had admiration.

By midmorning, when Indian Jim came off the mountain and walked into her camp, Ruth's newfound appreciation of nature's power had diminished considerably, being overruled by her consternation over the damage to her camp and project. Once she had stabilized her center tent pole and set the rest of her furniture upright, she hung bedding in the sun and lay her damp journal and books to dry on the rock table. It was the first time she had unsealed the boxes of books that Cally had sent a week before Ruth came to the canyon. They had belonged to Ruth's father; Cally said he'd left them when he went back East and she was tired of keeping them around all these years.

Ruth kept a suspicious eye on the cloudless blue sky. She set up the shelves by the fire ring that had blown over and cleaned her pans and utensils of sand. The burlap cooler had fallen beneath the pine, where she left it for the time being. She wanted coffee in the worst way with her makeshift breakfast of sardines, but there was no wood yet dry enough to burn, so she gathered up twigs from a dead bush and placed them in the sun. As she restored her camp, she considered where to begin on repairing the concrete project, an intimidating prospect. Most of the sand mixture had been washed off the board, leaving hardening chunks and lumps stuck to the bottom. The network of rivulets covering the ground of her foundation could be filled in and raked over—perhaps raised, since so much dirt had washed away, but the larger channel would be difficult to erase, since the cement it carried had caked the earth tight. And the sink around the boulder was already hardening in place. Turning from her frustration with all the work it would take merely to get back to where she'd started, Ruth picked up the water bucket and headed to the spring. She would find a way to start a fire for coffee even if she had to burn blank pages of her journal.

Another shock came at the wash bank when she nearly put her foot down into empty air. The path leading down the bank into the wash had been completely erased, along with a good portion of the bank itself, which had been sliced off by the flood. But the sight of the spring gave her even more pause. She remembered hearing water running in the wash before she fell asleep; now she found it had risen high enough to cover over the spring's grass and small pool with sand and debris. And nothing of her chicken wire garden remained, not even the small rising where she had planted seeds. All was gone, carried away by the flash flood, which had deposited a pile of rounded rocks in its place. Such indifference to her survival seemed a betrayal. "Goddamn it, I'll not leave this place. You'll not make me. Do you hear?" Ruth shouted toward the bluff, which bounced the words right back at her.

She retrieved the shovel from camp and began digging away the sand. It was a few minutes later that she looked up to see Jim descending the bluff, a bedroll strapped to his knapsack. Her gladness was tempered slightly by embarrassment that he might have heard her yelling earlier. She was glad to see anyone right now, she told herself, though she knew she was especially glad it was Jim walking toward her, sunlight adding silver streaks to his dark hair. She jammed the shovel upright in the sand and stood watching the way he moved lightly over the landscape.

"I'm surprised your tent withstood the storm," he said, nodding toward the knoll. His lips held the hint of a smile.

"It didn't," she told him, "but it kept me dry, or mostly so. One side ripped loose from the baling wire and everything tumbled," she added. "I'd offer you coffee, but my spring seems to have disappeared. I've a whole tubful of water in camp. I guess I could clean out the pinecones and twigs and whatever else the wind blew into it."

"Looks like you lost some of the wash bank."

"And my garden. But that wasn't the worst of it," she said, and told him about the damage to her concrete mix and foundation.

"John planned on bringing up the crew once we got out the next load of onyx. Still will, but in a day or two; they were repairing the road to get the load out when I left the mine. I came over the mountain to see what happened on your side. They'll have to do some fixing on the stretch of road up to your place to get the truck here, too. I could see from the mountain where the flood took out whole sections." Jim looked up at the clear sky. "We watched it building for a couple days, but weren't sure what was coming. Early in the year for that kind of storm."

"I thought they were just heat clouds," Ruth said.

"Not when they get those flat black bottoms. Then it's time to look out."

"I covered the mix just before the rain came, but the tarp didn't hold," she said.

Jim nodded. "Why don't you clean that water for coffee? I could use some. Meanwhile, I'll get rid of some sand here. You'll have your spring back in an hour or so." He took hold of the shovel Ruth had left standing. "Water's already trying to fight its way through." He pointed to a spot about two feet from where she had started to dig, where the sand was so saturated it was beginning to flow outward. Ruth wondered how she could have missed the spot.

She was still struggling to light a fire when Jim climbed the bank of the wash and went over to examine the ruined foundation. Finally, with a few strips of cardboard left from her shredded food boxes and the twigs she had dried earlier, she managed to get a small flame going. She built up the fire before setting the coffeepot on and went over to join him. One glimpse of the depression surrounding the now visible ridge of the boulder and Ruth's spirits sank like the earth packed around the rock.

"The rain cemented it in place," Jim told her. "That's a good thing. You wouldn't want the loose dirt dropping down like that once you had the cement over it. It would weaken the foundation."

"I stomped the dirt down. It felt solid to me," she said.

"The rain showed you different. Helped pack it down."

"Could be," Ruth said, trying on the point of view that the rain had actually been a help. Then she thought about all the work wasted making the sand mixture. "Took care of a lot else, too."

Jim used the shovel to chip away at the drying clumps on the board. "You made some strong cement here," he said with a subtle grin. Ruth picked up a rake and worked with him, filling in the eroded fissures. When he used the shovel to loosen the dirt in the main escape channel, she did not object, but imitated his actions, pounding up and down along the gully, softening the soil the way a cook would tenderize meat with a cleaver.

Later, over coffee, she told him about the conflict with the cowboys and the encounter with the bear a few days before. She liked the careful way he listened to her, as if he were taking in her words the way sand takes in water.

"You can take care of yourself," he said when she finished. "But there's a lot of work to be done here. You should let us help you. It's a neighborly thing people do for each other out here. The cowboys shouldn't give you as much trouble once you're built. You might borrow one of John's shotguns and keep it on hand, though, just in case."

"I like to do for myself," Ruth said, nodding, "but I see now the foundation's a big job alone—like John said. Even without a thunderstorm. So I've no objection to accepting help—just so I'm a part of the crew."

"There'll be plenty for everyone to do, including you." His smile held an understanding of her that went deeper than Ruth liked. She said nothing, but rose to pour another cup of coffee.

"Would you like to see those inscriptions while we wait for John?" Jim asked when she sat back down. "I could take you there in the morning."

Ruth's flash of excitement faded as she looked over at her ruined work.

"We've done all we can do for now, and it'll be another day before they get here," he continued. "There's only one more thing for us to do tonight. Make some biscuits. Didn't you want to show me how good you can make them?"

Ruth smiled at the prospect, feeling her spirits lighten. Surely she could spare the flour for that. "I'd be delighted," she said. "Do you think you can find enough dry wood to make coals?"

The biscuits turned out to be Ruth's best yet, and she was most pleased with herself as the two of them sat at the campfire later, darkness softening around them. "What made you come here?" Jim asked, sometime after the second cup of after-supper coffee. "Such a long way from where young women usually go."

"My life, I think," she said, realizing she didn't know exactly. "Sometimes I get the feeling I was meant to be here. But that's silly, I guess. Yet I seemed to recognize this place the moment I saw it, as if I had been looking for it a long time without knowing." In the protective darkness, Ruth found herself telling Jim of her background in El Paso, of the feud between her aunt and mother, and of Cally's hushed past. She continued, describing the finishing school and her escape, hitching back to El Paso to become a flapper, her training as a nurse, and the move to the West. She told him not only the facts of the events, but also her struggles and confusions along the way. When she had spilled herself out, she stopped, feeling like someone who had taken off clothes for the first time ever and wasn't sure what to make of the warm air on her body, without shame but with an uncertainty that felt tangible in the night.

Neither spoke for some time. Finally she said, "And you? Where did you grow up? You've been somewhere besides the other side of that mountain."

"I was born there," he said, "on the Black Canyon Reservation. When I was eleven some people—Mormons—came and took me away to raise. It was right after my grandmother died. They gave my parents money, shoes for my brother and sister. We were very poor; my folks did what they had to.

"They were good people, the Mormons, meant well. They wanted the best for me, just as my parents did. Sent me to good schools. Tried to teach me their values. I kept my mouth shut and did what they said, as my parents had told me to do. I learned to talk and act like a Mormon, but I was never one of them. I sure didn't look like them. And after all that education what was I to do? Even with a college degree I was still an Indian."

Jim stopped talking, and they sat with the sound of crickets. An occasional shooting star. Somewhere down canyon, coyotes began to howl. Ruth remembered the woman who had hissed *squaw* at Cally, the undisguised disdain and hatred in the woman's voice. She thought about the secrecy and shame associated with her mother's background.

"So I came back home. You could say I escaped, too," he said, after a while. "My father was dead by then—of cancer or alcohol, I'm not sure—and my mother had severe diabetes. My brother had been killed; my sister had married a white and left the reservation. But still it was home. It was where I wanted to be. And my mother needed me. After she died, I had a bout with alcohol for a while, but it didn't help for long. Then one day I found work with John here on this side of the mountain. That was three years ago."

They sat for a while longer, watching the campfire flame change to liquid embers, comfortable in the warm evening. Jim was easy to be with, Ruth thought, though she missed the excitement she felt with Matt. . . . She stopped herself. She would not dwell on such things. Then Jim rose and stretched. "I'll camp up there on the mountain, just above the spring," he said, "if that's all right with you. We can get an early start that way."

He was in her camp as the sun came up. After coffee, they packed some jerky and the biscuits left from the night before, filled canteens in the spring, which had now recovered, and started climbing a long ridge that led up the side of Rocky Mountain. The ridge was fairly rocky and steep, the surface hard-packed, except near the sides, where draws led off and the mountain sagged into soft rivers of sand, as if it were dissolving as they walked. Her boots sank in, at times, and the loose, pebbly sand closed over them, pulling her a few inches back down the mountain with each step. After crossing one such draw, Jim stopped in the shade of a pinyon ahead of her and motioned for her to rest.

"The granite's wearing away there," he said. "Decomposing fast." Ruth let her feet slide out from under her and dropped down beside him. The granite wasn't the only thing decomposing, she thought. A sharp jab in one buttock caused her to lean to one side; she reached down and extracted a pine needle from her pants. She wriggled in her blouse to ease the tickle of sweat trickling down between her breasts, and waited while her breath began to come easier and her pounding heart slowed.

The green spot that was Glory Springs appeared minuscule far down in the canyon below. She was surprised how high they had come so fast, already deserting the pinyon for taller pines. When she climbed alone, Ruth set her own pace, as she did now everywhere in her new life. She uncorked her canteen and took a long, deep drink, restraining herself from allowing water to pour down her neck and into her shirt. Instead, she rationed out a mere handful to pat over her hot face.

"The rest of the way's not so steep," Jim said, regarding her. "And there'll be water near the top."

The climb did become less steep afterward, but more rocky and less direct, forcing them to skirt huge tangles of manzanita and thick clumps of scrub oak. At one point Jim held up a hand, and they stopped so he could listen, though Ruth heard nothing other than the drum in her chest. "I think we surprised a doe," he said. When they rounded the next knoll, Jim showed her the animal's track.

"But how do you know it was a doe and not a buck?" Ruth asked, unconvinced, looking at the set of V's at her feet. The size of the print and the noise told him, he said, and bucks usually make more crashing as they go. They bent to examine the track, and Jim showed her how the ridges were still sharp and the ground underneath still tight from impact, explaining that the way the tracks came down side by side again and again showed how the deer was bounding up the mountain.

They climbed for about an hour more, until Jim led her into a passageway concealed between mammoth boulders, where weather had sculpted a near tunnel. They stepped out the other side into a small valley. Ruth blinked, for a moment not believing her eyes; how could a place so strangely beautiful be hidden high on the mountain?

A few feet from her, a small stream flowed down over smoothed pink-marbled rocks to form a small lake. Beside the stream rose a wall of the same colorful rock, embedded with large chunks of shiny flakes that mirrored the sunlight. Willows and tall grasses grew along the far rim of the pond. Ferns grew thick beneath tall pines and huge oaks that overhung the rocky outcrop. Hugging the rocks was a rounded lean-to, made of pole-like branches and covered with skins, and boughs and mud. A hawk floated out from the mountaintop and sounded a shrill cry.

"No wonder you stay up here." Ruth walked farther out toward the pond and looked around. That he trusted her enough to show her his camp touched her. "It's a world unto itself," she said, at once realizing that a similar attribute drew her to her own place, though his was far less accessible. She squatted and put a finger in the water, found it cold but not frigid. "But the inscriptions," she said, turning back toward him, "are they nearby?" Jim said nothing, but looked toward the rose-colored rocks.

She followed the trail of his eyes. It took a few seconds for her to realize that some of the marbling she was seeing was geometrical, that mixed in among the natural rivers and swirls of color were hundreds of shapes etched purposefully into the stone.

Walking closer to the rock, she could make out some of the shapes. Many appeared to be animals: coyote or wolf, some definitely deer with antlers, some of those hugely pregnant. Still other figures looked to be large lizards. She also found human shapes, and swirls, intricate mazes, and sun circles with outward rays. There was a figure with what seemed to be a huge penis, beneath him another figure with large breasts, from whom a smaller figure was emerging. For a long time Ruth walked under the rock face, running her hand over the hard surface, trailing her fingers along the grooved lines of the forms, worn smooth by time, as if the feel of them would bring her closer to deciphering them. Instead, it deepened their mystery, and she found herself no closer to answers that would interpret the past than before. The lives of the early people here stayed as closed to her as the mystery of her mother's past, impenetrable as the etched stone. She was left with only the future to make sense of.

The next day when John Olsen and his miners arrived at Glory Springs, they made short work of Ruth's foundation. The six men accomplished with ease in a day what would have taken her four to complete. And probably with better results, she admitted. She helped them, worked hard too, making a total of seven on the project—which was one reason it was superior to her own efforts, she reminded herself. Glad as she was to have it finished, she was left with a sticky beholden feeling, although she knew there were no better people to be beholden to.

They all assured her it was common neighborly practice, as Jim had said, part of a tradition of house raising. She knew that was true, yet she suspected that the practice might also give them neighborly say-so in other areas of her life, some stake in her life that she didn't want anyone to have. It was that feeling of obligation that kept her from refusing when they insisted she accompany them back to the Olsens' for supper at dusk. Ruth knew she should have been more grateful for their thoughtfulness—and for the hearty food Kate prepared, which she did enjoy immensely.

After supper John drove her home, armed with a few supplies Kate sent to replace what the bear had eaten—Ruth couldn't even tell her story without Kate rushing in to help. But there she was, being ungrateful again, instead of being glad she could now have sugar with her oatmeal. It would be more than two weeks before her next allowance check arrived at Matt's store, which served as the post office for the community as well. She was grateful also to know that the Olsens would be taking her into town for supplies, and so she needn't rely on Matt Baxter. His affections turned out to be thin indeed. But that was a matter she was no longer concerned with.

On the way back to Glory Springs, John suggested that, because of all the lumber she had ruined on the rock, she build the bottom half of her cabin with stones from the wash—which were certainly in plentiful supply.

The next morning as she stood in front of the freshly poured slab, the sunlight of a new day filtering through the pinyons, Ruth felt the canyon take hold of her. Her uneasy feelings dropped away as she remembered how ruined she had felt after the storm. Now the damage had been repaired; what did it matter how? She squatted and touched a finger to the drying cement. Yesterday on a whim, when they finished the slab, she had removed a boot and pressed her bare footprint into the concrete of the cabin doorway. The surprise and chagrin of the miners, who had only just smoothed the surface, had embarrassed and almost stopped her. This morning she was glad she had not stopped. She admired her footprint, the round scoops of toes and heel seemed as much her mark on the land as the barred-heart brand was for the cattle ranch and cowboy she had come to hate. Her soleprint and the slab beneath it sealed a contract between herself and the place she had chosen.

Over the next few days, Ruth settled nicely into the routine of summer days, mixing small batches of concrete each morning and adding layers of stone wall for her cabin. Once she had collected rock and sand and piled it near her foundation, her work did not take up all of the day, but left her time during the afternoon to read or to explore the mountains around the canyon. She especially enjoyed the days Jim would appear, usually early enough to help her add a few stones. Then the two of them would set out together, the Indian taking time to point out as they went various kinds and features of animal tracks that were new to her. Soon she was able to distinguish bobcat from coyote and to know whether the tracks were old or new, walking or running, though she was far from the understanding Jim had. Yet she was fascinated by what she learned and intrigued by this man who was as fluent in the language of the land as he was in words. Jim knew vegetation, too, and showed her plants that she found quite tasty mixed in with other dishes; she became particularly fond of the tender, arrowhead-shaped leaves of lamb's-quarters. The watercress near the willows was a favorite, too. While the plants fulfilled some of her need for greens, Ruth shot rabbits regularly to supplement her meat, and she had three cans of Hereford corned beef and two of stew left the afternoon before the Olsens were due to fetch her in for supplies.

She decided to bathe and set out clothing that afternoon, since her neighbors were due to arrive early the next morning. As she hauled buckets to fill her tub, Ruth found herself imagining her encounter with Matt at his store the next day. "Good day," she would say politely to him. "Could I have my mail, please?"—all traces of familiarity absent from her voice. Then, "Thank you, Mr. Baxter." When her fantasy progressed to include his response, Ruth would catch herself and erase the scene from her mind.

As she soaked in the tub, memories gathered over her with the soap on her skin, and when she closed her eyes to pour rinse water over her lathered hair, she found Matt's face in the darkness behind her eyelids. She turned in early, then tossed until she thought her cot might tip over. She got back up to resolve in her journal that she would quit this silliness, for "the man was not that likable" to her. Why should she be stuck on the way his eyes examined her, the promise of sun on his light hair? If they had bedded just once, she wrote, perhaps she would be able to forget that one quick moment when he pressed his body against hers.

The sight of Matt Baxter's Model A down by the bend the next morning rocked Ruth back on her heels. Impatient with the lateness of the Olsens' arrival, she had looked up at the sound of the motor, expecting to see the flatbed. Instead, the modern tan shape swept away her guard. She almost took off running toward Rocky Mountain. Then she dropped down into the camp chair, rose quickly again, ducked, and dashed into the tent, where she paced, picked up the piece of mirror, glanced, paced again. When the car pulled in front of her camp, Ruth was still unsure what to do.

"I'll be right there, John," Ruth called, when the motor quit in front of her camp. She took a deep breath, grabbed her sweater, and stepped out of the tent, letting her face settle into an expression of surprise as she looked over at Matt's car. She stopped and stood without speaking as he climbed out of the Model A.

"Hello, Ruth," he said, walking around the slab toward her.

She waited quietly until he came near. "I should have known that wasn't the sound of John's motor. He's coming, you know, to take me to town."

Matt shook his head. "I stopped on the way up and told him I had your supplies with me. They sent up a few vegetables again. When I left them, they were on their way down to Juniper Valley. That Indian went with them."

"Jim," Ruth said. "His name is Jim."

"Okay, Jim, then." Matt looked over at the slab and the layers of rock around it. "So you're making your house of stone now?"

"I'm not sure why you're here," Ruth said. "I wasn't expecting to see you anymore. I can make my own arrangements."

"I told you I wouldn't let you down, Ruth," he said, looking back at her.

"That's already happened."

Matt gazed down at the ground. He began rubbing a pine ant into the sand with one foot.

"And May?" Ruth asked. "I trust she's getting stronger again, with Lily's help."

"No." Matt looked up again as he spoke. "That hasn't happened. She's worse than before . . . before you came. If it weren't for . . ." He closed his eyes and looked away.

"You shouldn't have left her, then, to come here today."

Matt pulled at a strand of hair above his ear. "Lily Rose is with her. Ruth . . ." He reached down and took her hand. "I had to see you again. I know it's wrong, Ruth . . . if only we hadn't . . ."

Ruth let him keep her hand. The cold sweat on his palm strengthened her. "It might be wrong—or it might not," she said, "but it has nothing to do with May's getting ill. Have you taken her to a doctor?"

He let her hand fall and reached back up to pull at his hair. "Dr. Bendall thinks she might have to go back to the sanatorium if she doesn't improve. I don't know what I'd do without Lily's help. She's a fine girl, Ruth, honest. She practically ordered me to make this trip, knowing how much it's been on my mind."

"How sweet of her," Ruth said, heat rising to her cheeks. "So I have her to thank for these groceries. We'd better unload them, then, so you can be off." She began walking toward the car.

"Ruth . . . ," Matt said, starting after her. "That's not what I meant." He came up beside her as she took hold of the door handle and covered her hand with his. Pulling her fingers away from the lever, he turned her to face him. Suddenly his arm whipped around her waist to jam her body up against his. "It's wrong, we both know that. But I can't stop thinking about it, Ruth," he whispered into her hair and neck. "The way it felt to press up against you that night. I can't forget . . . I have to have you for my own."

Her breath caught as he crushed her into the side of the car, bending her back against the fender. Ruth thrust him away from her, escaping from the heat of his embrace and from the tingling chills she felt as his lips moved against her neck. "Stop now, for godsakes, since you think it's so wrong." She straightened the front of her blouse. "I don't want you blaming me for it."

He grabbed hold of her arms, but she put her hands up to his shoulders and held him away from her. "Wrong is wrong, Ruth," he said, hoarsely, his chest heaving. "I didn't make the rules."

"Rules? How can you talk about rules? What have they got to

do with the way we feel . . . what harm would we do?" She dropped her hands from his shoulders. "I don't care about rules. If I minded rules I'd still be . . ."

"Don't talk like that. You don't sound like . . . like any woman I ever heard talk." He gathered her to him. "But the devil knows I want you . . . oh, how I want you. Whatever you are."

When she turned her face away, his teeth bit gently into her neck. Ruth felt herself dissolving. "If you don't think it's wrong, why are you fighting it now?" he whispered, snaking a hand under her skirt. He pressed himself against her leg, and she felt him fumble at his pants. Before she could push him off, his fingers reached down and slipped under the rim of her underpants. Her resolve was rent with the edge of cloth that first gave, then came apart. Before she wrapped her legs behind him and pulled him into her, Ruth glanced quickly into the branches of the pinyon above her and over at the bluff across the wash. Then with her backside against the cold tin fender of the Model A, she rode the man hard toward that place where all men merged with the rest.

Ruth's experience in El Paso had taught her the cost of freedom from her monthly nuisance, and she had not failed to rinse herself with vinegar and herbs each time Matt left. Yet her relief was great the day her curse returned. The fact that she had only two of the new Kotex pads left and would soon have to resort to rags as she had used in her early years did not dampen her gladness, nor did the inconvenience that Matt was due up again tomorrow. Pads would not be included with her supplies, either, for she could not bring herself to list them.

After breakfast, Ruth mixed her daily batch of concrete and sculpted a layer over a small space of wall, jiggling each rock to fix it in the mudlike texture. The cabin walls had now reached waist high, and it gave her much satisfaction to go through a doorway to reach the interior. The strenuous work helped to stem the cravings in her, for at the slightest provocation her body would remember its wild pleasures, her lust opening up to a vast array of possible partners. Sometimes she found herself imagining how it would be with Johnny Lee or some of the others, the sounds and smells of the men, the size and shape of them—already she had experienced substantial differences. Her intense urges both pleased and frightened her.

By the time the sun bore down overhead, Ruth had set the last of her day's stones in place. She stepped back to survey her work, then moved next to the fresh section of wall to measure its height against her body. Today's new layer, about four feet long, had raised that section as high as the cage of her ribs. Pleased with her progress, she sat under the pinyon and drank from the cooler. When she saw Jim's figure descending a ridge on the mountain, she felt as if she'd been waiting for him. Ruth had missed the Indian, for he had come only once since Matt began making his visits, and they had spent the day following the cattle trail up the *cienaga seca*. She had been preoccupied the whole while, her body overruling her head at every chance, not only with bawdy memories, but also with revived appetite at the sight of the muscles of Jim's back and the movement of his buttocks beneath his cotton trousers. More than once she had to avert her eyes to keep her thoughts clear. Sometimes she had not.

Her shirt tied up under her breasts to let the currents cool her, Ruth drank from the dipper while he approached. Even in the shade of the pinyon the still air gave little relief, the heat bound up with the ringing din of locusts in the cottonwoods across the wash. Ruth remembered the cool pond behind Jim's place and wondered why he had left it to come to her oven of a camp—at least it had become one the last few days, until she sometimes felt like one of the biscuits she baked. She did not untie her blouse as he came near, his own shirt hanging down around his waist, hair knotted behind his head and held tight against it with a bandana. Her hair had grown too long for this heat; if she had better scissors, she would reinstate her flapper cut for the summer and get it off her neck.

Ruth held out the dipper as Jim walked up and set his rifle against the pine. He nodded, then drank, watching her as she settled onto a small rock beside the tree. "Thanks," he said, hanging the ladle on the side of the tin container. He slid the knapsack from his shoulders and sat on the ground beside her, leaning his back against the truck of the pine, and closed his eyes. Neither of them spoke. A deerfly droned by. Ruth quit wondering why he had come. It didn't matter. Whatever the reason, it felt good to have him there, and she had the odd sensation that they'd been sitting beneath the pinyon for a long time.

"Kate said to tell you to come down and help yourself to whatever is in her garden," Jim said, when some time had passed. "That was a few days ago, before we went up for a load of onyx. Maybe, when it's cooler, you'll want to walk down with me to get the vegetables. John or I will drive you home." He opened his eyes and smiled. "It's cooler there in the willows by the Olsens', you know. We could even stop and find a place in the stream to soak."

Ruth considered the wavering mosquito larvae she'd seen stuck to rocks where the stream calmed, the forests of fuzzy mosses that now inhabited the bottom of each small pond. Sweat trickled down her neck, finding its way under her collar and into the waiting pools beneath her breasts. "Why not go now, then," she said, "while it's still hot?"

Time flowed by unhurriedly, barely moving in the heat. "Okay," Jim said, finally. "That's a good idea." Ruth nodded, but didn't move from the spot. She had remembered during the interval that she was cursed. Should she defy the medical books? The notion that her condition should keep her from cooling her heated body angered her—as did the potential of bloody water spreading out around her and dribbling down between her legs to stain her pants as she rose from the water while Jim looked on. But she could not tell him this.

Jim pulled his knapsack onto his lap. "My magic bag," he said. Reaching inside, he extracted a cloth and unwrapped it. "Lunch," he said, holding some out to her.

The jerked meat was dry and tough, with a gamy taste, and a bit salty. Each bite required a great deal of chewing before she could swallow it down with hot water from Jim's canteen, the two of them being too lethargic to make the journey to the cooler for lukewarm liquid. But the food filled and promptly strengthened her.

Before leaving, each filled a canteen and wet a shirt in the scanty runoff from her spring, Jim first, who then turned his back and walked toward her camp, while Ruth soaked hers in the coldest water dripping from the bank, then slipped her arms back in the sleeves and covered her bare breasts with the chilled cloth. Her nipples flared up under the sudden cold, and with them her awareness of being half exposed and alone with this man, though he had never shown any sign of regarding her as anything other than a friend.

Their clothing had dried by the time they were halfway to the willows, so when they finally reached the beginning of the stream a ways up canyon from the Swedes' they sank down on the shady bank, parched, welcoming even the moist smell of decay beneath the willow trees. The steady stream had exposed layers of debris from other epochs, the preclay revealing slices of pebbly pink sands left by floods, along with darker tiers containing the packed roots that had gathered in quieter eras. Ruth sat on a rock and splashed her arms and face, took off her boots to soak her feet where the stream slowed and eddied into a small pool rimmed with watercress.

"You can bathe here," Jim said, getting to his feet. "I'll be just on the other side of those willows downstream."

Ruth waited for the lap and splash that told her Jim had entered the water, before she undressed, rolling her pad and underwear up with her pants. She waded out past the rocks into the waist-high water. The bottom of the pool was sandy under the soft moss that her footsteps loosened to float up and murk the clear fluid. When the shock of the cold on her hot body eased, she squatted, letting water flow over her shoulders. Bits of blood floated up to mix with the debris, dissolving and washing away in the stream's flow. Ruth kept still until the water cleared. She closed her eyes and for a long while savored the cooling liquid that pronounced every pore on her skin.

She had heard no sound of Jim and looked about should he be hiding somewhere to watch her. And if he were, she wondered, remembering the sight of his bare shoulders, how bad would that be? She stood upright, then, aware of the thrust of her breasts, her nipples lifted to let the sun reheat them, the wet ends of her hair dribbling cold water down her back. She reached down and broke off a sprig of watercress, began nibbling at its tangy leaves.

The cowboys' horses neighed before they appeared, in time for Ruth to squat back down and hide from the riders who came into sight on the road a few yards away. The watercress and brush between the pond and the road nearly concealed her. Then one of the cowboys looked over. He pulled his buckskin to a halt. The other continued on. "Well, looky what we got here," Ruth heard the first say. The other cowboy turned his horse and rode back.

"What kind of a fish do you suppose that is, Charlie?" the returned rider asked.

"Don't know for sure. But I think it's some kind of cattle-hating fish. What do you say we get closer and find out?" Charlie Stine swung one leg over the saddle and dropped down, hanging his hat on the saddle horn to expose a tangle of orangy strands to the sun. Bobby Key remained fidgeting on his horse.

Ruth fumbled in the sand near the edge until her hands closed around a slick rock. "Don't come any closer," she said. She felt absurd giving orders from her lowered posture and was afraid the tone of her voice announced that fact.

"Hey, Bobby, it's a talking cattle-hating fish," Charlie said, walking toward her. "I'm gonna see if I can catch it and have it for dinner."

"Stop right where you are." Jim stepped out from the willow. "What do you think you're doing?" He kept his rifle lowered, though Ruth could see his finger on the trigger. Stine saw it too.

"Looks like it's an Indian-loving cattle-hating talking fish," Stine said. "I mighta known."

"I think you better just get back on your horse and leave right now."

Stine snorted. Jim cocked the hammer and raised the rifle. For a moment Stine stood glaring, then turned and sauntered to his horse. Jim followed behind him, waiting while the cowboy replaced his hat, mounted, and the two rode off. While Jim climbed the knoll to make sure they left, Ruth rose and stumbled out of the water, her teeth chattering and her hands gone blue. She dressed behind the willow, remaining chattery, the warm air and sun failing to revive her.

"I'm sorry, Ruth," Jim said, when he came down from the knoll. "I was half submerged and didn't hear them until you did. And I didn't think I'd have much effect walking out without pants or the rifle."

"They were the same two who drove up the cattle, the ones I told you about," Ruth said, her teeth banging against each other to cut hunks from her words.

Jim nodded. "The Texans. They're new around here, only the last year or so." He walked over and set down the rifle, took hold of her hands and rubbed them. "Here," he said. "You need sand." Ruth glanced down at the .22 and back at the road. "They won't be back," Jim told her, "at least not today."

Jim lay Ruth facedown on the sun-soaked sand and covered her hands and arms with its warm blanket. He sat beside her and kept watch while, pressed against the heated ground, cell by cell, Ruth's body began to calm. When she could breathe easy again, they walked on to the Swedes'.

Both Olsens overpowered Ruth with huge hugs as she and Jim came into the yard. Kate at once invited her for supper. John's face clouded and his jaw clenched when they told him about the behavior of the cowboys. "Those two a bad lot, ya," he said later, over a meal of cornbread and sweet goat chili. "I warn them good next time they come by here." Ruth sat with the Olsens at the long table with Jim and four other miners, who spoke among themselves in Swedish and sometimes to Ruth in English with thick accents. Only Ingmar, a large man about thirty, spoke English as well as Kate and John.

"Some of the women said Johnny Lee was trouble, too," Ruth said, remembering Lily's words. "But he seemed a different sort to me."

John nodded. "That boy he okay, John Lee. Too much fun in him sometime. Too much liquor, too," he said laughing. "Shoot mouth off sometime. Don't mean harm. But the two today different story."

"Ruth could use one of your shotguns, maybe the twelve-gauge," Jim said. "She needs more than a twenty-two around with them coming through." He picked a moth out of his chili, flicked it toward the open door, and swiped the bottom of his bowl with cornbread. The moth flew back to join others banging into the lanterns at the ends of the table.

"I told you, Rute, this canyon no place for woman alone." John rose from the table and pulled a shotgun from its rack above a cabinet. "But you here now. Shotgun, it good idea." He held the gun out to her.

Ruth pushed back her bowl and took hold of the big shotgun, having no doubt that she might need it. "It's good for shooting quail, too," Jim said. "If you want to add them to your menu."

"I'll pay you," she said, despite Olsen's shaking his head and holding up a hand at her words. "When I get my check tomorrow. Matt will bring it with the supplies." She turned to Jim. "But I don't think I could kill those cute quail with their little topnots, Jim. A whole crowd of them come every morning to drink at the spring."

John and Kate exchanged glances. John Olsen shook his head again. "I take you to town," he said. "Baxter, he take the wife to San Bernardino."

"To the sanatorium? Did she have a turn?" Ruth asked, careful to keep her voice even, her face controlled, aware that the couple knew every trip Matt had made up past their house in the last two months. Each time he had stopped to offer them some different excuse, he told Ruth, some item he had forgotten to bring the time before, but she knew they must have questioned the frequency of his visits. "He told me she was improving." She felt Jim's eyes on her. In truth, she was not surprised at May's decline; though Matt had claimed May was again gaining strength, Ruth had suspected all along he was fooling himself.

Kate got up to fetch the enamel coffeepot from the woodstove. "Ya, Baxter send word up with Ingmar and Olaf two days ago," she said, setting the pot on the wooden table, "when they were in town. Said to tell you." She turned back to the stove and unlatched the oven door.

"Aye, Baxter say wife took ill," Ingmar said.

"I go into valley with you in three day," Olsen said, pouring hot coffee into his mug and passing the pot down the line.

"You need more food now, Rute?" Kate asked, carrying over a steamy strudel from the oven. "I got everyting you want."

"You sure do," Ruth said. She breathed in the aroma of the pastry. "I have plenty until then, Kate, especially with all the vegetables you keep giving me." She took the pot that came her way and filled her cup to the brim. Kate's pastry was indeed a consolation, but it could not override the sick feeling Ruth got at the mention of May's condition.

"Maybe she's just gone in to be evaluated," Ruth said.

After the dishes were done, Jim drove Ruth up canyon to her camp. When the flatbed's headlamps fell on the tent as they pulled up, she noted that the flap had gapped open. Inside, she struck a match to the new kerosene lamp Matt had delivered. Everything was as she had left it, or at least it appeared so at first. Then Jim noticed a small lump moving under the blanket on the cot. He motioned for Ruth to stay put and threw off the cover.

The two of them jumped back as the snake shot out toward them, dived off the bed, and wriggled under the chest of drawers. Ruth reached under her mattress for the .22. "It's just a racer, Ruth," Jim laughed. "But they do move fast enough to make your heart stop."

"But that reddish color—I thought it was a rattler." Ruth sank down on the mattress. "I wonder how it got in here."

"I wonder too," Jim said. "Let's look." He picked up the lamp and went through the flap. "That's what I thought," he said as Ruth followed him out. Even in the weak light cast by the small lamp, Ruth could see the ground was pocked with hoofprints. "They were here all right."

Checking further, they discovered that Ruth's water containers had been emptied, dumped over the stone walls into the interior of her cabin-to-be, and the rope that hung her burlap cooler had been frayed by knife so that it would fall at the slightest addition of weight or movement. By the time they got to her spring to find the chicken wire torn away and the new zucchini and tomato plants she had transplanted from Kate's garden trampled, Ruth was choked with fury. "How could they? How dare they?" she spat. "If they come back, I'll shoot them on sight." She swallowed hard. "Bastards!"

"They're bastards, all right," Jim said. "Dangerous ones. At least Stine is. I'm not so sure about the other—but he goes along." He set the lantern down and knelt beside Ruth, who had begun to pull off fragments of leaves and broken stems and prop up the rest with twigs, and helped her repair the little they could; then they replaced the chicken wire to protect what was left.

Before leaving, Jim showed Ruth how to crack open the shotgun and put in the shells, reminding her that the kick would be much stronger than the .22. When he was gone, she sat at her writing table and filled several pages of her journal with angry words, then more pages to explain to herself why she needn't feel guilty over May's deteriorating condition. When she finally blew out the lamp and lay back in the dark, sleep was slow to come. The day's events had doused the flames of sensuality that had raged for the last two months. Now each sound that disturbed the quiet night reminded her of the cowboys' threats. They had violated her home; what else might they do? That fear chilled her more than had the images of cougars and bears materializing from dark outlines those first nights in the wild. This was not a peril to be explained away as an imagined danger.

T he morning before the Hudsons' party, Ruth set each stone in place with a jaunty little half-dance. The day had taken forever to arrive. After she finished the last section of stone, which raised the entire layer to just above her breasts, she began hauling water for her bath. Ruth had first heard about the event when the Swedes took her to town. It was just as well that Matt had not been at the store that day when they picked up groceries. He had gone to visit May in San Bernardino, leaving Lily Rose in charge of the store, and the girl did not indicate that he had left a note for Ruth. Every day, she had half expected to see his Model A appear around the bend, until John Olsen had told her Matt was gone. Between bouts of guilt and lust she found herself wonder-ing what he would do when May returned from the sanatorium, since it would no longer be appropriate for Ruth to nurse her. She would ask him at the Hudsons' dance tonight—assuming he would be there. Local gatherings were such occasions that folks had been known to leave deathbeds to attend.

Ruth had received letters from Cally and Myrtle when she was in town. There had been some scandal involving Cally and the mayor, her aunt wrote, without going into details on the trouble, and for that Ruth was grateful. Myrtle warned her not to believe the "shameless hussy," who had once again brought such disgrace to the family name. As for Cally's letter, it was intended to remind Ruth that El Paso was where she belonged and that she should return immediately. No doubt Ruth's allowance check was dearly missed. Only at the very end of the letter did Cally make oblique reference to the scandal, cautioning Ruth to beware of rumormongers and small-minded people. Once she read the letters, Ruth used them to start her evening campfire.

The Olsens arrived midafternoon to fetch her. With the summer heat upon them, the event wouldn't start until just before dark. Like most families in Juniper Valley, the Hudsons had electricity—which made possible outdoor lights and a late start of the potluck. The Hudsons' house was roomier than John and Kate's and more equipped for social gatherings. Tables with benches were set end to end behind the kitchen so that all could be seated around what appeared to be one long picnic table, with dishes of food down the middle. Ruth had brought her own contribution this time, a pot of rabbit stew. The dancing would take place after dark, inside on wooden floors where the light was good.

Because the Hudsons' place sat back against several piles of boulders, with many hidden spaces for parking, it took some minutes before Ruth could determine that Matt had not arrived. Then she joined the women on the porch and watched each approaching trail of dust on the dirt road, while children played kick-the-can in front of them. The sun lay low on the horizon when the familiar shape of the Model A finally came into view. She remained seated beside Kate as Matt pulled up, observing as he walked around the car to open the passenger door. First Lily Rose, then her mother exited the automobile.

Ruth noted a tightness in Matt's jaw as he greeted her that was not present when he spoke to others gathered on the porch. He avoided her eyes. He and the two women he brought were only staying for the potluck, he told Martha Hudson as they came up the steps. "We'll leave before the dance. I'm making another trip in to San Bernardino early in the morning, and Lily Rose has to mind the store." Ruth listened closely as he answered Mrs. Hudson's questions about his wife's stay at the sanatorium, his voice brittle beneath the words.

"This must have been a shock. You thought she was getting better," Ruth offered. He looked at her, then, and nodded slowly, his pupils shrinking to tiny dots in the pale blue of his eyes. He looked away.

"Even her doctor had said she was improving," Lily Rose added. "You mustn't blame yourself, Matt. You did everything you could."

"Did I?" Matt said with some bitterness.

Ruth knew it was not himself he was blaming. "What made the doctor believe her improved?" Ruth asked, thinking of her own intuition in the matter.

"Ya, doctor not always know," Kate said, her usually robust face pale. "She die at twenty, my Sarah. I told them, but they not listen."

"May hid the worst from us," Lily said. "She didn't want anyone to know. She made sure even Matt didn't know."

"And if my Lily Rose hadn't come across those bags of soiled tissues, no one would have known until she was dead of it." Mrs. Rose reached over to pat her daughter's arm. "Thank God you cared enough to investigate."

"Mother!" Lily said. "You shouldn't . . ."

"All that blood," Matt said. He bent his head and covered his eyes with one hand. "I never knew."

"I'm so sorry, Matt," Martha Hudson said, her leathery face gone soft with pity. "How long had that been going on?"

"We don't know, Mrs. Hudson," Lily said. "It could have been for some time."

"She wasn't coughing up blood when I left," Ruth remarked.

"I would have known. Even the fevers had left her. She was much stronger." She noticed Matt was staring at her, his face empty of expression.

"Are you sure, Ruth?" Lily asked, a bit of mettle showing beneath her sweetness. "She was very good at hiding things."

"I would have known," Ruth repeated. "I'm sure"—though she couldn't help remembering May's words that morning in the tent.

"Rute is nurse. She know if someting wrong," Kate told Lily. "That morning after the dance, Rute worry about her." Kate looked over at Matt. "Rute knew what to do."

"Maybe she shouldn't have left May for that godforsaken wilderness," Mrs. Rose said. "Then the poor woman might never have worsened."

"I told you she was improved when I left." Ruth got to her feet. "May no longer had need for a nurse. That's why I left," Ruth said, though she knew there was more to the truth, not just the flirtation between her and Matt but the fact that she'd only taken the job to come west and could hardly wait to leave and begin her own life. "I'm going out to see John," Ruth told Kate. She could not bring herself to say "excuse me" to the rest, as she knew was expected. Except for Kate, Ruth didn't care whether they excused her or not.

She walked around the house and out past the crowd of men near the tables, toward an opening in the cluster of boulders, and slipped out of sight behind them. Two ravens rattled their throats and barked at her from the top of the rocks, then flew off. She flattened her back and shoulders against the stone, reaching behind with shaking hands to grip the rough granite. The rock's surface felt solid beneath her fingers. If only she could absorb its stillness to quiet her heart. She took deep breaths, swallowing hard to quell the welling rage and shame. Who were they to pass judgment on her? She should just give them something to pass judgment on, march right back to the porch and slap Matt's sheepish face, grab Lily by the throat and shove her face-first into one of her mother's creamy casseroles.

So now they all accused her—all but Kate. It stood to reason that Matt found it convenient to blame her for his failure to his wife. Well, maybe she had asked for that. It was unfair, but it was the way men usually operated. She'd seen it enough times over those years with Cally. But, God, she hated to compare herself with her mother. She wasn't about to follow that twisty path.

Then why was she fooling around with a married man, she asked herself? Ruth couldn't say that she loved him—she had never loved any of them. But that didn't keep it from hurting when he disregarded her. She was unable to find an answer beyond the fact that he was there, and he attracted her. Maybe that was all there was to it. But, be that as it may, she reminded herself, their couplings had nothing to do with May's worsening. May had never known what went on between them. Ruth was sure that Matt hadn't told her. She wondered for a moment if Lily Rose suspected, might have hinted at it to May, then dismissed the idea; someone as naive as Lily, who knew nothing beyond the inside of a living room, would never entertain such a thought.

Ruth had no desire to go back and face the politeness inside—a civility that was as cool to her as it was warm to Lily. But what was she to do, hide out in the rocks until Matt left? Surely Kate would miss her eventually and come out to find her. Ruth walked on, skirting the backside of the boulder and heading down a path that led toward the interior of the cluster. She had gone only a few yards in when she nearly tripped over a leg that suddenly shot out from a cove in the rocks. She peeked around the corner to see Johnny Lee tipping back a flask, so engrossed that he noticed her only when she spoke.

"What are you doing out here, Johnny? I hope you don't intend to keep all that moonshine to yourself," Ruth said. Maybe there was a way out of her dilemma.

Johnny looked up at her and grinned, pulled on the handlebars of his moustache. "Why, just having myself a little drink or two before dinner. Helps the food go down." He took another swig and held out the flask. "Well, come sit yourself beside me, you sweet thing." He patted the ground next to him with his other hand. "There's nobody I'd rather share with than you, Ruthy."

Ruth settled against the rock next to him. It felt good to find someone glad to see her. She tipped the flask up and took a healthy belt, relishing the sharp burn as the liquor made its way toward her stomach. She took another and passed back the flask. "I forgot how good you do that for a woman," he said. "Haven't seen you drink since . . . well, I guess it was the last dance here at the Hudsons'."

"That was the last whiskey I had," she said. "But I feel in the mood tonight."

"I hear tell you had a run-in with a couple Heart Bar boys," Johnny said. He made a depression in the sand with the flask and left the liquor between them.

"More than one run-in." Ruth felt heat rise to her cheeks. "Then they went through my camp while I was gone and wreaked havoc, deliberately ruined my new garden—the one I had to replant after their cattle stomped out my first one. I was counting on those vegetables. I'll give those cowboys a piece of my mind when I see them." She raised the flask to her lips again.

"That might well be tonight," Johnny Lee said. "They're big trouble, all right, those two. We wouldn't hire 'em over at Mound Springs when they showed up in the area about a year or so ago. Don't need that kind of headache."

"That why you and Stine were fighting at the Swedes'?"

"Nope. There doesn't have to be a why with Stine. I just have to pound that devil every chance he gives me." Lee swigged more whiskey. "How do you think the food's comin' along?"

"Who cares?" Ruth took back the flask from him. She was feeling stronger already.

"Well, I do, kinda. Us cowboys need to eat something besides beans, you know. And they got everthing a man could eat just waiting over there on that table." He waited for her to drink, then took the flask and screwed on the cap. A cactus wren sang out just as the sun vanished behind a red glow above the mountain horizon. "But know what I like best about eatin'? That way you can drink even more before you fall down," he said with a wide grin. "And we got some dancin' to do, darlin'." He got to his feet and reached out a hand to her.

Ruth laughed despite herself. She allowed him to pull her up, stood for a moment until her dizziness passed. "Just one more," she said, "before we go."

He looked reluctant but handed back the flask. "Easy, girl," he said. "Don't worry. There's plenty more in my saddlebag."

Ignoring him, she took a long drink before returning the whiskey. She heard Kate calling her name. "That means it's time to eat, I bet," she said, slipping her arm through the crook of Johnny's held out for her as they walked back toward the crowd.

Ruth sat next to Johnny on the bench, across from Kate and John. She had noticed Matt seated by Lily and her mother down at the far end of the table and made a point of not glancing his way, though it wasn't long before even those next to her became blurred with dim light and whiskey, as did conversation and the differing tastes of the foods on her plate. Sometime during dinner Kate said she was feeling poorly and that she and John would have to leave early. The two of them tried to talk Ruth into going with them instead of staying the night at the Hudsons'. But Ruth was feeling exceptionally fine by this time and was not about to miss the dancing. The evening was just beginning to get exciting. After Johnny Lee walked over to tell John Olsen that he'd "ride lil' Ruthy home if'n she wants to go," the couple gave up and headed out.

Ruth didn't see the Heart Bar crowd ride in when she and Johnny Lee walked back behind the boulder for an after-dinner shot or two, didn't notice them alone at the table when she and Johnny returned and headed into the house to dance. She did notice Lily Rose and her mother waiting in the car while Matt conversed with some men on the porch. Ruth went inside and vowed to think no more of him, but he came up beside her when Johnny went to get her a glass of water.

When Matt whispered her name, she turned to look at him. "Just look at you," he hissed. "You look like a drunken slut." The mixture of hatred, lust, and jealousy on his face seemed to knock her back against the wall she'd been leaning on. Then he turned away and was gone, and Johnny was there with a glass of water. Then they were dancing to the fiddles, and she was having trouble keeping on her feet during the peppy steps of fast tunes, Johnny Lee steadying her so she did not fall. It was her disequilibrium that knocked her against Charlie Stine as Johnny spun her around.

"Watch where you're going, squaw woman," he said. Ruth heard him clearly, but before she could respond, Johnny had pulled her away into the whirl of dancers again. For the rest of that tune, she kept hearing Stine's voice repeating those words in her head, a dark stillness in the blurred world of motion around her. When the song ended, Ruth broke away from Johnny and ran toward the door, where she'd seen Stine last, searching all the bleary faces for his as she went. She would kill that man. Another dance began and Johnny followed, catching hold of her and trying to pull her back onto the dance floor. She wrenched herself from his grasp and marched toward the door, Stine's voice and Matt's expression fused into a hot poker to goad her.

· Ruth found Stine on the porch with the rest of the Heart Bar cowboys. She didn't hesitate, but cut through the small crowd, pushing the men between them aside until she stood staring straight up into his face. "What did you say to me in there?" she demanded.

"You heard me," he said, pulling his hat brim down.

"Say it again, then. I dare you." Ruth stepped a few inches closer to him. The men around them shuffled and guffawed.

"I don't like to repeat myself," Stine said.

Ruth pushed at his chest. "Say it," she yelled. "Say it, you son of a bitch. I double dare you." Behind her she heard Johnny calling.

"All right, then, squaw woman. I said to watch where you're going," he said calmly, steadying himself. "And careful where you put your hands." Stine leaned over and stuck his face next to hers. "Squaw woman," he jeered.

Ruth struck him with all the force she could pack into her fist. It was enough, along with the surprise of it, to knock the man against the porch rail. His hat flew off into the dirt. Before he could recover and turn on her, she felt herself being pulled back and swung to the side, and would have fallen had she not crashed into the wall beside the doorjamb. Johnny had removed her and jumped in, in her place. Furious at being rescued, she strode back toward the men, grabbed hold of Johnny's arm, which was now pounding Stine's face, and tried to pull him away. "He's mine," she yelled. "Get away."

Maybe it was because the cowboys who pulled her off were laughing at her that she began trying to punch them instead. Then the porch was crowded with men, and everyone was shouting and arguing. Martha Hudson was peeking out from the doorway, along with the other women behind her. Larry Hudson was trying to hold Ruth still and quiet her. "What did the man do, dear?" Hudson kept saying, and "Why don't you go inside now?" Someone had pulled Johnny Lee off of Stine, who lay on the porch groaning. Johnny brushed off his chaps and walked over to her.

"Come on, Ruthy, I'll take you home," he said. "He won't bother you for a while."

"What did the man do, Johnny?" Hudson called as they walked away. "Don't you think you should just take the poor woman inside?" He stepped off the porch after them into the moonlight as Johnny pulled Ruth up behind him on his horse. He wrapped her arms around his waist.

"Now hold on tight, darlin'," he said, and kicked the horse.

Ruth clung to the wiry body in front of her, while wind whipped back her hair. Each gallop of the horse threatened to toss her body out into the night. The events behind her became hazy and dissociated, swept away by the huge animal power that thrust her body up again and again. Sweat trickled between her legs where they rubbed the beast's back.

After that, the night grew holes, blank except for a flash or two that came back when she half woke the next morning, her eyes sealed against the light: she and Johnny on sand somewhere while the horse drank; the two of them bending to drink water like horses; more whiskey; Johnny pulling at her clothes; her pushing him away; back on the horse again, then down; her throwing up; Johnny leading her somewhere to lie down. She fought against the consciousness restoring these memories, but the early sun was drilling heat into her face; she turned over, but it drilled harder into her back. The boulder she'd buried seemed to have risen and attached itself to her shoulders; it was all Ruth could do to crawl into the shade behind a juniper and fall back asleep. When she woke again, her mouth dry as sand, her head felt a bit less dense; she looked around—first to find the water she craved, then to question her surroundings and the fact that she had been left sleeping on the bare ground. Neither Johnny Lee nor his sorrel was anywhere around. Attempting to piece together what had happened from the few flashes left made her brain hurt more, and her heart and dignity as well, so she quit trying and concentrated on finding water.

She managed to sit up, her head growing more massive as she rose and throbbing violently. But she began to recognize the landscape; though she had never seen it from quite this angle, her outhouse was not ten feet away. When she reached the privy, Ruth realized her underwear was missing and the top of her dress had come unbuttoned.

The distance to the water cooler seemed insurmountable, but her need was great. By the time Ruth reached it, her head was screaming, and she could hardly drink. Her stomach kept wanting to hurl up what the rest of her body demanded. From the tent, already swollen with the sun's excess heat, Ruth retrieved a pillow for her sore head so she could lie in the shade of the pinyon, and fell into another strange semi-sleep for several hours. By late afternoon her body had begun to revive, and with its revival came a further deepening of memory. She lay under the tree, her mind clearing while her eyes followed the motion of the pine branches in afternoon breeze. Odd fragments of recollection came to her. She remembered coming to, finding Johnny's hands on her breasts. He was slamming himself between her legs, where she had been open and enjoying him in her stupor. She had bent her legs and shoved him off.

She recalled him crawling back for her, apologetic, mumbling her name, his face drunken and desperate in its desire. In the half moonlight she saw the flash of belt buckle around his knees. The shine of skin on his thighs. She had met him halfway, pushing him over sideways and backward. Then she rode him, plunging, the way she had ridden the horse, galloping his body into the night. Anger had put a sharp edge to her lust, bursts of pleasure exploded inside her. She had never felt more powerful and had meant to ride the man into the ground. Like a lion, she would devour all of them, every last one. Again and again the man pushed himself up into her and she rode him down. Someone was laughing, shouting out, "Ride 'em, cowboy!" There was a point where Johnny had cried out, but she had kept pounding on. A voice was laughing and sobbing at the same time. She felt him struggling under her as he yelled for her to stop, calling her names when she pressed on. But she did not stop—not until he lifted and pushed her upward and she was catapulted into the night.

Well, Ruth thought, I guess I got carried away. A dark laugh bubbled up as a hiccup, and a vise gripped the sides of her head. She closed her eyes. Not that she thought any of it funny. But it was better than worrying about the stories that mouthy cowboy would tell about her. Getting to her knees, Ruth put a hand on the trunk of the pinyon and pulled herself to her feet. She finished unbuttoning her dress, let it fall to her feet, and stepped out of it. She needed to bathe herself, but hauling water was out of the question. At least she still had time to use the vinegar and herbs.

Ruth ate a few beans cold from the can and drank water till her stomach sloshed. She didn't allow her mind to dwell on anything beyond her own thirst and hunger, the calls of quail watering at her spring, crickets warming up in the bushes at sunset, a coyote beginning to yip in the distance. Gradually, the canyon reassured her.

Gathering her .22 and the shotgun from under the back edge of her outhouse, where since Stine's last visit she had taken to hiding them when she left her camp unattended, she set both beside her cot—as if she might use them to chase away any other memories that crept up on her. But when she blew out the lamp and lay alone in the tent, moon illuminating the white canvas, she was visited by the question she had avoided earlier: Just who was this woman she was becoming, this woman so out of control? What would become of her? Ruth had been thrilled to leave behind the constraints that had been placed on her in El Paso. But what was to replace them? She had spent her whole life fighting others' attempts to control her. Now that no one else was around to control her, Ruth wasn't really sure she knew how—or why, or when—she should control herself. And the more she broke the rules, it appeared, the more rules she was willing to break. That could be as bad in its own way as ending up being someone like Mrs. Hudson or, worse yet, Mrs. Rose. It was the old choice between Cally or Aunt Myrtle all over again. Ruth was neither, would be neither. But what then, how was she to know how to be, even here in this place where she could be free? Or was she truly free? she wondered. Were there things that this place itself required of her?

Ruth woke the next morning filled with worry over Kate. In a dream she couldn't remember the details of, she had seen Kate's face pale, all jolliness gone from her eyes. As Ruth built a fire for coffee, she made up her mind to walk down after breakfast to see if Kate had recovered from her ailment. Ruth felt much recovered herself, her mind clear and fresh again, her body filled with energy. And she was ravenous. Her thoughts from the night before now seemed unreal. What was done could not be undone— and why should she place restraints upon her inclinations? Wasn't that exactly what made women the submissive creatures she despised?

While she waited for water to boil, Ruth inspected the rock walls of her cabin. It seemed strange not to start her day by mixing concrete, but when John Olsen had come up to get her for the dance, he told her not to add another layer. "Is good, Rute," he had said, walking around the rectangle, bending now and again to eye the evenness of the structure. "Fine level." He nodded in approval. "Build rest with wood now. I come and get you started." The two of them had surveyed what remained of her building supplies, which was everything but the cement and the planks she had used on the boulder.

She would need to learn new skills to finish her cabin. Laying the rocks had been backbreaking work, but simple. Constructing walls and a roof with wood would be more complicated than nesting stones in cement. This time, Ruth decided as she started down the road toward the Swedes', if John suggested the help of his men, she would accept at once. He had at least offered to get her started.

Ruth arrived at the Olsens' to find Kate's face still as wan as the night of the dance, though the woman claimed that she felt her old self. "It was someting I eat," Kate said. "Too much. Ya, I try everyting." Her good humor had certainly returned. John Olsen, along with Jim and the miners, had taken a load of onyx down to the valley to sell. She had hoped to ask John when he might be up to help her with the construction, but Kate assured her that John had said he would come up to help soon. "Now, come," Kate ordered her. "Time for the coffee."

Afterward, the two of them walked to the garden, where she helped Kate with the weeding. The uninvited thrived also in the dark, rich soil. Kate raised the small dam to let stream water run into the rows as they worked. In Ruth's small patch at Glory Springs, the spring runoff rose on its own and flowed from the little pool to saturate her garden soil sometime during each night, and then the soil became dry again during the heat of the summer day. When they had weeded and watered and picked the ripened vegetables, the women returned to the house. Kate heated up a stew with goat meatballs and vegetables and made biscuits for lunch on the outdoor stove beneath the cottonwoods that she used during the day to keep the house cool.

Ruth had been waiting to ask Kate about the Sarah she had spoken of that night at the Hudsons', wondering if that memory had been the cause of her feeling poorly, but she struggled with just how to ask. Finally, as they sat at the window watching a nanny trying to fend off twin kids from her teats, Ruth blurted out, "Tell me about Sarah, Kate. Who was she?"

"It was long time ago. Twenty year. Before we came to this canyon." Kate said after a short silence, her face and body drooping as she continued. "She was our only child, Sarah. When she gone, we came here." She pushed up from the table and shuffled toward the pantry, which tunneled from the kitchen into the hill behind the house. Ruth waited until Kate returned with a tin box. Setting it carefully on the table, Kate unlatched the lid and opened the box.

The girl in the photos she spread on the table was as blond as Ruth was dark. Not a frilly blond, like Lily Rose, but sturdy and as capable as Kate. Ruth put her hand on Kate's arm. "She was beautiful," Ruth said. "And strong. I'm so sorry, Kate. It must have been . . . been so hard."

Kate's face looked tired as she gathered up the pictures and locked them back in the box. Her face had aged ten years since Ruth asked her question, and she was sorry she'd stirred things up.

"It was the cancer," Kate said, placing a hand on her breast. "My mother and sister too. I told them. But Sarah . . . she was the hardest." Kate took the box back to the pantry.

Though Ruth had intended to leave after lunch, now she could not, and she and Kate spent the rest of the afternoon outside in the shade of the cottonwood, Kate telling stories about her life in the old country as they prepared a huge chicken stew for John and the miners to eat when they returned. Chopping vegetables as she listened, Ruth admired the way Kate had been able to retain such a generous and caring nature despite a life that would have warped a lesser person out of shape, the way it had Cally, giving her a mean and selfish edge that Ruth had been the recipient of time and again. Kate's spirit was as abundant as her body.

As for Ruth's stories, it took persistent probing on Kate's part to get her to begin telling stories of her own growing up. Once started, she could not stop, and the two women were still deep in conversation when the flatbed drove into sight, and neither of them had heard its approach.

Ruth ended up staying for the stew she had helped to prepare. The miners, even John, brought back with them the odor of whiskey on their breath—just the smell was almost more than Ruth could stomach after her own adventure. It was during their stop at the Red Dog Cafe, a thinly disguised speakeasy like the Lone Star, that they'd run into Matt Baxter, who told them that May had weakened even more. Her condition was so serious that Matt was returning to San Bernardino to spend some days near her. Ruth felt a rush of sympathy for the woman. It was a revelation to find that her thoughts were for May and not at all for the husband she had coveted and now disliked intensely. Ruth pictured herself begging the dying woman to forgive her—and no doubt May would. Ruth would not confess, of course, since she still hoped May knew nothing.

Jim had arrived with the miners, but disappeared soon after they unloaded. Ruth was pleased to see him return shortly after they sat for supper. He nodded and sat at the table across from her. Ruth smiled, then turned her attention back to John, who was talking about their work in the low desert mines during winter. She'd felt her cheeks flush at Jim's glance and could not look back again. His eyes had shaken loose the memory of her night with Johnny Lee, only now she was sure Jim had observed it all. But that was impossible, she knew—simply a product of her imagination and the guilt she tried to disown. But what was it about this man that tortured her conscience and left her with a shame she could not escape?

The moment he spoke, asking how her damaged garden had survived the cowboys' trampling, all tightness left her. "Between the two of us, I think we saved about half of it," she said. "Lost most of the squash. All but two plants." She took a breath and met his look full on. It contained no disapproval.

"The story's around town that you showed those cowboys a thing or two that night at the Hudsons'," Jim said, smiling. The miners around him were smiling at her too.

Ingmar patted Ruth on the back. "Ya, hear you was tiger after him."

"A lion, actually," Ruth said. The miners laughed out loud. Only John looked at her with concern.

"You keep shotgun handy, Rute?" he asked.

"By my bed."

Jim glanced over by the door. "Then I hope you brought it

with you today," he said. "You might run into those two on the road again sometime."

Ruth shook her head. "You're right, though." She must get into the habit of bringing the gun with her, though she hated the idea that their threat should place such a limitation on her freedom—that even in her own canyon she could not travel safely. And that damn gun was heavy to carry.

Before Jim drove Ruth home, John Olsen assured her that he would be up in a few days to get her started on the rest of her cabin, and even though she sensed some mystery in John's demeanor, she trusted him and left feeling lighter inside than she had felt in some time. She looked forward to being home and to having soon a real house of her own. Small and primitive as it would be, Ruth knew the stone structure would stand strong for a long time. To have neighbors like Jim and the Olsens was fortunate. She realized, as the truck bumped its way up the rut road, that she had no desire to see Matt Baxter again. And who knew what else lay ahead for her; she could see no more of the future, she thought, than she could see ahead of her on the dim path illuminated by the truck's headlamps, the vague shapes of shrubbery looming for an instant, then folding into the darkness the way events melt back into the times surrounding them.

CHAPTER NINE

Ruth took the east ridge up the mountain so she would have an unobstructed view of the road between her place and the Swedes'. But when she reached the high ridge, she saw no sign of a flatbed inching its way up canyon. Blood pulsing against her temples from exertion in afternoon heat, she flung herself down under a pinyon. A week had passed without her seeing a sign of John Olsen, and her patience had worn as thin as a page in her journal. Jim had walked up three days ago to take an inventory of her construction materials, so she was sure Olsen did plan to help her. But she wanted to get on with it. For the first few days she'd counted herself lucky to have time to climb around and explore, to hunt fresh meat for her table each night. But she tired quickly of the novelty, finding it impossible to concentrate on exploration when her overriding concern was for completing her cabin. She found nothing more aggravating than waiting, and it was only her determination to have a cabin that would last that kept her from attempting to finish the place herself.

Ruth poured a dab of canteen water in her palm to wet her face, then peeled off her blouse so the light wind could reach the sweat on her torso. She was about to remove her boots and lie back beneath the pine when she noticed a rider in the canyon below, just the other side of the bend down from her camp. Reaching for her .22, she placed it across her lap and tried to make out more details.

Before the figure disappeared behind the ridge, she determined that he wasn't riding Stine's big buckskin, but a small sorrel—like Johnny Lee's. The man didn't seem large enough to be Stine, either; his frame appeared wiry—also like Lee. But why would Lee be returning after what had happened? Ruth slipped on her blouse as she rose, gathered up the rifle and canteen, and started down the mountain, buttoning her blouse with her free hand.

It was some time before she got another clear sighting of the man. By then he was already parked in a chair at her camp, tipping back a flask while his horse grazed near the spring. The closer view confirmed that he was indeed Johnny Lee. Better Johnny than Charlie Stine, Ruth told herself as she stopped on the way down for the shotgun she had concealed underneath a scrub oak. But she didn't want to see either of them, not anyone but Jim and John Olsen—and the crew of miners she hoped John would bring.

Lee rose when Ruth walked into camp, smiling hugely beneath his moustache. An empty whiskey bottle sat propped against the saddle on the ground beside him. He paid no attention to the two guns she was carrying. "Why, there you are, little darlin'. I wondered where you'd got yourself to," he said, snaking an arm around her as she walked. Each word he spoke floated toward her in a cloud of whiskey breath.

Ruth shrugged him off and claimed the chair he had vacated, sitting with the guns erect between her legs. "Don't be like that, sweetheart," Johnny said, squatting in front of her. He took her hand. "I'm sorry I ran off like that, Ruthy. But you like to of scared the bejesus out of me. Never before have I seen a gal like you." He pulled her hand toward his puckered lips.

Ruth shoved his hand away. With her foot, she pushed him over on his backside, his hat bouncing between them. The man cried out, then got to his knees and reached around to his back pocket for a small glass flask. "Almost broke it," he said. Unscrewing the cap, he brought the container to his lips, but stopped without taking a drink. He held the flask out to Ruth instead.

Ruth shook her head. "C'mon, Ruthy, I know you like this stuff. I 'member the things you like," he said with a sloppy smile.

"Why did you come back here, Johnny?" Ruth got to her feet. "What do you want with me?" She stepped around the man and his hat and walked to her tent with the firearms.

"You know what I want with you, Ruthy. You know why I came back," he called after her. Laying the .22 on her bed, she cracked the shotgun. The shells were intact. She slammed it shut and flicked off the safety. Lee was standing, hat held in front just below his waist, when Ruth charged out of the tent with the shotgun.

"You can get right back on your horse and leave," she told him.

"Now, darlin', you don't have to be like that." Lee put on his hat. "Shucks, I don't want nothin' more than to do the right thing by you. I want to marry you, gal." He stood before her, grinning wider than ever.

"What are you talking about? I'm not marrying you, Johnny Lee."

"Sure you are, Ruthy. Wouldn't be right not to, after what happened between us." He tipped back his hat with the back of a hand. "'Course, it all scared me at first. Didn't know what to do with all that—comin' from a little thing like you. But I'm ready for you now."

"I don't know what you're talking about. Now, go on and get out of here."

"I'm not going nowhere without you, darlin'. I'll ride you down to the preacher right now, or we can wait for mornin'."

Ruth brought the shotgun up to her shoulder. "You're riding off, all right, but not with me."

Johnny pulled the flask from his hip pocket and unscrewed the top. "Go ahead," he said, "shoot me if you want. My life's in your hands, Ruthy." He raised the flask and took several swallows.

Ruth took aim. Johnny blotted his moustache with the back of a hand and looked at her. "Sure you don't want some?" He held the flask out to her, then took another swallow himself. Ruth lowered the gun.

"I knowed you wouldn't shoot a man who loved you," Johnny said, stepping toward her. Ruth moved back fast.

"Don't press your luck," she said. "I want you to leave, Johnny."

"Say you'll marry me first."

"I won't marry you. I told you that."

"But you have to, sugar darlin'."

"No, I don't. I won't. Now get out of here."

"Nope," Johnny said, straightening his hat brim. "You'll have to shoot this cowpoke first, drag my carcass off."

"That can be arranged," Ruth said, raising the shotgun. Johnny grinned, crossed his arms, and looked at her, teetering on legs spread wide apart.

"Oh, for godsake," Ruth said, walking past him toward the campfire. "Stand there like an idiot, then. I'm going to fix myself coffee and something to eat."

Ruth set the shotgun beside her and piled the kindling into the fire ring. Johnny Lee stumbled after her, bending occasionally to put in a stray stick, all the while keeping up a barrage of slurred nonsense meant to persuade her. She lit the fire and filled the coffeepot from her water bucket, then pulled the rabbit she'd shot that morning from her cooler and began to braise it, stymied as to how to rid herself of this drunken cowboy who only stopped talking long enough to slug down more whiskey. His behavior might well have been funny, if it weren't so annoying.

Likable as he could be, Ruth had no desire for a repeat of the other night—how desperate and drunk she must have been—let alone a lifetime with him. Look at the complications that just one encounter had wrought.

Johnny Lee collapsed into the camp chair as Ruth worked. Gradually, he began to wind down and soon quit talking completely. Between belts he sat staring off at the mountain with glazed eyes. When Ruth served up two plates of food—thinking to sober him out of his delusions—and pulled up the other camp chair for herself, he didn't respond. His plate of rabbit and beans stayed untouched on the top of Ruth's flat rock table.

Ruth was half finished with her plate when Johnny Lee rose from the chair and staggered over to the rock table. "Iff'n you don't say you'll marry me, I'll cut this here finger off," he blurted out suddenly. He had her carving knife in one hand.

"Don't be crazy," Ruth told him. She turned her head and continued to chew the mouthful of food she had taken.

"Marry me then?"

"Put down the knife, Johnny."

"Not'll you say yes." He pressed the knife against his left index finger.

"I'll not." She kept her head turned away as long as she could stand it. When she looked back, she found him sawing small cuts into his flesh, his face screwed up with pain, squinting as if to see through the dimming dusk or an alcohol fog. "Goddamn it, Johnny, stop that stupidity!"

He kept cutting.

Ruth rose abruptly from her chair and lunged for the knife. Drunk as he was, the cowboy sidestepped her movement and lifted the knife out of her reach, leaving the hand with the wounded finger on the rock to support him. "Say it," he said.

Ruth looked down at the bloodied finger, sliced open just above the knuckle. "You're a fool, Johnny Lee. A drunken fool," she said, wincing and turning away as he brought the knife back down to make several snapping chops at his target. Ruth swung back around and ran straight for him, knocking him over sideways.

"Now whadcha do that for?" he mumbled, fumbling to his knees, then collapsed back onto the dirt. He crawled forward toward the fallen knife, fell again, took in a breath, then lay still. "Ruffy," he slurred. "My lil' Ruffy." When Ruth walked around to pick up the knife, his eyes were closed. Soon he began to snore.

His lil' Ruthy, indeed. The arrogance of that assumption was as crass as Matt's blaming her for May's worsening. Staring down at his injured finger, Ruth was seized with pity and anger—and intense relief. Still, Johnny had a good heart. And the man could dance, she'd give him that. At any rate, the finger appeared not to be bleeding much, from what she could see of it in the fading twilight. She had no desire to tend it at the moment; nursing had never come naturally to her.

Ruth threw a couple of chunks of pine on the fire and poured herself a cup of hot coffee. She settled into the camp chair, then had another thought. She removed Lee's flask from his back pocket and dumped the remaining shot of whiskey into her cup. The smell of it no longer repulsed her. After she drained her cup, Ruth lit the kerosene lamp and examined Johnny's finger. It pained her to see how his last hacking had further mutilated the flesh around the original cut.

Lee's saddlebags held another, bigger bottle of whiskey. She poured some over the cut, then soaked the finger in water. When the crusted blood softened, she used a damp cloth to clean the wound the best she could while he groaned and resisted from his stupor. White bone was clearly visible at the heart of the slice. The cowboy yelled out and opened his eyes when Ruth painted the injury with iodine, but was asleep again by the time she bound it with a strip of soft bandage. Storing the leftover rabbit in the cooler, she refilled Lee's flask and set it beside him, before pouring a sizable shot into a fresh cup of coffee. She stashed the bottle among her underwear in the tent.

At daybreak Ruth heard the cowboy stirring. After some initial groaning and shuffling around outside the tent, all was quiet, so she dressed and pulled back the tent flap to see if he had left. His saddle remained beside the chair. Craning her neck, she saw him down at her spring, washing his face in the pool she drew water from, which annoyed her greatly. She peed, then built a fire for coffee before he climbed the wash bank. "Guess I got a little drunk last night," he said, coming up beside her. He looked down at his mutilated finger.

"You should keep the bandage on. That's a deep cut," Ruth told him.

"You're not gonna marry me, huh?"

Ruth shook her head. She turned to measure out coffee.

"I might as well go, then," he said.

"Suit yourself. Have coffee first, if you like. Water'll boil soon."

Lee picked up his saddle and carried it to the wash. Ruth had just stirred coffee into the water and pulled the pot off to settle when he led his sorrel up the bank. Neither of them spoke as they sat drinking coffee. His second cup, he doctored with whiskey, then held it out to her. She refused.

"There's leftover rabbit in the cooler if you're hungry," she said a few minutes later as he drained the last of the cup.

"Naw, it's too early for food," he said. "I'll take a hunk with me if you got enough."

She wrapped one leg in waxed paper and put another on the grill to heat for herself, since she was running low on oatmeal. "You want me to rebandage that for you?" she asked as she handed him the rabbit.

"I'll manage." He turned and walked toward his horse. "But thanks for the food." He put a foot in the stirrup and swung the other leg over. For a moment he sat looking down at her. "I don't understand you, gal, I swear. I thought we had somethin' goin'. Makes me wonder just what kind of a woman you are, anyway." He spurred the horse to a trot toward the road, then galloped nearly to the bend, where he slowed to a trot, then a walk as he disappeared at the apex.

Ruth took in a deep breath, feeling the canyon expand at his absence. She ate the rabbit leg, finished off the pot of coffee, and was just wondering what to do with her day when she heard the drone of an approaching motor—a large one, from the sound of it. From the bank of the wash, she verified that the motor belonged to Olsen's flatbed. Not only did the flatbed round the bend, but two Model T's followed behind as well. The moment she saw them, Ruth understood. She would be having a house raising! No wonder John had been so mysterious about it all.

Men spilled from the truck and other vehicles like ants from a hill, unloading materials as they came. A few nodded to her. John Olsen gave a wave from beside the flatbed's cab, where Jim was filling a crate. Ruth wanted to hug them both. Besides Olsen's crew, there were Larry Hudson, Jake Tunstall, Vince and George Talmadge, Bob Thompson, and several men whose names Ruth couldn't remember. Amazed as she had been to see all the men, she was even more astonished when Martha Hudson and Jane Thompson climbed out of the automobiles and began lugging a crate toward her campfire.

"Morning, Ruth," Martha Hudson said as Ruth walked up to greet them. The Thompson woman nodded as they carted the crate past Ruth to her rock table. Their polite coolness puzzled her; had they come to the house raising just to snub her?

"Martha. Jane," Ruth said, nodding back. "This is a real surprise. I hardly know what to say."

"I can imagine," Martha said. "It doesn't appear that you were expecting us."

"No one had told me you were coming. Not even you, Jim," Ruth said to the Indian when he appeared with another crate of foodstuffs and dishes. "I was expecting only John and maybe the rest of his men."

"John wanted to surprise you," Jim said. "We weren't sure if we could put it together."

"Certainly, that cowboy, Johnny Lee, we passed on the way up was unaware anyone was coming," Jane Thompson said. "Robert tried to talk him into returning to join the work party. He appeared uninterested . . . seemed insulted to be asked."

"Well, Mr. Lee hasn't been seen since Ruth rode off with him that night. So the house raising must have surprised him," Martha said. "It appears Ruth has seen him, though," she added.

"He's in the canyon often," Jim said, "like other cowboys. Rounding up strays."

The two women glanced at each other. Jane Thompson reached into the crate and brought out two loaves of bread. "I'll bet," she said, setting the loaves on the rock table. "No telling what goes on this far from the civilized world."

Ruth swallowed hard and looked away from the two women. "Kate didn't come?" she asked Jim.

"She said her stomach was troubled again. But she sent up a pot of quail stew and the pastries," he said.

"The men do have to eat after all the hard work," Jane Thompson explained, as Jim walked off to join the others gathered next to the cabin walls. "That's why we're here instead of at May Baxter's funeral."

Ruth put her hand on the rock. "When did it happen?"

"May passed away three days ago. Such a shame. She was a lovely woman." Martha Hudson's face took on a somber cast as she turned from unloading the crate. She looked at the ground and shook her head. "A good woman," she said. "The very best." She pulled a handkerchief from her dress pocket and dabbed at her eyes.

"The burial is in Los Angeles," the Thompson woman said, putting a hand on Martha Hudson's shoulder. "Personally, I think the house raising should have been postponed so more of us could make the trip in. Martha and I both have family there, you understand. Los Angeles is our home."

"That would have been fine by me," Ruth said. "After all, I wasn't even aware anyone was coming."

Martha straightened and turned back to her food duties. "That's why Agnes Rose isn't here; the Roses have accompanied poor Matt to the service."

"Of course, they've closed the store for now. Agnes said Lily will open it again when she returns . . . run it until the man can get over his grief." She turned to Jane. "Oh, he looked so stricken. As if it were all his fault."

Ruth rekindled the fire while the women continued to discuss details of the event that Ruth did not care to hear—the color of Lily's dress, the look on Matt's face, the terrible loss the community had sustained. She didn't know how to extricate herself, so she hauled a bucket of fresh water, filled the coffeepot, and collected more wood for the fire. Just as she was ready to slip over and watch how the men were constructing the rest of her cabin, Martha Hudson said, "I don't see, Ruth, how anyone can possibly live in this place." The woman shook her head. "Even when your shack is built, you'll never have running water or electricity. It's beyond me why you decided to stay in this wilderness."

"If you ask me, the isolation here is unnatural. You have no one to help you if something happened, nobody to talk to. Any normal person would just go plain crazy," Jane Thompson said. "Whatever do you do with yourself . . . between visitors, I mean? Isn't it boring?"

"I'm never bored," Ruth said, her voice tight with the effort of having to explain. She looked over at the developing cabin. "Constructing the walls has taken most of my time so far. But I like to explore the mountains when I'm not busy. Sometimes I follow animal tracks—Jim's showing me how to read them. He can tell all kinds of things from just looking at a track," she said, forgetting herself as she remembered. "I like to sit and watch the birds and animals too. The canyon is full of squirrels and chipmunks and rabbits and . . ."

"Such pests—you must have snakes, too . . . and mice. How annoying."

"And even lizards in your camp. Those creepy things give me the chills," Jane Thompson said.

"You better move quickly, then, ladies," Ruth told them on a whim, as the sweet sound of hammers echoed off the bluff. "Because there's one right there on the rock near Martha's arm."

Their reaction would cheer Ruth the rest of the day, even if one of Martha's casseroles next to the crate did get knocked off the rock and the bucket of water Ruth had hauled got kicked over by Jane Thompson's left foot when she stepped in it. In all the ruckus, neither of the women saw any sign of Ruth's lizard. But Ruth knew lizards move fast—and there could well have been one. She was not sorry in the least.

The incident freed her to inspect the cabin's construction whenever she liked and to stand around and watch the section of wall develop above the stone ledge, then rafters and a roof go up. She found it difficult to study the workers' methods, with all the hammering and sawing and measuring going on at the same time. No one seemed interested in answering her questions, except Jim, and she could see that even he would rather work than explain. Finally, John Olsen chased her out, saying that they wanted her to wait and see the cabin when they finished.

The women had pulled the camp chairs into the shade, rising occasionally to tend the food on the fire. Ruth joined them, relating stories of living in the wild that she knew they'd detest. She pointed out the "clothesline" where she hung her rabbits to skin them, going on in detail about the process. While they were enjoying a drink from her water cooler, she showed them the green patch of her spring and bragged about the clean water, with very few bugs and water skaters to clean out when she filled her buckets. Only once, she told them, had she found a dead chipmunk in the pool. There weren't too many bears this low down on the mountain, either, she said, like the one she'd found in her tent. After that story, Ruth was delighted to see how their eyes kept constant vigil on the mountain. She could not understand just why, with their city ways, they would choose to live out on the desert. Even with running water and electricity, the area was still rife with wild creatures. The women seemed to have no liking for anything outside their modern homes. She supposed that if people like that had their way, there would be no desert, but a mere extension of cities like Los Angeles. It was not so much that they were women, she discovered, that made them so different from her; it was some ingrained attitude, as if they were of another species altogether.

The house-raising was completed well before sunset. By that time Ruth was so impatient to see the results that she could no longer sit—or even stand, for that matter—so she busied herself with mixing biscuit dough and filling another coffeepot and water bucket. She knew John Olsen and Jim were coming for her almost before they took the first step in her direction. The two men waited with the rest of the workers while she stood outside her newly hung door and took in a deep breath. Then she swung the door open and stepped inside. The concrete slab and rock walls she had spent so many hours making had been transformed completely. With just the addition of a bit of wood and roofing paper—window frames, too, though there was yet no glass for them—the place had become a home. She was nearly overcome when she saw they had installed a small two-burner woodstove, which must have come up with the truck. Rust adhered to her palm as she swept her hand across the iron surface. The men had followed her inside and watched as she fought the great wave of gratitude that enveloped her. Ruth did not bother to hide her struggle, knowing that it was in part their payment. She turned to face the group, seeing a pleasure on their tired faces that intensified when she swiped at her eyes and told them, "Thank you. Thank you so much."

Her gratitude was so genuine it extended itself to the women as well—at least it did at the moment when she walked back outside and glimpsed a softening in their expressions, some interest in how much the house-raising had meant to her. "Thank you, too, neighbors," she said, and meant it. She wondered if perhaps, after all, there existed a connection deeper and more important than all the differences between them. Then the moment passed, their faces tightened, and things went on as before.

The men, who had been helping themselves to bread and casseroles throughout the afternoon, now settled down to Kate's quail stew and the pot of chili and beans Martha and Jane had prepared. Ruth fixed two batches of biscuits and a big pot of coffee to accompany the meal. When all the cups were replenished and her second batch of biscuits off the fire, she dished herself out a plate and sat down on the ground between John Olsen and Jim, who were already to the point of mopping up the last of their food with a biscuit.

"Jim bring up glass for your window few days from now. First we haul load of onyx," John said as Ruth settled in between them. Ruth leaned over and hugged his shoulder.

"You know how much I appreciate all this, John. I don't know how I can ever repay you," she said.

"You neighbor, Rute," he said, shrugging off her obligation, though she could see he was pleased. "Work hard you do. I glad to help."

"Thank you, too, Jim," Ruth said to the Indian, who had been watching them without speaking. He nodded in response.

"I heard those two giving you trouble earlier," he said quietly, his eyes flashing to the women in the camp chairs.

Ruth looked into his face, past the question she saw there. "Thanks for that, too," she said.

"There's talk, Rute," John told her. "You know that."

"I don't care. It's none of their business," she said. Neither man responded.

"He came up drunk yesterday wanting to marry me," Ruth said, softening. Their silence had nudged her. She brought her voice down lower. "Did you see his finger? He threatened to cut it off if I wouldn't say yes. Then he passed out. I like to never got rid of him." John laughed and patted her back. He rose and walked toward the food beside the campfire. When Ruth looked back at Jim, he was smiling. He touched a finger to her upper arm and when she glanced down she saw he was making a bridge for a ladybug to climb from her to him. With the bug aboard his finger, he raised it and the insect flew off into the air.

"You will be careful, won't you, Ruth?" he asked, when the beetle had left his hand. "I don't want anything bad happening to you."

Ruth was never sure whether it was his care with the insect, the feel of that touch, the sound in his voice, or maybe the way his eyes seemed to pull her into them, but something about that moment connected and bound her to him. His eyes remained on her, and she felt some deep stirring in her center that drew her toward him. It was a new and strange sensation, as if she were barely able to force her body to stay where it was, seated next to him, close, but not close enough. She felt heat in her cheeks as she wrenched her eyes away.

CHAPTER TEN

The cabin seemed cavernous compared to her tiny tent, and Ruth felt an odd reluctance to sleep there that first night, staying another night in her old surroundings to prepare herself. One of the men, she wrote in her journal, had measured the cabin at 13 feet 5 inches by 19 feet 2 inches, all of them laughing at the idea of someone building a structure of such uneven dimensions. But Ruth had seen no need to measure when she laid out the form for her slab; she simply marked out the area that best fit under the pines. She didn't know why they should think even measurements would be more suitable. Suitable for whom? she wondered, content with a method that suited herself.

The following morning Ruth cleaned up the construction scraps—collecting a sizable pile of kindling for her new stove—

and began carting furniture into her cabin. The bed, chest of drawers, writing table, and chair that had crowded the tent left the room still looking bare. She stacked the two boxes of books beneath her writing table and the crates of groceries in the far corner, then went out to look through the larger remnants of lumber, hoping to find enough to construct a makeshift shelf. The only usable wood turned out to be the sheets of plyboard John Olsen had left, but that was meant for building a shelter around her open privy seats, which he said she would need before long. With the days still hot, Ruth had trouble believing cold weather would soon move in, though twice lately she had pulled up her extra blanket during the night.

She didn't see Jim again for five days and had put the incident at the house-raising firmly from her mind, concentrating on settling into a life that didn't involve hours each morning spent constructing her dwelling, dividing her day between exploring crevices of the surrounding mountains and the pages of books in the boxes. They were difficult books, but interesting, written by men with foreign names that she wasn't sure how to say. She thought it a strange delight to come in from her wild canyon and lie on her cot, reading about people in crowded European cities—which is what she was doing when she heard the flatbed motor.

The sound brought blood rushing to her head. It must be Jim with the windowpanes. She jerked up from the bed, her heart picking up where it had left off a few days before. She paced the length of the cabin twice, then walked out into the yard, down to the spring and back again before the vehicle came around the bend. By then she had regained control of herself and had started to lay wood in her campfire to occupy herself.

With a smile to acknowledge her, Jim extracted two burlap-wrapped panes of glass from the cab of the truck and leaned them against the house. He returned to the cab and brought back something bundled in his red shirt. "For your house," he said, holding out the bundle and pulling aside the shirt so she could look.

Not many things had surprised Ruth as much as the olla Jim

handed her, nor pleased her as much. It filled the space in her arms as she cradled it against her, running her hand around its round bottom, following the circumference that curved up to its narrow neck. The fluctuating earthy colors closely matched those of the shards she found, the small thrill of each discovery now culminating in true wonderment at the whole vessel she held. "Is it real?" she said. "From . . . from somewhere around here?"

"I found it in the rocks near the petroglyphs a few days ago," he said, sliding his arms into the sleeves of his shirt. "Usually I leave them be, but I think you were meant to have this. It was probably used for carrying water, maybe grain. It's an old one."

"What can I say?" she said. "I've never had anything so . . . so special. I'll never be able to repay you."

"Your eyes repay me," he said. "Watching you hold it."

Ruth sat down carefully in the camp chair, holding the olla tenderly on her lap. "I love it," she said, staring down into the dark opening inside the neck.

"I have something else, too, for your house. Something more practical," he said. As he walked back toward the truck, Ruth thought she could be content for the rest of her life, just sitting with the ancient pot, pondering its origins and the people who had used it here in this canyon.

The table Jim brought over was small and irregular, but lovely, fashioned from the trunk of an oak that had been sliced and sanded smooth. "I used to make these to sell from the reservation," he explained, running a hand over the table's surface, "before I came here." He carried the table into the cabin and situated it beneath a window. "You'll need a chair or two," he said, stepping back. "Some shelves also." Ruth propped the olla against the pillow on her cot and came to stand next to him.

"I can get wood for the shelves in town," she said, "if John will take me again."

"He's driving Kate in to the doctor in a few days. You could go with them then."

"She's still ill, then?" Ruth asked, ashamed that she had forgotten all about her friend's distress. "How bad is she, do you think?" she asked as the two of them walked outside and Jim began unwrapping the glass.

"Some days fine. The next day she doesn't eat much. She keeps shrugging it off, but John's worried about it, I can tell."

Ruth nodded. "I'd like to help you put in the panes, so I'll know how it's done," she said.

"Then I'll do one while you watch, and you can do the other if you like," he said, grinning. "But remember, you won't be watching an expert. I've only done this twice before."

"Twice more than I have." She sat cross-legged on the ground to watch.

The pane wouldn't fit properly until Jim gouged out wood on one side of the frame with his knife. Ruth had the opposite problem when she got to her window—a gap between the glass and the frame in one of the far corners. Inverting his example, she jammed in a slice of wood and generously puttied over it and the edge of the glass. Except for more putty on the pane and a less-than-even strip of it around the glass, Ruth's looked as good as his, or so she thought, being that she'd managed to do it herself.

"I wonder if making clay pots was easier than putting in windows," Ruth said, as they washed putty from their hands in the runoff at the spring. "I'll bet it was more fun."

Jim shook water from his hands and wiped them on his pant legs. "Why don't you try it and find out?" he said. "There's enough clay in that bank to keep you busy for a long time."

"Really? That's what they made them from?" Ruth walked over to the ledge behind the spring and dug in with one hand, scooping out a gooey gob that felt like silken mud between her fingers.

"The whole bank is clay, even the white, dry stuff way up there. If it's too slick, you add sand or debris to stiffen it so it holds its shape," he said, watching her knead it into a ball.

Ruth squeezed her clay and patted it firm. "How do you know all this?" she asked.

"My grandmother," Jim said. "She was a potter. I used to watch her work before they sent me away to school. We would walk up Black Canyon to gather clay at the place she liked best. I liked to copy her, making clay snakes and coiling them into my own little pots the way she did. But the elders stopped me when I was still very young. Boys weren't supposed to do women's work. Today, no one would know that—or care."

"Show me," Ruth said, noticing how his speech had become more Indian-sounding when he told his story, "how you make clay snakes into a pot. There's no one to stop you here." She held out the clay. "Except yourself."

Jim rolled small sections of the clay into thin strips between his palms. With his thumb he made a depression in another section and began coiling the strips around it. "This is the way to do it," he said, as he built part of a doll-sized jar. "Then you wet your fingers and smooth it all around, inside and out. Or you can use another piece of pottery to smooth it. All it takes is practice." He squeezed the clay back into a ball and fitted it back into the bank.

With the sun low on the horizon, Ruth invited Jim for a simple supper of canned stew and biscuits. She still used the campfire to prepare her meals, having developed a fondness for living outdoors, continuing to eat and sit out almost as much as before, when the heat of her tent had prohibited her from being inside. She loved having the land open before her as she rested in the shade under the pine or ate her supper watching sunset display its dazzle of color. She liked to linger as the light faded to a dusk that sucked all color from the landscape. Then night began scattering stars overhead—a few at first, then so many that the darkness seemed ready to burst into illumination, as it sometimes did when a round moon rose to saturate it with milky light.

Ruth was relieved that she and Jim had fallen naturally into their old friendship, as if nothing different had passed between them. And maybe it had not, she thought, as Jim set the coffee-pot on the grill. Nothing in his manner indicated a change. She stepped back from lighting the fire, wondering if it could have been some mood of hers that caused her to imagine the whole thing, when another ladybug dropped down onto Jim's shoulder, becoming nearly invisible against the red cloth. Ruth reached out, meaning to imitate Jim's bridge, but the insect flew into her open hand, its tiny black legs tickling the skin of her palm. She laughed and held the bug out for Jim to see. It whirled up in a fiery blur and flew into the air.

"There's a place where they congregate, usually in spring, but for some reason they're doing it again this year. It's on the mountain above my place," he said, "a kind of ladybug land. Would you like to see it?" Ruth laughed at the picture his words placed in her head, a city of little red bugs. "I can take you in a couple of days," he told her. "I have to set swedges for John first. I can come get you afterward." She nodded, though she wasn't sure what she was agreeing to—certainly not the busy bug city that came to mind at his words.

When Jim left, Ruth set the olla on the writing table and took out her journal. She turned the pot slowly, examining the shifts in shades of reds and browns around its sides, trying to put into words the lines of dots and stripes of paint added with an adept fingertip. She ran her finger along the rough patch where a small chip was missing from the olla's lip. She could see why Jim said it was very old, painted before brushes were used and the designs became more intricate. What was the woman like who made this, Ruth wondered in her journal, so long ago? Was she old or young? Had she children? Did she live on the pinyon nuts and acorns that Jim said were diet staples, the way Ruth used beans and potatoes?

Ruth found words, for the first time, for the experience with Jim at the house-raising. She had never felt so drawn to a man as at that moment—and in a way that was not entirely sexual. It was that, too, she admitted, but something else she didn't understand. It puzzled her that the attraction was so completely erased tonight, as if she had wholly imagined it. Yet she'd had the sense, she wrote, when she studied his familiar features in tonight's campfire light, that he was holding something in abeyance, that at any time he might look over at her in that same way and it would all come back as real as before. Or was her imagination in control again, the way it had been with other men? When she turned off the lamp and lay on her cot in the darkness, Ruth realized that she hadn't thought of Matt in several days, and now that she had, she felt nothing but indifference.

The next morning Ruth woke wanting to get her hands back into the clay. She had dreamed so vividly of her fingers manipulating the silky mud that she was surprised not to find it coating the skin of her palms. In her dream, she had been refashioning the rocks in her walls, changing them to ollas as she shaped them. As soon as her coffee water was on the campfire, she walked down to the spring with a bowl. Unsure of which texture of clay to use, she dug samples from different areas of the bank and carried them back to her camp. After breakfast she rolled and flattened coils of clay, unrolled, kneaded, rewet them, added various kinds of sand and debris to some and worked them again. Before she realized, it was midafternoon.

She had moved indoors when the heat hit, snacking on old biscuits as she worked. Now at the writing table with a shapeless pile of clay beside the olla, she wondered how someone got from amorphous mass to shapely vessel. Making pots was definitely not easier than putting in a windowpane. But it brought more satisfaction, she thought, as she rolled clay snakes between her palms, afterward winding them into layers around a small shape visible only to her imagination. When the coils were a few inches high, she wet her fingers in the dipper and began pressing layers together to even them, trying to make the outside of the coiled olla as smooth as the one Jim had made, as smooth as the sides of the olla he had given her. The process was long and tedious. When she finished, her clay jar looked nothing like the olla. It reached only about a third of the olla's size, its shape was askew and the surface bumpy, even after much wetting and rewetting and rubbing with her fingers. Spots on its sides and near the bottom were left so thin from overworking they felt like the canvas of her old tent flap. Yet Ruth was happy with her crooked pot. She set it and the other olla on the top of her chest of drawers, where she could view them from her bed, and went out to start her evening campfire.

That night Ruth dreamed again that the huge rock she'd buried rose up from beneath the concrete, shards of cement falling around it. This time it did not disturb her, for in her dream she had realized it was really an olla, and had wrapped her arms around its rounded sides, while hot tears ran down her cheeks. It had come back to greet her like an old friend, never to be parted from again. And then the house surrounding them had become an olla, not like the dream of the night before, when individual rocks were clay pots, but the whole of it became one olla, a continuous flow of substance that contained herself and her olla rock, as alive as she had sensed when she fought its presence on her homesite but now not her enemy. The dream fluid coursing down her face had began to pool around her feet, allowing sunlight from her open door to mirror itself in the liquid and infuse the space inside with such light as she had never seen. The very walls seemed made of light. *I, too, am an olla, and know now the purpose of my tears,* she had thought in her wonderment.

Ruth awoke enveloped in the awe of her dream, tears wet on her face. On the floor beside her bed, bright sunlight streamed in from the crack under her door, bouncing up from the cement floor to illuminate the clay vessels she had shaped the day before. Overlaid with the images of the dream, the room came alive with joy and light. "So this is my place," her own voice whispered inside her head. The concrete by the door where the rock lay buried appeared as thin as spots in the walls of her clay pot, and seemed to throb with force. For a moment, she thought she heard a drumming come from the ground, then realized it was only the sound of her own heart.

All day, Ruth felt a strong sense of anticipation, as if something important was about to happen. She made two pots by afternoon, neither much better than the first, but felt content when she set all three out in the sun to dry. All the while she kept a suspicious eye on the white billows that had been growing each day above Rocky Mountain, their airy forms mirroring the solid mountain's shape. When she went inside and opened her book, Ruth found herself in the seedy streets of London nearly a century before, and she stayed there until the day cooled. Then she went out to her garden to pluck her very first small zucchini from the bush that had survived the onslaught of hooves. She admired the tiny green globes appearing on her tomato vine. Already, birds were trying to peck at them through the chicken wire. A new tunnel had been started outside the wire fence. Twice, she had rocked over tunnels dug by rabbits, in the end making a meal of the creatures to save her vegetables. Now she guessed she'd be obliged to dispatch another rabbit soon to go with that next squash already burgeoning beneath the leaves.

Indian Jim came for her early the next morning. Ruth heard the crunch of his footsteps outside the open cabin window, the quiet sounds as he built a fire. She lay back against her pillow to enjoy the comforting sounds of his movement, not rising until the smell of coffee wafted in. Wishing for the first time that she had an indoor bathroom, she walked out to the campfire, where he was examining the clay pots she had placed on the rock table. He looked up at her, his eyes admiring. "You have the knack," he said. "I'm not surprised."

"But they're terrible. It was fun making them, though. I'll keep trying." She took the one from his hands. "Look how uneven it is. I can't seem to get it right."

"You will," he said. He picked up her last piece, where she had actually managed to bow out the sides a bit. "Look what you've done here without any help at all."

"But you helped get me started."

"And we better, too, soon as we put together some food." He set the pot back on the table. "Get started up the mountain, I mean. Before the heat comes in—or before it storms." He looked up at wisps above the mountain. "So far there's just been a lot of noise up there, but today may be different."

They tanked up on coffee, ate biscuits and jerky, then headed up the ridge across the wash. To save time, Jim took her straight up the bluff, not a route she would have attempted alone, she thought, as Jim reached down a hand to help her across one of the steeper stretches on a narrow ledge. When they reached the top of the bluff, Ruth realized how high they'd come so fast. They continued to climb, keeping to ridges that weren't closed off by thickets of scrub oak and manzanita or rugged piles of boulders. As they went up, the pinyon and juniper thinned and ponderosa began, then predominated, mixing with fir and huge oak trees. Clouds formed feathery pillows above the mountain, cushioning their climb off and on from the sun. Finally, they topped a ridge, and Jim pointed across a deep ravine to a peak that seemed higher than the rest.

"There. That's the place," he said, panting. "At the very top." Sweat glistened on his face, breaking into trickles down his neck when he bent to unscrew the cap on his canteen. "But we have to go down into the ravine and then up that steep slope to get there. It won't be easy. That old quartz mine up there where the trees start has made the whole mountainside loose. But it's the only way from this side of the mountain."

They chewed more jerky, then slid down into the ravine and started up the open strip of rock and sand on the slope, which was in other places furred thick with buckthorn, scrub oak, and manzanita clustered as tight as coils of wool on a sheep. The going was slow. Ground dissolved under their feet as they climbed, pulling them back a step or two for every three they took forward. Chunks of rock that appeared solidly anchored came loose in their hands when they took hold. Even Jim, who was agile as a mountain sheep on the cliff, was here as helpless and ineffective as Ruth, ascending and sliding back, ascending again and sliding back. About halfway up the slope, on their hands and knees like comic supplicants, they looked over at each other and began to laugh — at first a light chuckle at the absurdity of it, then more forcefully as the realization dawned that they had been completely humbled by the mountain, stripped of any sense of their own importance. Ruth felt hefty grains of sand in her boot, down her shirt and pants, in her hair, and she was afraid to think where else. In a spasm of belly laughter, she fell flat on her stomach and hugged the warm, decomposing granite to keep from sliding down further. Okay, I got the message, she thought.

She was still laughing when she felt Jim's hand cover her own, squeezing it until the fine, rough pebbles impressed the cracks between her fingers. When she turned her head, she saw that laughter had left his face. His look captured her breath and sent a hot current into her belly. She could not move as he inched toward her, though her insides squirmed against the ground. Somewhere in the distance came the faint grumble of thunder. With one hand he turned her toward him, sand streaming from his clothes and hair as he rose over her slightly, fragments of rock embedded in moisture on the dark skin of his cheek as his face moved toward hers. Jim's eyes never left her own, and when his mouth made contact, the power she'd sensed in his look took hold of her. They began sliding down the river of sand, lips locked in a language that Ruth would have traveled off the end of the earth to learn. They stopped briefly when she felt a sharp rock against her buttocks, but he turned her on top of him and they journeyed on, safely attached to the dissolving mountain, coming to rest, finally, after the flow turned them to one side somewhere near the bottom of the slope. A wave of sand and small rock washed over their faces.

They rolled apart, panting, passion changing to laughter in the deluge. Still laughing, Ruth shook her head to knock tiny rocks out of her ears, then turned away to spit sand and wipe dirt from her eyes, along with the moisture of happiness and mirth. They looked back at each other, then up at the distance they had lost, and became convulsed again with laughter.

Jim reached over and brushed grains from Ruth's cheek. He looked up at the peak. "We better get started again," he said, so flatly that they broke into another fit. When it died, Ruth was about to ask whether they should give up for today, but Jim stood and pulled her to her feet. "You'll be glad when you see it," he said. Then he grinned and looked down at her mischievously. "We can wait," he said. "This is not the place."

So they started up the mountain again, Ruth reluctant, feeling unrequited and unmotivated to attempt the frustrating climb-and-slide slope just to see some ladybugs, which, after all, were plentiful right where she lived. Yet she went along, not convinced, but trusting Jim's judgment enough to participate. Besides, what was she to do, pull him back to her as she had the cowboy in her drunkenness and ride him down? That did not fit what had passed between them.

They battled their way up. Near the top of the slope, they

passed the depression left from the mine, then the rock underneath became more solid and the dirt stayed put when they stepped on it, and soon they were back in forest, with duff underfoot. Jim led her toward a grove of fir just below a cluster of rocks that crowned the top, stopping when they reached the perimeter. "Go ahead," he said, nodding toward the trees. Puzzled, Ruth stepped forward.

She had taken a few steps when she began to see, and the spectacle was so strange and unexpected that she stopped suddenly where she stood. Never had she seen such a thing. Bright red against the green fir needles, ladybugs beaded solid the trunk of each fir tree and adorned most of the branches, right down to the smallest twig. It seemed to her that there must have been a million little beetles, all unmoving, attached like living jewels from some enchanted kingdom, encrusting each trunk and twig with brilliant color, spreading even into thick clusters of needles. She and Jim walked slowly through the grove, marveling at the magic display. When they came out at the foot of the pile of rocks just at the top, to Ruth's further surprise, even the sides of rocks were bejeweled with the same small red dots. Carefully, they moved around to the far end of the rock pile, where there were no bugs, and took a path to the very top.

Except for the rumbling cloud above them, the peak felt like the top of the world. Below them, the mountaintop flattened, dipped and swooped up into several lower peaks and small valleys. On three sides the mountain dwindled away to desert, trailing its ridges outward as they diminished in size until they reached the flatland below. To the west, the mountain dropped down too, but wrinkled into the San Bernardino range, punctuating it like a huge exclamation mark. As they ate biscuits and jerky, Jim pointed out Black Canyon and its reservation embedded in the tangle of canyons and showed her the peak above the onyx mine, at the end of the North Fork off Rattlesnake Canyon. The blue-green lake near Jim's camp at the petroglyphs was visible in a crevice not far from them. When the thunder became more pronounced, accompanied by bright spiderwebs against the dark belly of cloud, they went down the other side of the peak, making an easy descent across a trail of uncluttered ridges toward the cove of Jim's camp.

The ball of sun slid out from the cloud above as they arrived at the camp, though more clouds were swelling madly behind and had swallowed it whole again by the time they had swum the length of the pond and come out dripping in front of Jim's lean-to. Ruth pressed her front up against the sun-warmed rocks behind the lean-to, absorbing their heat through her wet clothes. She turned, spread her arms, and snuggled her back onto a dry granite surface. Behind her she heard the high-pitched scolding of a chipmunk, its call as repetitious as excited bedsprings. The peak at the top had vanished behind a gray curtain, and a wind had come up, quivering the pond and sending shivers up her spine. Jim came toward her with a blanket, the muscles of his chest swelling beneath smooth skin as he held out the red-and-black patterned fabric. He was saying something, but a clap of thunder drowned out his words. "The rocks are warm," she said, her teeth chattering just a little. "I'll be all right."

"They'll not be warm for long," he said, looking up. "It's about to pour down any minute. Let's go inside." He took her arm and pried her from the wall as a drop splashed her nose. Another hit her arm.

"I'm already wet," she protested, as he wrapped the blanket around her shoulders and led her toward the shelter. "A little rain won't make much difference."

He stopped in front of the lean-to and looked at her. Drops began crackling the oak leaves around them. "You have to get out of those clothes. I'll make a fire." He pulled back the skin flap and ducked under. A huge crash of thunder pushed Ruth in the door just as the deluge hit. She tightened the flap behind her.

Inside, the dwelling was compact and efficient, its bent willow pole frame covered with animal skins and boughs. Squatting with his back to her, Jim piled wood near an overhanging boulder that served as an extension of the structure and left a space for smoke to exit without rain entering. Two flat sitting rocks were situated beside the small fire ring. A section of floor on the far side of the lean-to had been heaped with forest duff, spread over with fresh willow boughs and sprigs of sage. The fragrance mixed with the juniper woodsmoke, filling the room with a pungent aroma. Ruth sat on one of the two stones, feeling shy and clumsy, while Jim built the fire. She could have undressed behind the blanket, but she took off just her boots and socks, feeling as if now only her cold clothes held her together. If she took them off, her shape would be changed forever. Not until a flame blazed up did Jim turn to look at her. When he did, Ruth thought she might melt to become part of the rock she sat on.

He took hold of her hand and led her to the willow boughs, easing her back against the leaves. Under her back, Ruth could feel the ground give, the soft history of trees make room for her. Above them, the shapes and shades of animals bound together as shelter, deer and coyote and mountain lion, the tightly joined seams visible between them. Ruth felt herself caught up in some great undercurrent, as if this small refuge itself were being carried on the mountain's river of dissolving rock. Jim bent over and kissed her lips softly. "You're so cold," he said, and began to undo the buttons of her blouse, one by one. His eyes stayed with hers, while rain drummed the skins overhead. She felt more quiet than she could remember, finding an excitement so deep in her it hadn't yet reached the surface. She watched his eyes travel over her body as he revealed it, his face loose with desire as he unbuttoned and peeled her wet pants down from her buttocks, her legs, her feet. Then her underpants. He kissed the small bump of her belly. "So cold," he said, lifting her shoulders to pull off her blouse. "We'll warm you."

The Indian kneeled beside her shivering form, his hair a darker shade against the brown skin of his shoulders. When he undid his belt and dropped his pants past his knees, Ruth saw his sex rise out of the dark tangle of leaves like a budding yucca. She nearly gasped at the wonder of it, could not keep her hand from reaching out to touch. They remained looking at each other, neither moving, except to quicken their breath.

When they came together, it was without awkwardness, the rhythm of their movements choreographed in an ageless dance, and when he entered, Ruth knew him as she would know another self. Each touch sent her spinning outward into air and brought her back again to her senses, heightening her pleasure until she thought she might burst with the deliciousness of it. Even her skin was singing. Then as they followed the ancient steps laid out for them, she felt herself stumble, and opened her eyes to find him watching, waiting for her, his dark hair falling into a curtain around their faces. She felt her life shift with their connection. Eyes in contact as intimate as their bodies, they smiled as ecstasy enveloped them.

CHAPTER ELEVEN

It was ten days later that Ruth returned to the cabin she'd aban-
doned in the canyon, and nearly a week before she even thought
of going—and then in terms of getting things she wished she'd
brought with her, things like a change of clothes and her own
brush. Not that she had much need for clothes, with the two of
them spending the greater part of each day unclothed around
the lake, or inside the lean-to when afternoon rains came. The
showers dwindled after the first two days, and they moved outside completely, even sleeping out under the stars, entangling
under the blanket to ward off the cool, high mountain night.
Each day they found new places and new ways to make love, in
the water, on rocks, on the sand at the edge of the lake, standing
and sitting or somewhere in between, they explored each other's

bodies and pleasures as they had once explored the land around them, and as with the land, the discoveries they made seemed endless. They dressed only to hunt rabbit or quail for supper or to gather pine nuts, or when the chill of evening set upon them. With clay from a spring that fed the pond, and by copying Jim's every detail, Ruth was able to fashion an olla larger and more shapely than she had made in the canyon. Together they constructed a campfire kiln so she could sometime fire the three pots she had left drying in the canyon.

Ruth felt herself growing into new habits. This was the life she had been looking for, she told Jim one morning when they wakened to a pink, sun-washed dawn. He reminded her that it was not a life for winter and with a little half-smile called her his naked savage. She mock-attacked him, then, climbing astride, whooping and pretending to shoot him with an arrow, then to scalp him with an invisible knife. But he turned his head and lashed out his tongue to lick the nipple whipping his cheek, lifting his pelvis to rock her; thus he was saved from uncertain death.

It was, in the end, concern for Kate that pulled them out of their idyllic state and sent them down the mountain toward Ruth's cabin, where they spent yet another day and night before they gave in to their worries and walked down canyon. As they sat in front of the campfire the night before they left, quiet as they roasted open pinyon cones and ate the sweet nuts inside, Ruth sensed that once they left this place and went back to everyday life, they would never again regain such blissful ease together. She didn't know why she should think that, and didn't want to confess her worry to Jim, in case saying the words would make what she felt more real, make it come true in some way. So she watched campfire sparks pop and leap toward the stars, only to fade and fizzle, and tried to shut out all that pulled at her— anxiety over Kate, the need for food supplies, some vague urge to move on with things. The two of them had used up Jim's small supplies of flour and coffee, and hers were low also. She still had vinegar in the canyon, though Jim had had none. The two of them couldn't just stay on the mountain and exist on pinyon nuts and game, she told herself. Even their supply of bullets was low. When Jim spoke, she found he had his own concerns.

"What will we do, Ruth," he said, "you and I? An Indian man and a . . . a white woman."

She looked over at his craggy features, the wavering flame fickle in its highlights. "What difference does that make, except for the man and woman part?" Ruth reached over and took his hand. "And I'm not all white woman, anyway. I told you about my mother. Besides, what do we care what people think? I certainly don't."

"A rumor about your mother doesn't make you an Indian." He turned his face to look at the fire. "You're white. That will make a difference to everyone else. I heard about what Stine called you at the Hudsons'."

"I'll be proud to be called squaw woman," she said, squeezing his fingers, "if it's on account of you. But it's none of their business. Why worry about what small-minded people say?" She rose from her chair and began feeding the fire with small branches.

"Their minds may be small, as you say, but their effect is great. It follows me wherever I go off the reservation. That's why I'm here hammering wooden pegs into rocks to make a living." Jim got to his feet as she tossed on the last branch and turned her toward him. "That's not true, entirely," he amended. "This life is what I want. But it would be good to have a choice." For a moment they stood facing each other. He reached down and touched her cheek lightly. "I just don't want their mean notions to affect you on my account."

"People already have notions about me, even without you. But I welcome their knowing about us. I think I'll send out an announcement."

"So lovely," he said, breaking into a smile, "and so damned stubborn."

"Would you want me any other way?" Ruth felt her chest swell with a surge of power.

He shook his head. "But I smell trouble ahead," he said, pulling her into a kiss that in a few seconds had them struggling out of their clothes again by the fire. They stood naked in the fire-light watching each other, restraining their impulse to come together. Ruth stared intensely, as if she were etching each detail of him into her heart, the flow of muscle beneath the bronze skin, the strands of hair she remembered trailing over her skin, tickling, whenever he kissed his way up her body, the dark, eloquent eyes, the way his face dropped down abruptly at the cheekbones to the mouth that had left its imprint on her own. When mere sight caused more ache than either of them could take, they merged more ferociously than ever before, and Ruth felt herself straining to breathe his very smell into her, to inscribe the feel of his touch onto her skin like the fingertip paintings on the olla, listening to his breath and soft moans as if she would carry them always in her ears to mix with the sounds of birds and wind in the pines.

Neither slept much that night, each waking often and pulling the other as close as two beings can get and still stay separated by skin. They made love once more at dawn, then rose to fix coffee before heading down canyon, walking side by side into the birdsong morning. Down by the bend they stopped to watch a mother fox nosing a kit up the sliding bank across the wash, while the rest of the litter waited at the top. Then the little band trotted off toward a snarl of oak and buckthorn covering the knoll.

Just before they reached the North Fork, Ruth heard the sounds of cattle mewling and the pounding of many hooves. "Must be the fall drive," Jim said in response to her inquiring look; it appeared he'd been aware of the animals for a while.

"Heart Bar?"

He nodded. "They're moving them to the desert until spring."

"Seems a little early," Ruth said. "The days are still warm." As they came around a bend, she could see cattle pouring across the road out of the North Fork and rumbling down the wash in front of them.

"Maybe. But it's well into October and they have to get them out before the snow starts." He stopped beside a scrub oak growing along the rut road and took hold of a branch. "You see how thick the acorns are? And the cones on the pinyons are plentiful. Squirrels are gathering already. My grandmother used to say that means a hard winter." They stopped to watch the procession, then walked on, stopping again when they came to the fork to wait for the cattle to pass. When the main herd had gone by and only a few steers were left meandering down the gully, Ruth and Jim crossed and continued down the road beside the wash. They were nearing the willows when they saw Stine galloping toward them through the brush.

He reined in his big buckskin directly in their path, then, with a smirk, touched his spurs to its flanks, and pranced in circles around them, the horse puffing and snorting as it lifted and swished its tail. They kept walking, Jim moving to position his body between Ruth and the trotting horse. He kept the rifle trained on the ground, though Ruth noticed he had flipped off the safety. This time Stine had a pistol strapped to one hip as well as the rifle on his saddle. When he tired of riding rings of horse nuggets around them, the cowboy whipped off his hat and whacked the animal on the rear with it, then raced off whooping into the wash, his orange-red hair smoldering in the sunlight. It took Ruth a moment to realize he was trying to imitate an Indian war cry, though Jim's face told her the fact hadn't escaped him for a second.

When they arrived at the Swedes', the Olsens' flatbed was not in the yard. From Ingmar and another miner who were out milking the nannies, they learned that John had driven Kate into San Bernardino a few days ago, after waiting some time for Ruth and Jim to come down and make the trip with them. "Ya, should be back now," the Swede added. "We need a load before we go to winter mines," by which he meant, Jim explained, that they had one more shipment of onyx to make before they all left for the mines on the low desert for the winter.

"The whole herd of miners leaves for the desert just like the cattle," Jim said, with a little laugh as they entered the house.

"You too? And John and Kate?"

"John and Kate, yes. I go home for the winter," he said, "usually." He looked down and touched her arm. "Maybe I won't go anywhere this year." They decided to walk on into town for a few of the supplies they needed and to see if there had been any word by phone of Kate down at the store. With any luck they'd find themselves a ride back.

Carrying empty knapsacks, they followed the trail up a ridge on the small mountain that ran parallel to the base of Rocky Mountain. Jim said this would cut the miles by road in half. The trail was old, said to have been used by Indians and then Mormons long before the present rut road for cars existed. As they climbed, he sometimes stopped suddenly when she came close behind so she would smack against him and he could turn and kiss her. Sometimes he motioned her on ahead, then lunged out playfully to grab her as she passed. When they were nearing the top of the ridge, Ruth looked down at the cattle now making their noisy way down the canyon below them. On the bank of the wash, Charlie Stine and Bobby Key sat on their horses looking up the mountain.

It was early afternoon when she and Jim reached the store. So caught up in her happiness with Jim, Ruth hadn't thought once about the awkwardness of the situation until she stepped up onto the wooden porch. It was the first time she had seen Matt since the night of the Hudsons' dance. She expressed her condolences at May's death, saying she hadn't known until folks came up to raise her house. He accepted with cool politeness and handed her two letters, one from Cally and another envelope that she knew would contain her allowance check. Her mail had been there nearly two weeks. No one in town had heard from the Olsens, he said, avoiding Ruth's eyes and ignoring Jim altogether, though Jim had been the one who asked the question. Matt hadn't known about the Olsens' trip in to see the doctor, he said, since they had not stopped on their way to San Bernardino.

Lily Rose came in from the back room carrying a pile of empty flour sacks. "Ruth," she said, laying the sacks on the counter and stretching out a hand, "how good to see you. Have you come in with the Olsens again?" Lily seemed not to notice Jim.

"Apparently the Olsens went in to the doctor's some days ago. Ruth's come to inquire if we've heard from them," Matt told Lily as she came to stand alongside him.

"We've both come to inquire," Ruth said, turning toward the shelves, where Jim had already begun to select items. "And to get a few supplies, since we're almost out of everything." Ruth walked up to the Indian and took hold of his upper arm. He smiled slightly, despite himself. She didn't have to glance up to see the look the pair at the counter gave each other. After a silence, Ruth heard footsteps, then the back door shut. When they brought their items to the front, only Lily remained in the room, busying herself with rearranging canned goods on the shelves behind the counter.

They kept their packs light, each buying a small sack of flour, some coffee and lard, a few canned goods, and a couple of boxes of shells, for they were not sure whether they would go back over the mountain or keep to the road and hope for a ride. Yet neither of them much cared which way they traveled, as long as they traveled together, and they walked along the wide dirt road feeling carefree under their burdens. Dust devils spiraled skyward in the distance, churning apart in the air at the top. Beside the road, Joshua trees shook spiny arms at them in the strengthening wind. Two cars passed on the stretch of road that led to the trail at the edge of town, but neither car carried anyone who lived in the rimrock country that skirted the base of Rocky Mountain.

Ruth stopped to kneel and bury her nose in the velvet petals of desert primrose that bloomed on the sandy shoulder, finding a sweet earthiness in the flower's faint fragrance. The delicate, papery petals asserted themselves in tender defiance, one last burst of transformed earth before the ground froze over. Ruth loved the feel of powdery pollen that clung when she dipped in her fingertips and traced them over her cheeks.

"The bees will think you're a flower," Jim said, squatting beside her as she lifted her head from a cluster of blossoms. "Your whole face is streaked with yellow. I wonder if you taste like a flower." He took hold of her face, his tongue darting out, bee-like, to taste her cheeks, as she squirmed and giggled, moving his lips down till he reached her mouth. He sampled its flavor with a sweetness that no honeybee ever imparted.

They moved apart at the approach of a car, which happened to belong to Jake Tunstall, from out in the rimrock. He said he'd carry them as far as the mouth of Rattlesnake Canyon, a short four-mile walk to the Swedes'. Even before she got in, Ruth could smell whiskey, and the way Jake simply approximated the road told her he had been at it a while. He kept up a steady barrage of slurred song as the car's tires slipped in and out of the ruts, half the time two on one side crushing brush on the roadside, while the other two squirreled in the sandy middle hump. If the mesa hadn't been fairly flat and free of boulders, they would have asked him to let them out, or would have started walking one of the times the car got hung up on sage or sand and they had to get out and help him push it back onto the road. Even with four miles left to walk, they were glad to be let out at the canyon's mouth.

The sun was gone by the time they got to the willows, and dusk had come with a round moon rising as they walked into the Olsens' yard. The miners had put together a stew with goat and vegetables from the garden, though it was lacking in spice and the meat had not been braised first. Tired as she was, Ruth did what she could to rescue it, and she and Jim made fresh biscuits that the men seemed grateful to have. The miners had become so used to Kate's skills, they hardly remembered how to cook without her. Their anxiety for her return in some small part, Ruth suspected, had to do with their eagerness to have a decent meal. Throughout the day, concern for Kate had stayed with Ruth, though there was no use speaking of it or dwelling on it. She was certain that Jim felt the same. Now, as they sat with the miners at Kate's table, her absence spoke loudly for itself. No one joked, as they had while preparing supper, about Kate's needing to be there to keep them from starving; they merely ate in silence or talked of things at hand—the billy that fell from the rocks the day before and broke off half a horn, the row of squash decimated by rabbits digging under the fence and avoiding the traps.

"That Stine today, he ask too many question," Ingmar told them, nodding his head as he spoke. "Want to know when you been at Rute's place. How long. Where John gone. I not tell him nothing." He rubbed at his moustache. "Not like that fellow," he said. "Mean look to him, ya?"

A goat wandered in the open door and jumped up on the end of the table, trying to get his head in the pot of goat stew. Another poked a head inside the door.

"Cannibal," Ingmar said, and they all laughed, but no one chased the goat away until Ruth got up to bring over the coffee-pot. While the men were pouring, she shooed the goats out and shut the door. The evening had begun to cool anyway. The place was deteriorating without Kate; Ruth could see several small yellow poolings near the door that told her chickens didn't always get chased out either. The men were so used to spending time outdoors that they didn't seem to know where the boundaries lay, much like herself. But she surely would know to chase the chickens out.

"Do you think they'll be back?" Ruth asked as she sat back down. "The cowboys, I mean."

"In spring," Ingmar said, "when they drive cattle back again."

"We'll see them here in a few days," Jim said, "on their way back up to the Heart Bar. But they'll go up the North Fork, shouldn't come by you."

"The first time they showed up at my place, they came looking for strays that had missed the fork and wandered up my way," Ruth said, filling her cup.

"That only happens in the spring, when they drive the herd up canyon to the Heart Bar. But the cattle stay down in the desert until then."

"Good riddance," a miner said.

"But," Jim added, "if they do come your way, it won't be the cattle they're after." He placed a hand on her forearm. "Keep that shotgun handy in case I'm not there."

Some of the men had begun conversing in Swedish as Ruth and Jim talked. From the tone, she sensed it was about the two of them, though she had no way of knowing for sure. Others joined in and soon she could tell the conversation had moved on to places far from the canyon, the men laughing and telling stories. Ruth enjoyed listening to the foreign words, the different rhythm of the sentences, and the abrupt shifts that turned the sounds around, somewhat like the German that she used to enjoy hearing Karl speak. Its sound was quite different from the Mexican spoken by workers at Aunt Myrtle's, different yet from the sounds of Mexican Indian languages she'd listened to on the streets of El Paso. Ramon had taught her to say a few Mexican phrases before she was sent away, but she could never make them sound like he did. She wondered what Jim's language was like, if he would speak it for her.

Since they had rested, and since the moon was so bright, they decided to walk the rest of the way to her place that night. The miners promised to fetch them as soon as John and Kate returned. Ruth wore one of Jim's long-sleeved shirts over her short-sleeved blouse to keep out the cold, though the air warmed once they got past the willows and water. "I think it's time we get you some winter wood in," Jim said as they walked along. "And that shell built around the privy shelf as well."

As much as she appreciated his use of "we," Ruth didn't much like the idea of someone else building her privy, even Jim. She was ready to protest until he added, "I know I sure don't want to sit out exposed while I'm here."

"When will that be?" Ruth asked, looking down the stretch of open road in front of them, where moonlight pooled in dips and ruts between the shadowy brush along the sides. "When will you be here with me?" As they walked along, Ruth thought about how much she had yearned to be alone in the canyon. It gave her freedom to do as she pleased. Yet Jim's presence was not an intrusion. She never longed for him to be gone, as she had others, even Matt. Jim's proximity didn't take away from being alone with her canyon but added a dimension, as if he were a way into its wildness. It wasn't simply the way he shared his knowledge of its mysteries, or the way he had of matching his ways to the land around him, but more that she loved him in exactly the same way she loved the wildness around her, with its rocks and streams, its deer and bear and burgundy-streaked sunsets.

Minutes went by before he answered, both of them thinking over her question. They were nearly to the far bend when Jim said, "I'll be here whenever you want me to be here, Ruth, though for your sake I shouldn't be." The quiet canyon swallowed his words, leaving only the wavering voices of a few crickets still braving the chill evening and the steady crunch of footfall on the sand.

"I want you with me as much as you want to be. But don't tell me you shouldn't be," Ruth said finally. "Who are those people to tell us what we can do—should do? What they think is not important. I know what I want, don't you?"

He took hold of her arm to stop her, and she turned to face him, his face half in moon shadow. "While there was still community among my own people," he said, "it would have been important to me what the people in the tribe thought. That is a difference between us. But these are not my people."

"They're not my people either." Ruth shrugged him off and crossed her arms. "White people don't have tribes, just a lot of people living close by who like to stick their noses in everybody's business and tell them how they should live."

"All cultures are like that, not just yours. Surely you must know that with all the books you read. It's not just ourselves we're responsible to."

"It is for me." Ruth started to walk on, then swung back. "And how can you talk about being responsible to people who treat you the way they do?" She heard her voice go shrill. "You think you owe them anything but contempt?"

"I don't, but don't you?"

"Me? Owe them?"

"The house-raising, the trips to town for groceries."

"But that was all John's doing. He's different. I don't mind being responsible to him and Kate," Ruth said as they walked on.

"Then what do you think John would say about us being together? You think he would clap his hands in celebration?"

"Of course he would. He . . . he told me right off how smart you were, how he likes you."

"Yes, he likes me—and he lets me work for him. But this is another matter, this . . ?"

"He'd never say anything against us being together."

"He already has . . . not directly, but he let me know how he feels."

Ruth stopped again, the peaked cabin roof broadcasting a sheet of reflected moonlight ahead of them.

"He worries about what people would say—for my sake, like you do," she said, moving on. "I can't believe it's more than that with John."

"Maybe not, but he's the one who told me what was said at the Hudsons' after he left. He said people were talking already. And that was before . . . before . . ?"

"Before we were lovers."

"I told him we were just good friends," Jim said as they walked up to the front door. "But I knew I wanted more from you, that there would be more. He knew it too."

Ruth struggled the key into the padlock, turned it to snap the hook open and pull it from the latch. "So what was the more you wanted, then? My body?" She gave the door a shove and looked up into his face, dark against the moon behind his head.

"Not just that," he said.

"What, then?"

"Just what you've given me," Jim said, brushing the hair back from her forehead. "The rest of you." They stood in the doorway looking at each other, his hands gripping her upper arms. "There are words in your language for what's happened between us, but they cheapen it. Silly words compared to what we feel. My people have some that are better, but I see now that even they are not enough." He stopped and spoke sounds to her that she did not understand, but she pleasured at the way they felt in her ears. She smiled and he said them again. "I don't know how to explain what that means," he told her. "Something in the spirit of another self—'man who finds the woman living inside him with woman who finds the man dwelling in her,'" but that doesn't really come very close."

"They're nice-sounding words. Say something else."

When he spoke again, Ruth listened with her tongue, drinking in the movements of his mouth; she could almost feel the slidey sounds coming from her own lips, carrying forth the same lovely thoughts into the air. "Mmmm, what did you say?" she asked when he stopped.

"I said tomorrow we have to make a shithouse and bring in firewood before we freeze to death." Ruth gave him playful push and stepped through the doorway.

The next morning they went to work, first building the frame for the outhouse, then heading up a draw in the afternoon with an axe and a saw, to a place where Ruth had come across three dead pinyons, one of them blown to bits by lightning. They chopped and hauled branches the rest of that day and the next, falling asleep each night tired-sexless and tattooed with patches of black pine pitch wherever their bodies had been left open to air. On the third morning, Jim was ready to spend the day hauling down the rest of the wood they'd left hacked into stove-size pieces, but Ruth convinced him they could go back for it in days to come—she hadn't labored so many hours nonstop since her days with the boulder and the slab, and wanted to get back some of the easy time the two of them had spent before they went to Juniper Valley. So they took turns hauling water to fill the #8 tub, then went to work with kerosene on the adhered sap that threatened to become part of their skins, exchanging their scratchy blackened patches for red and tender ones that they uncovered and enhanced by scrubbing with paraffin, which they promptly removed with soap and water.

Free of the pitch, they stood in the tub and began lathering each other's bodies, laughing and tickling and pausing longer at strategic spots, so caught up in the frolic that neither heard the horseman approach until he spurred his mount up the bank of the wash and his partner rode up behind, neither man stopping until the horses' heads were hung over the tub. Ruth and Jim stopped cold in the moment, each still holding the other's soapy, dripping body as they stared at the cowboys. "How these thirsty horses gonna drink, Bobby, when this here water's full of garbage? Damned if it ain't that Indian and his squaw pollutin' up another water hole," Stine said. He kept one hand on the handle of the pistol on his hip. The air was saturated with the smell of sour liquor.

All Ruth could think was that the rifle and shotgun were in the cabin. What she said was, "You have no business here. Get off my property, Mr. Stine, right now."

Charlie Stine laughed. "'Mr. Stine,' is it? At least it shows respect. Well, you don't got nothin' to say about it this time, whore." As he moved his horse toward her, Jim leapt out of the tub and ran for the cabin door. Stine swung off his buckskin after him, Ruth pursuing them both until Bobby Key rammed his horse between her and the door, his boot catching her in the ribs. She went down just as she heard the soft thuds of metal striking flesh. Key was off his horse before she could get to her feet, kicking her off balance. She went down flat on her belly, where he pinned her tight, his legs kneeling on her thighs, his hands pressing her wrists against the ground. Thuds still sounded from inside her cabin. She could do nothing but watch from under the horse as Stine's arm lifted and came down again and again, as she stifled screams of outrage and horror.

By the time Stine stepped out of the cabin, fear for Jim had made her silent and cold in her anger, though she could do nothing to stop the flow of tears. "That damned Indian was going after a gun, Bobby. Can you imagine that?" he said, as he came through the doorway. "I had to defend myself. Their kind never learn. He was no different than the one who murdered my grandpap." Stine stopped when he saw Key holding Ruth down, a smile spreading over his face. "Let 'er up, Bobby."

"Don't know about that, Charlie. She'd be hard to pin down again. 'Sides, I kinda like the view from here."

"I said get off her." Stine gave him a shove. As soon as the man's weight lifted from her, Ruth was on her feet. "Well, looky here. You're makin' it easy for us, naked and all," he said, sending his eyes up and down her form in an exaggerated manner. "But too bad you had to get yourself all dirty when you was so nice and clean for us." Ruth ran for the door, but Bobby Key grabbed her from behind as she went past, lifted her, and trapped her arms at her sides. He looked down over her shoulder, his breath hot against her neck, "Jesus," he said. Stine walked around in front of her. She wanted to gouge out his eyes and squish them in her palms like grapes. "So you been givin' all that to an Injun, have you?" he said, attempting to get a hand between her fighting legs. "Guess I'll have to remind you what a white man's like—in case you forgot after that Johnny Lee feller." Like a striking rattler, he reached out and grabbed her breast, twisted and pulled, as if he would rip it from her body. She kicked out at his groin, but he moved aside and her bare foot merely brushed his leg. Key tightened his hold around her arms and ribs until she could barely breathe and clamped one of her legs between his while she kicked back at his knee with the other. Stine took possession of the free leg and jerked it out to one side, slapping her face from cheek to cheek at the same time. When he quit she spit blood at him, and he hit her again, harder.

"Can't hold on much longer, Charlie. Let's get on with it," Key said. He pressed his pelvis tight into her buttocks.

"Don't let yer horse out of the barn yet, Bobby," Stine said. He looked around, then pulled at the buckle of his gun belt, jerking out the pistol before the holster fell. He lifted Ruth's leg higher and shoved the cold metal barrel into the tender flesh between her struggling legs, pushing his face next to hers and exhaling putrid breath as he spoke. "You know what I like to do to squaw whores?" he said, applying pressure with the pistol. Tears came, but she did not cry out, thinking that Jim might still hear her. She could not bear to pain him further. Ruth did not take her eyes away from Stine's, sending her message clearly: I will kill you, she promised silently as he jammed the barrel deeper.

"Christ," Key said, his pelvis already rocking behind her. "Let's get on with it before it's too late."

All at once Key let go and moved his arms away, and Ruth felt Stine's fingers dig into her breasts, using them as handles to fling her to the ground by her cabin wall. A sharp pain sent light cracking through her brain, and the world went hazy and far away, where she could no longer see it. She heard ugly sounds in the distance, where there was pain and bad things being done to her, but it was all happening so far away it ceased to matter. Then came a loud noise, like the blast of a shotgun, a shout, then silence for a very long time.

CHAPTER TWELVE

Nausea overruled Ruth's dark place, and she managed to turn to one side and dry-heave, though her head was a wounded thing and her body throbbed and pushed her back into black space. But the urge to vomit kept needling her into a dazed awakeness that she fought with every bruised cell until it finally pried her eyelids up. In the haze she understood she was lying on the ground in front of her cabin, chattering with cold, though the sun shone down on her. Jim lay not far from her, near the door, his face turned away and his long hair fanned out behind his head. After several more dim bursts of consciousness, she began to crawl toward him to see if he was as cold as she was. The inches between them were long, and she had to pause several times for dizziness and retching before she could reach him.

Jim's skin gave off no warmth, but she hugged herself up to his body so heat could grow between them. She saw that there was blood matted in his hair, but could not remember why. Then someone was lifting her away from Jim, wrapping a blanket around her. John Olsen was there, though his face kept wavering. They were carrying her inside. On her bed. She tried to tell John not to forget Jim, that she knew he would be glad for them, but her stomach spasmed instead, and she fell back into the cave of her head's pain.

Ruth bobbed up several times more, gradually understanding that John Olsen sat in a chair next to her bed. The room still undulated behind him, but it became clearer and more still each time she blinked her eyes open. It pained her head to wonder what John was doing there, yet she hadn't the strength to question him. Slowly memories began to come to her, stinging pieces that squeezed tears from her eyes, left them trickling down her cheeks to fill her ears. Olsen reached out and took her hand. His red eyes looked into hers. He swallowed, but didn't speak. Ruth wanted to give voice to the fear inside her, to sit up and yell, "Jim, where's Jim?" But Olsen's look told her what she didn't want to hear.

She closed her eyes. "No," she whispered, her split lip reopening. "No." She felt John's lips on her hand, the sharp stubble around his mouth, his tears dropping wet and warm on her arm. She remembered the soft brush of Jim's lips on the same hand and heard a cry escape as she drew in her breath at the memory. Jim had become a part of her so quickly. Behind her eyes his face looked out from a thousand angles, his eyes meeting hers with an affection to match her own. She remembered standing with him in the doorway when they walked back from town, felt his hand brush back the hair from her forehead, just as John's was doing now. With a large, rough finger, Olsen wiped tears from under each of her eyes, wiped away her snot with his handkerchief. He lifted a glass of water toward her, and she turned her face away to refuse, though her tongue was dried fast to the roof of her mouth.

For some time anguish took precedent over the pain pounding

her head and the ache of her body; even those remembered fragments of her own attack held little meaning for her. After a while, when her quiet sobs eased and her breath spasms stopped, John rose and began stuffing the stove with wood. She heard him fill a pan with water. When he returned to the chair, she opened her eyes and forced out the words. "Tell me," she said.

"Ingmar went for sheriff in San Bernardino. He be back today sometime." Olsen looked out the window at the moving pine branches.

"No," she said. "About Jim." John looked back at her, but still didn't say anything. Ruth turned her head toward the wall as the tears came back. She knew what John would say but couldn't conceive of that truth. It seemed she and Jim had just risen from this very bed. But then she remembered him on the ground, his lovely hair spread out and streaked with red. After a few minutes, John went over to fix the coffee. When he came back carrying two cups and set them on the floor, she said, "Say it, John. I need you to say it."

"Jim dead, Rute. You know that." He swallowed and clenched his jaw. "He was good man. We get those cowboys. What they do to you . . . men like that not deserve to live." He twisted his fists, one on top of the other. "The whole world gone crazy," he said.

How could Jim be dead, gone so soon from smiling and alive with his hands lathering the skin of her body? Then she remembered other hands and sat up like a shot, pulling the blanket up to cover her breasts. "I'll do it. I'm the one to kill them," she said, imagining herself snapping back the trigger of a shotgun and watching buckshot tear through Charlie Stine's gut, splattering brains out of Bobby Key's skull, the way she'd seen it happen to rabbits after a bad aim. The image surged into her with a blast of black joy.

She registered the shock in John Olsen's face as he nodded and picked up one of the coffee cups, holding it out toward her. "It matter for the sheriff," he said. "I want kill them, too, but we let him handle it." He picked up his own cup and stood. "I go out now so you can dress," he said.

When he shut the door, Ruth set the coffee cup on the chair and moved gingerly out of the bed, her leg and back muscles stiff and sore. Her head swam as she rose. She looked down to see that her breasts were marked with dark streaks and finger-dot bruises, as were her arms and thighs. Dried blood was caked between her thighs. Keeping her balance, she shuffled across the room to the chest of drawers with small, careful steps. She dragged her clothes back to the bed and managed to put on a blouse and skirt and boots without socks, then started toward the front door, her bladder ready to burst. Yet it was a moment before she could bring herself to yank open that door, so afraid she was of finding Jim still on the ground in front of her cabin. But when she pulled it open, he was not there. Their bathtub had been emptied. Ruth looked around. Where had they put him then?

She saw John Olsen down in the wash heading for the spring with a water bucket; she would have to wait to ask him. Ruth began limping toward the outhouse she and Jim had finished, but got only as far as the edge of camp and stopped, easing down on a rock. She winced as her sore flesh met the hard surface. The difficulty of movement, her pounding head, made the privy too far to reach. She got up and hobbled around behind a juniper to relieve herself in a position that further aggravated her racked muscles—but more painful was the sting of urine as it left her. It was all she could do not to cry out and alarm the Swede.

By the time she found her way back to the cabin, Olsen was pouring water into the container that she'd moved inside. "Where is he, John?" she asked, stopping at the cabin door, one hand grasping each side of the wooden frame.

"The dugout. Ingmar, he carry him there till sheriff come. Dugout keep body cool." John slapped the tin lid on the water cooler and picked up the bucket. "I heat water for your bath on campfire, ya." Ruth pictured Jim's body lying in the darkened earth cave where Kate stored her meat carcasses and the photographs of her dead daughter.

"I want to see him," Ruth said, taking a few steps toward the bed and lowering herself onto the mattress until she could lean back against the pillow.

"They be here, Rute. Bring Jim back today."

"Today?" she asked, confused. It was not yet noon and they had just left. "How . . . how . . . can they be back?"

Olsen stopped beside her bed. He lifted the coffee cup from the chair and handed it to her. "Here. You feel better, Rute." She could not bring herself to drink. He sat watching until she brought the cup to her lips and pretended to sip the liquid that stung yet tempted her tongue, its flavor calling out to the life in her she would not heed. John Olsen touched her arm gently. "That good now." When she nodded, he rose, picked up the bucket, and walked the rest of the way to the door, where he turned back.

"It was yesterday, Rute, when they go to San Bernardino. It happen yesterday. You sleep a long time," he said, then walked outside, leaving the door open behind him.

Ruth set the coffee on the floor, but drank the glass of water next to it. Water, she decided, was not an enjoyment; she needed it to stay alive—and she wanted to stay alive to see to it that Stine did not. Her head a bit clearer, she wondered why Kate was not here with her, then worried about why. What else might have happened she hated to think. In such a world, anything might occur. After John had the water heating, she asked him.

"Ya," he said, sitting again in the chair next to her bed. "Kate in San Bernardino hospital. I bring her home next week."

"Is it cancer?"

John shook his head. His eyes sparked up as he said, "She have operation for the gall bladder. She be fine."

"I'm glad, John. Jim . . ?" Ruth stopped, blinked away the moisture that wouldn't leave her eyes, forced her tightening throat to swallow, then continued, "Jim and I were worried. We walked into Juniper to see if anyone had heard from you."

He nodded. "Ya, I stop at the general store for supply. Baxter tell me. I hear what Stine say at Lone Star—that he come after you. John Lee tell me. I drive fast as I can, pick up men to help. But too late."

"Are you saying he told people what he was going to do?"

"People say he yust had too much to drink. A bragging cowboy, ya. But Lee, he think different, come to tell me."

Ruth recalled Stine's remark about her and Johnny Lee. Lee couldn't have been too worried; he'd bragged a bit himself—and he didn't bother to check up, either. So Matt had heard too. She choked up again at the thought. What a conversation those drunken cowboys must have had at the Lone Star, except Stine didn't really get drunk, but mean. The image of Stine's hand lifting and coming down again and again inside her door jerked through her head like the silent film scenes she'd watched in El Paso movie houses. Oh, my poor Jim, what that bastard must have done to you, she thought. Her mind substituted another picture, one of Stine's belly blown open. After she shot him, she would take a knife to him, not to the scalp of his head, but lower, much lower. "How long before they bring Jim back?" she asked to settle herself. "Will the sheriff be here right away?"

John shrugged. "I hope so. Everyting a mess down there, Rute, in San Bernardino. After the crash." Nothing registered with Ruth, preoccupied as she was with seeing the proof of her loss, until John said, "Stock market crash, Rute, you heard?" But she had no interest in such fabricated abstractions, and no understanding that they could affect the real lives of almost everyone she knew.

By the time the bucket of water on the campfire boiled, John Olsen had dutifully filled the tin tub with buckets of water from the spring. He added to that more boiling water from Ruth's large enamel coffeepot, rendering the bath water a more comfortable temperature than the cold water Ruth had been bathing in all summer. Its very comfort at first caused her to refuse, but Olsen's concern, and her own knowledge from nurses' training, changed her mind. When Olsen shut himself inside the house, Ruth lowered her body carefully into the warm water, taking time to adjust to each level of smarting as she settled deeper. When she was immersed in the tub's soothing liquid and the stinging had quieted, another concern came over her. She had used no vinegar or herb after the attack, and for the first time she truly feared for herself. It was too late now, she thought, and the idea of rinsing her sore parts with vinegar made her shudder.

Ruth let the warm water clean her wounds, while sun warmed

her shoulders above the water. Birds flitted and chirped among the pinyons, and a squirrel with a green cone in its mouth ran down a trunk. High overhead, a hawk floated down canyon. But it all seemed removed from her, as if something invisible now stood between her and the world, encasing her in a glasslike bubble. The squirrel trotted toward the tub, stopping to raise up and use two front legs to readjust its pinecone. It stared right at her with tiny, beady eyes. Another squirrel ran toward the first, and the two tore off toward the wash. She recalled what Jim had said about needing to get the pine nuts before the squirrels did. They had filled two gunnysacks with cones. Now he was gone and the squirrels would have the rest to themselves forever.

Ruth pushed away the thought and stood, blotting her skin gently with the towel before stepping out onto the sand in her bare feet. She dressed again in the same skirt and blouse, realizing it would be a while before she could hazard the pants she usually wore. She wished she could examine herself in the small mirror in her chest of drawers, but that would have to wait until John Olsen left. After calling out to John that she was dressed, Ruth walked cautiously to the chair beneath the pine, avoiding the sturdy pinyon needles that tried to penetrate the thick callus layered onto the soles of her feet, the way memories of her attack wanted to penetrate every waking thought. She wouldn't let them, though. She'd had no way to stop the men from hurting her, but she could keep it from happening over again in her mind. She could still deny them the shame they had left with her, though doing so did leave a crust around everything else.

When Olsen came out to empty the tub, he tried to get her to eat some of the canned stew he'd warmed and to go in and rest. But Ruth wanted to be awake when the men came back with Jim's body. She positioned her chair so she faced the cliff on the mountain, putting the area of yesterday's scene behind her back.

The sun was midway to the horizon before they heard the sound of the flatbed engine. Ruth had dozed in her chair, but she jerked awake when the truck rounded the bend. Tears stung behind her burning eyeballs, and she had swallowed several times to dam them by the time the truck pulled up in front of her cabin. And there, behind the cab, she saw the red-and-black blanket—faded but similar to the one they had slept under in the hut. Wrapped in it were the remains of the only person in her life she had ever loved completely, proof that he would never again descend from the bluff to surprise her. Never fix biscuits with her, never kiss her lips.

"Olaf be up later with sheriff," Ingmar told Olsen as he got out of the truck. "I show him the way. They be here soon." He walked over and stood beside Ruth's chair, the others milling around her. The big Swede said nothing, but clamped a hand on her shoulder.

"Did sheriff get Stine?" Olsen asked.

Igmar shook his head. "Stine, he show up at Heart Bar last night. Rode off somewhere. No one seen him after."

"Key?" John Olsen asked. Ingmar shook his head. One of the men spoke in Swedish. "Posse out looking for them," Olsen explained to Ruth.

The men had brought a huge can of stew with them and heated it on the campfire, along with water for coffee, then sat drinking and eating as they waited for the sheriff to arrive, which didn't happen until just before the sun went down. Ruth refused all but the water offered her, though her stomach had started to make its demands known, and her continued dizziness had as much to do now with hunger as with her injuries. Yet she was resolved to ignore it.

Ruth observed the sheriff as he stood talking with the miners by the truck. She turned away when he inspected the bundle. The law officer was a large man, with a huge belly swollen over an oversized belt buckle that cut up into his stomach. He had a walrus moustache and a habit of chewing the inside of his mouth as he stood thinking, giving the impression that the bouncing gray bristles had a life of their own. When he and John Olsen walked over to confer in front of the cabin, Ruth heard for the first time a description of the scene the miners had come upon when they drove up that day.

She had understood that they found the two of them together naked on the ground, for she remembered wrapping her arm around Jim earlier. But she hadn't known that Jim had the shotgun under him, nor that there was a blood trail leading away from the front of the house to the wash and beyond. It didn't jibe with the picture she remembered, Stine's arm coming down and Jim left on the floor of the cabin. But now she wondered how Jim got back out in front where she last saw him. The sound of the loud blast came back to her. Of course.

Ruth explained to the sheriff what had happened, how she and Jim were in the yard when the cowboys came, how the men threatened them and Jim ran for the gun, with Stine going in after him. How they went after her when he came out. The men shuffled and looked away when the sheriff asked if she and Jim had been bathing together when the cowboys rode up, another part she'd skipped over as she told her story, but one that seemed to interest the sheriff. She nodded, took in a breath, and filled in the details of what Stine had said, though she didn't see that the cowboys' reasons were anything to consider. The sheriff studied her as she spoke, one hand massaging his chin. His mouth fidgeted, and his head bobbed subtly in a knowing nod. Ruth felt more than saw the shift; even in the dimming light Ruth could tell that his pale gray eyes were the deadest she'd ever seen.

"How long did you know the two men before that day?" he asked, studying her.

"I don't know, since sometime in spring—after I started my homestead. April, maybe. If you can call it knowing them." He continued to stare at her until she explained further. "The first time we met, their cattle trampled my garden."

"So you didn't know them in any other way?" He looked down at his boot, rubbed its sole in the sand and tapped its toe, then looked back up at her. "Like you knew the Indian, I mean."

Blood rushed to Ruth's head so fast her ears rang. The moment throbbed under his question. No one moved or spoke until the sheriff said, "I mean, it seems like a lot of damage for those boys to do for no reason at all."

"They bad men, I warn her . . . no good . . . no good," John Olsen started to explain, his face pained for her, but the sheriff raised his palm to stop him.

"I asked the lady a question," he said. "Let's hear what she answers." But Ruth was far from answering, her eyes fixed firm on the six-gun strapped to the sheriff's hip, ready to lunge for it at his next word and blow his simulated pregnancy to smithereens.

John Olsen came around behind Ruth's chair and set a firm hand on each of her shoulders.

"I ran them off with a rifle the first time they came here," she said, her jaw clenched and rage roaring into her ears that she had to say it. "Jim did the same once when they threatened us down at the willows. That seems like reason to me. They harassed us again a few days ago."

"Rute punch Stine at the dance once," John added. "Everyone see it."

The sheriff stood rubbing his chin and tapping the toe of one boot. "She didn't answer my question," he said.

It took all the restraint Ruth had not to jump up and claw him. She wanted to draw blood, even if it was simply with fingernails. Only the granite of Olsen's hands kept her from flying apart. "What difference would that make?" she said. "They killed Jim and . . . attacked"—she forced out the word to correct herself—"raped me." When the sheriff's moustache began to rise in a knowing smile, she swallowed hard and said, "But to answer your question, no, I did not know the men, either man, in, as you put it, the way I knew the Indian. The man's name is Jim, sheriff, Jim Daniel." But she could see it was too late to make him believe her—if he ever would have.

"Was," he said. "Was Jim Daniel." The sheriff strode over to the front of her cabin and squatted down to examine the ground. With a soft squeeze to brace her, John let go of Ruth's shoulders and went to stand over the lawman. She took in a breath and found she held together. Ingmar gave her a kindly nod.

"I have to establish motive, that's all, Mr. Olsen," Ruth heard the sheriff say in response to something John said in low tones. "I'm just trying to find out what went on here."

"Rute tell you that. I tell you what Stine say at the Lone Star,"

Olsen said, his voice raised, but strong with authority. Ruth imagined the sheriff chewing furiously on his inner lip.

"I'll check all that out later," he said. "But this is a serious matter, serious charges to bring against a man. I have to be sure first." He sounded almost reasonable until Ruth heard him say in a lower voice, "With a woman like that men are sometimes driven to do things they wouldn't ordinarily do."

"And what kind of woman would that be, Mister Sheriff?" Ruth said, rising from her chair with a force that surprised her and everyone else. She closed the distance between them.

"I was speaking to Mr. Olsen here," the man said, his face a steel wall. Even the moustache had stopped bouncing. Ruth felt the miners gathering behind her.

"You were talking about me. At least you could say it to my face."

"I'm surprised you'd want me to." He looked square at her. "The kind of woman that cavorts naked with Indians needs no further explanation," he said.

Ruth swung around and flew inside her house, heading straight for the mattress. The gun was already in her hands when John came rushing in behind her. From the yard came the loud voices of miners arguing with the sheriff. In one motion, Olsen held fast her arm with a huge hand and with the other took the rifle. "Give it back," she hissed, her entire body shaking, her blood an axe-thumping pain against the top of her skull. All boundaries of behavior lay behind her. What else could she lose?

Olsen shook his head. He tossed the .22 onto the cot and pulled Ruth into his arms, holding her fast as she struggled to free herself, as if that would loosen the grip of emotion about to overpower her. In the end, the turmoil was too strong for her, and, bit by bit, she gave in to it, sobbing into Olsen's barrel of a chest as he held on to steady her.

The next morning Ruth was grateful for the thin sheet of cloud dimming the sun's light, a physical presence that gave body to the shield between herself and the world. A warm wind whipped at what was left of her hair as she watched the men carry Jim's wrapped body to the grave at the foot of the bluff.

The rest of her hair she had hacked off and coiled inside her first small olla, and when the miners laid Jim in the shallow depression, she knelt and placed the rough clay pot into the space where his arms came together under the blanket. She almost stopped the men, then, when they lifted the shovels and stood waiting as John walked over to move her back from the edge of the grave, fighting her desire to unwrap the blanket and pull it back from Jim's face, sure that he would wake up; yet she knew well that he would not and that his face would not now resemble the face of the man she had loved. So she allowed Olsen to raise her and stepped back from the rim so the men could throw on their shovels of dirt, hiding the faded patterns that defined Jim's shape. When earth began to cover his face, she found herself drawing in huge, deep breaths against a sensation of suffocation, as if she now had to breathe for both of them.

After the crevice around the body had been filled and sand mounded over, the miners covered the loosened earth with rocks brought up from the wash until several layers were piled over the site, so that nothing could dig Jim up. Olsen and the miners had wanted to construct a coffin, but Ruth could not bear to encase him, and they had agreed to use the rocks instead. Once the burial was complete, they went across the wash to roast slabs of John's billy kid over Ruth's campfire. John Olsen had tried hard to persuade Ruth to have supper and stay the night at his place in the willows, but she would not hear of it, nor would she allow anyone to stay with her another night.

"It too soon for you to be alone, Rute. You need be with others," Olsen said late that afternoon as the men sat eating around the campfire; Ruth, weak from no food, remained stalwart in her fast. "You not ready yet," he said. Ruth glanced at him, then back up at the bluff, as if she expected to see Jim suddenly rise up and ascend the rock face.

"Those cowboys might come back, ya," Ingmar told her. "You need we stay."

"The sheriff thinks Stine went back to Texas and Key with him, remember," Ruth reminded him, referring to the conversation John Olsen had with the sheriff when he returned earlier that morning. Ruth hadn't wanted the lawman there for the burial, so they'd waited around for him to leave. In the end, Ingmar had to make Ruth's request clear to him before he would go, which he did in an ugly humor.

"But you eat nothing," John Olsen said. It was as if he had become Kate in her absence, seeing to it that Ruth was fed. "Not good lose your strength. Jim not like it." Ruth took long drinks from her water to fill her stomach. The smells of food and coffee were getting to her; it had been nearly two days now since she had eaten, three if she counted the day of the cowboys' attack. The wind had cooled and increased in the gray afternoon, and she was finding it hard to resist the thought of hot coffee. But what would it say about her love for Jim if she ate so easily, as if nothing had happened?

"I'll eat," she said. "Soon. I'm not ready yet."

"I stay one more night," Olsen insisted. "Then I go." His tone told her no amount of arguing would change his mind, and Ruth was surprised to find herself glad of it.

The setting sun broke through a crack in the cloud, painting a sheet of red over their heads, and when Ruth looked up from the bluff, she found the color disturbed by huge black birds circling silently beneath the glowing surface. Buzzards, hundreds of them in spirals along the length of the open canyon. Before the others had seen to stop her, Ruth went in for her .22. She stepped out the door and aimed into the moving targets.

"Rute," John said, rising from his chair. "Buzzards go south for winter. Stop at willows for water. They not after Jim." But her shaking finger had already pulled the trigger.

Ruth's bullet lost itself in the sky and the buzzards continued their slow spirals without disruption. Afterward, she saw that they were indeed gradually moving away down canyon, and most were out of sight soon after the sun disappeared. A few that weren't dropped down into the cottonwoods behind the spring to roost, the weight of their huge bodies sending some of the weaker branches crashing to the ground.

Ruth moved her chair to the bank of the wash and kept watch

over the grave until long after the black birds had blended into the dark. Despite more assurance from John Olsen, and from the miners before they left, she kept expecting to see the creatures flap big, whooshing wings over to the pile of rocks and sweep the stones aside, digging ugly beaks deep into the earth to get at Jim's body.

"You need go back home, Rute, to El Paso," John said later that evening, after the others were gone and the two of them sat inside, Ruth at last allowing herself one cup of coffee and a small piece of goat meat, choosing one that had been charred tasteless. "This no place for you, now. Maybe you come back when things over."

"But this is my home, John. I have no other," she said, surprised. "This is the only place I want to be. Jim's here."

"But you have family, Rute, in El Paso. They take care of you."

Ruth stifled a laugh. Take care of her, indeed. Besides, she felt it might kill her to leave this place now. Where in Texas, she wondered, did Stine run to? Texas was a big place—huge and ugly. She would ask around when she got stronger. "I might go back, but not now. And not to stay," she said.

Her answer seemed to satisfy the Swede, and he got up to lay out the mat he'd brought to sleep on. Ruth knew he would wait for her to make a trip outside before he settled down for the night, so she went out to pee near the bank of the wash, finding it slightly easier each time, both to squat and to release the fluid. The afternoon's wind had turned chill, and there was now a dampness in the air. Thin, high clouds diffused light from the waning moon and spread brightness across the canyon; Ruth stared hard at the gravesite but saw no hovering black shapes above it.

When she returned, John Olsen blew out the lamp, and Ruth lay back in the dark cabin. The images of Jim's body being lowered into the ground, the dirt thrown over his form, the dark birds spiraling against a bloodred sky loomed large in the room, kept alive by Olsen's prolonged snores. Ruth's eyes stayed hot and dry. Then other images came to take the place of the first,

comforting her as they nudged her toward sleep. She saw the
wide-open El Paso plains, a rotting body with buzzards circling
purposefully above, while a few on the ground dug big beaks
into flesh just below a bright patch of orange hair.

CHAPTER THIRTEEN

Once Kate and John left tomorrow for the winter mines, Ruth would not see them until spring. The couple would have been gone a month ago had it not been for Kate's need to recover from surgery. Then the word came down that the desert mines would stay closed this year because of the crash. Yet a week ago they received new information that excavations would start on schedule—though wages had taken a cut—and the Olsens had spent the last few days preparing for their yearly move. Ruth expected they would be up today to say good-bye, and no doubt leave her more food. Kate had wanted to leave a nanny with Ruth for the winter, but Ruth would not accept it. They also tried to force several laying hens and a few pullets on her, claiming that they needed her to keep them. But Ruth knew they always took the animals with them. John insisted on driving her to town to get stocked up before the snows hit; already there was a thin coating of white at the top of Rocky Mountain. Ruth herself had lost all interest in addressing her needs—which was why the Olsens insisted—but she had hoped letters from El Paso would be waiting for her at the store, so she allowed them to take her. Yet no mail awaited her.

Ruth had gone along with several of the Olsens' plans for her, wanting to be grateful, though the most she could manage was a sense of obligation not to appear ungrateful. John and Kate cared for her—whether she wanted them to or not—and were more family than she had known in El Paso, where she had simply played a role in ongoing dramas. Now, because of the Olsens she walked and ate and spoke as if she were really herself and not, like the crusty locust shells she found attached to trees, emptied out. All that remained of her was the lust to obliterate a man with orange hair. All the softness inside her was gone, replaced by hate. It had been a blow to find no letters at the store yesterday. In her correspondence to Aunt Myrtle three weeks ago, Ruth had enclosed another letter, this one to her uncle Ben, asking the lawman if he could find out where in Texas the fugitive Charlie Stine had gone. Ruth had written to her aunt for that purpose alone; it had been a silly letter, really, meant to disguise any sign of Ruth's trouble, and mentioning casually at the end that she had told the local sheriff that she would personally ask her uncle, the well-known El Paso police chief, for his unofficial help in a matter—so would Aunt Myrtle please give him the letter? The enclosure to her uncle detailed the matter further—but left out Ruth's involvement in it. And, of course, Ruth had told the local sheriff no such thing, knowing he could care less if Stine were ever found and certainly would never share with Ruth any information he gathered. But Stine's escape was real enough and would be listed in the proper bulletins, where her uncle could verify the information. Since she had not revealed the name of the fictitious sheriff, Ruth hoped her uncle would be forced to go through her to answer the fictitious query.

Other than the loss of considerable weight, and a temporary

loss of strength, Kate had come back from her illness much her old self, and for that Ruth really was grateful. The woman had said nothing about Jim or the attack when John brought her to see Ruth that first time, but had taken Ruth in her large arms and rocked her. Ruth felt some slight stirrings then, yet since that day with the sheriff, her eyes had stayed as dry as desert sand and as parched as she felt inside.

It was midday by the time the flatbed rounded the bend, with Kate and John in the cab and the miners on the back. Kate had prepared a supper as well; one look at the bounty of strudels and bread told Ruth that Kate had spent the morning baking, which accounted for the returned paleness of her face. Guilt peppered Ruth's armor, angering her, until Kate reached out with abundant arms and cushioned Ruth's steely form inside them.

"Strudel for you. Make you strong," Kate told her, reaching into the basket she had set inside on Ruth's table. Ruth closed the door against the November gusts, while Kate piled kindling into the stove. The miners had gone up the draw for the rest of the cut wood, and John and Ingmar set to work constructing a shelter over the wood supply that she and Jim had piled high alongside the house. Ruth watched their industry with some dismay, not knowing what else she could do to discourage such well-intended intrusion.

"You be glad, Rute," Kate said, laying a hand on Ruth's back when she saw her watching the men out the window. "When cold and snow come." How could Ruth tell her that the weather outside could never be as cold as she felt inside? She merely nodded and spread her lips into a smile so forced she thought her cheeks might crack.

Kate patted her and went back to filling the coffeepot with water. Ruth put Kate's big pot of chili to heat on the back burner, dreading the nausea she expected to feel at the smell of food. While the pots were heating, Kate set Ruth's two chairs to face each other in front of the fire and sat in one of them. "Come sit, Rute," she said, patting the other chair. Ruth made her legs obey.

"I so sorry for what happen to you," Kate said, taking Ruth's hand, her face so full of feeling Ruth could hardly make herself look at it. "You be okay. You young woman, life ahead of you."

Ruth looked out the window. Stine had taken whatever life she had in her. The only way to get it back was to find him. She didn't care what happened after that. John himself said the man didn't deserve to live. Even so, Ruth couldn't imagine herself living afterward. Her former exuberance seemed to her as silly and excessive as the way she used to glamorize the men she was attracted to. Before Jim came along. He alone stood solid in his worth. And now he was buried like the boulder.

"Rute," Kate said, giving Ruth's hand a soft squeeze, "I wish I could stop the bad happening. But no one can. When Sarah die, I want die too." Kate's face brimmed with suffering. "But I have to go on."

"But were you ever the same, Kate?" Ruth said. "I mean, was it still you, really?" She stood up and walked to the window looking out onto the bluff. "Was the Kate that went on really the same you?" Ruth walked back and sat down again. The woman was looking down at the floor, her eyes fixed far away. "Sometimes I think, Kate, that you made the whole world your daughter—always making sure we're all fed, as if we are all your children."

"Specially you, Rute," Kate said, looking up. "You just like Sarah—full of life."

"But I'm not. I'm not full of life." Ruth jerked up from the chair. "Stop saying that." She didn't want that kind of love. It didn't belong to her; it belonged to their dead daughter. And love brought its own entrapments—even the best of loves, like Jim's—which is why she had been cleaned out inside, like the rabbits she had dressed out. A carcass ready to be cooked and eaten.

Ruth looked back at Kate's face. It had been easier to ignore Myrtle's concern born of duty and spite for Cally, and to disregard Cally's self-centered mothering. Ruth understood those things. But this kind of caring caught her off guard, obligated her in some way she couldn't defend against.

"It take time, Rute," Kate said, getting up from her chair. At the stove, she lifted the lid from the chili pot, and the spicy smell wafted across the room as she stirred. Ruth found the aroma appetizing and wondered if she might even eat for the first time in days. Almost hopeful, she considered for a moment not sending her letter to Cally with the Olsens, but decided she wouldn't take the chance: if her fears were justified, she would need Cally's mysterious herb—too much was at stake now to trust to fate. And she would send a reminder to her Uncle Ben that the information about Charlie Stine's whereabouts was still needed.

When the men came in, Ruth poured coffee into the cups Kate had laid out on the table, distributing them once the bowls of chili had been ladled out and the men seated on the cement floor to eat. Ruth found it easier these days to put aside the unpleasantness of being beholden; there were now far worse things to keep out of her reach. John and Kate ate without conversing, as if leaving Ruth weighed on them, but the miners joked about their having to get out before the snows came, and told her how the snow would be so huge it would close over the windows, and how she would wish the privy sat right outside her front door. Ruth appreciated their lightening the situation, but she wondered if such a winter were really possible here in this canyon. The miners' descriptions, Olsen said, were exaggerated, but old-timers had told of hard winters. They weren't leaving because of the threat of snow, he told her, but because the snow on Onyx Peak made mining impossible for the winter months, so they had in recent years worked the salt mines in the lower deserts. Several snowfalls of a few inches each were normal, he said, but some winters could get extremely cold in the canyons below Rocky Mountain. "Canyon no place for woman alone," he added, as if he hadn't already said that many times, trying once again to talk Ruth into going to El Paso for the winter.

She had no care whether or not the snow buried her and her cabin completely—the idea of being encased in ice seemed appropriate. Yet she wanted to be able to walk out to Juniper Valley and get word of Stine's location from Uncle Ben. She would go after him—even if she had to hitch a ride again, as she had when escaping from the girls' school. And the response from Cally could be crucial. Not knowing the contents of the letters she handed them, the Olsens seemed eager to mail them—the correspondence with Cally alone might have caused them to drag Ruth away to the mines if they'd known, so she allowed them to think she was considering a return to her family's comforting arms. And she might well return to Texas if she could learn the cowboy's whereabouts, though no one there would comfort her, as the Olsens thought. That family had no capacity for comfort, even if she should need such consolation. But she did not.

Once the supper mess had been cleared away, and Kate and John had given her several hugs and several more warnings about keeping in a supply of water that wouldn't be frozen, and wood inside for the stove and many other details that Ruth couldn't keep track of even had she wanted to, and Ingmar and the other miners wished her luck through the winter—and she them—the group gathered up and drove off. By then it was well past dark, and Ruth stood outside her front door watching their headlights illuminate the brush along the road as the vehicle traveled to the bend and out of sight. Then she was finally alone, opening up to the mournful whine of pines while cold wind harassed the few whips of hair left on her shorn head.

CHAPTER FOURTEEN

Ruth's decision to climb Rocky Mountain had come of a sudden, after weeks of clouded days, both inside and out, where she had warmed herself by the embers of her hatred for Stine. Then she had woken one morning from a dream where the olla of her house shattered to pieces around her as she used her arms to shield her face and head from heavy shards that kept cracking down on her. A nightmare no less real than her life had become. She had been relieved to find the rock walls around her intact, though she shivered in vivid dream residue and pulled up the covers under her chin. Ruth closed her eyes, and memories came to her of the days she had sat naked in the sun with Jim, coiling clay into ollas that they pit-fired a few days later. The two clay pots were still up in Jim's house of boughs and skins. She pictured them there, side by side, where they left them on Jim's red-and-black blanket—if his spare shelter had withstood the wind and storms that buffeted the mountaintop as Ruth watched from her window. Too much of her time she spent staring out that window at the bluff, as if the winter face of the mountain, with its frequent cap of foreboding cloud and rush of flurries, contained something for her. Her memories of those brief days with Jim were dimming until she had trouble believing them. Only her hatred remained real and constant. Until this morning, when the dream of ollas and a warm red blanket appeared like a tangible answer for her to seek from the mountain.

Ruth put her good pair of wool slacks over the ones she'd worn for the last few days, and another flannel shirt over the one covering her cotton undershirt. Each layer went on easily, her clothes now hanging loosely. An extra pair of socks made her boots a bit too snug, but she knew they would stretch as she walked. With her wool mackinaw covering all that, it took some doing to move her arms and she felt like a child's stuffed animal. Even warmly dressed, Ruth knew she took a chance climbing the mountain with the storm that seemed to be developing. This morning's clouds were not just a helmet capping the peaks, but gray racing rags overhead that spit an occasional flake against the windowpane in warning. To ignore the risk gave her a sense of satisfaction, as if she dared the world to care less about her than she herself did. It was a way to take back control and defy her body's betrayal.

Her nausea had subsided in the weeks since the Olsens had left, leaving a raging appetite in its place. That appetite seemed a hunger other than her own, and she had stood firm against it, not wanting to give in to the needs of anything alien inside her. As yet no curse had come to her, and the continued tenderness of her breasts long after the bruises had faded convinced her that her fears were justified. But still no word—or herb—from her mother, though she had twice made trips into Juniper Valley to check her mail. It angered her that such a plague, like the damnable curse she now longed for, was not one visited upon the men that caused it. Even more insidious than her bodily changes

180

was the growing change she felt in her thinking; already she had to resist impulses to protect and care for herself in ways that were not natural to her. And she had to fight an overwhelming desire to sleep more, to eat foods that didn't usually appeal to her. The condition had not gone this far the time in El Paso. It was as if something had taken root in her and was now wanting to take charge completely. At times her thinking was no longer her own, though she could still distinguish it through blurred lines. It galled her to know that she had struggled for so long to escape the control of those around her, to control her own life, and now found control wrested from her from the inside. Only Cally's remedy could save her, and each time Ruth returned empty-handed from town, her hatred of Stine deepened. She had not yet heard from Myrtle nor her uncle—had expected at least some word or gift for Christmas last week, but received nothing from anyone. And according to Jack Hudson, who gave her a ride back to the mouth of the canyon on her last trip, the sheriff had found no trace of Stine. As if he were actively looking. Unless she heard something soon, she would be forced by weather to wait until spring to go after him. She also learned, for the first time, that Bobby Key had been found dead of buckshot. It was believed that Jim had crawled outside and shot the man before he died and that given the trail of blood leading away, Stine might have been injured as well.

Ruth walked to Jim's grave before she left, welcoming the bitter blasts that blew under her coat collar, even as she tightened the opening against them. She squatted and stared down at the pile of stones, fragments of mountain that covered over her lover. Reaching out, she placed her palm on the cold surface of a rock. A snowflake landed on the back of her hand, and she watched it melt into her skin.

The few flakes that sputtered down in the canyon became a light gauze around her as she traveled up Rocky Mountain, though only a thin sheet of snow covered the ground, the rest swirled into tiny drifts against rocks or pooled under the bottoms of brush. She hurried upward before the snow stuck enough to hide the familiar features she was following toward

Jim's camp. Yet the flakes continued in fits and starts, not serious enough to hide the ground completely, but deepening to almost an inch from earlier snowfalls near his camp.

Rushing clouds thinned overhead and a patch of blue looked ready to show through just before Ruth reached the pile of boulders that guarded the entrance to Jim's camp, then thickened again as she slid through the opening between the rocks, and the lake came into view, its surface mottled with dull frozen patches. She stepped in further and caught sight of the whitened exterior of the hut front. Hugging her back against the cold boulder for support, a few stray flakes feathering against her face, Ruth fought an impulse to turn and flee from this place that had offered up a man to love and took him away quicker than it gave him, the way a stroke of lightning at night offers up a view of the world, then snatches it from you so fast you aren't sure you really saw it. Ruth wondered now if anything she felt those few days had been real. But she had come this far and so strode boldly across the clearing and undid the flap of the hut, the way she had once jumped abruptly into the cold water of the lake to get the shock over as quickly as possible.

Emptied of Jim, the shelter appeared forlorn. Bits of chewed pinecones lay strewn on the red blanket around the two ollas. Inside one of the ollas, Ruth found a small stash of pine nuts, where a squirrel had stored a portion of its winter food. She knelt beside the bed, took her hands from her jacket pockets, and put an arm around each of the ollas. Their rough surfaces felt warm against her frigid palms. Emotion surged up at their touch, roared out of her chest in harsh shouts, and somewhere in that tempest Ruth gave over and lost herself. It wasn't until she stood outside in front of the petroglyphs, one olla lying in shards among the snow-covered rocks, the other half buried in a drift, that she came back to herself. Snow was falling in a heavy curtain around her, the icy tinkle of colliding crystals soft against the rocks. The landscape had been glossed over with a thick coat of white. Where she had been and for how long she didn't know, but she dropped down and began gathering up shards, then let fall the pieces and rushed over to find the other olla intact. Jim's olla had somehow missed the rocks and survived.

Bone-chilled and shaking profusely, Ruth took the pot tenderly in her arms and carried it back into the hut. Hands red and white with cold, her fingers could barely manipulate the wood as she piled kindling and logs into the fire ring. She dug out a match from Jim's coffee can supply and struck it on a rock. Beyond exhaustion and emotion, she wanted simply to be warm and held out her palms to the fire as it blazed up. When the flame took hold fully, Ruth turned her back and sat stupefied in its heat, her mind blank as the snow-coat outside, no emotion or thought left in her. After a while, she crawled over to the blanket and under it with the olla, curling her body around the clay container.

A dim, blue-gray light permeated the hut when Ruth opened her eyes. The fire was out and her face felt like ice above the blanket. Crawling to the door, she pulled back the flap, squinting against the glare of surfaces brighter than the air around them, daylight fast draining away into night. Ruth leaned out and measured the snow with her hand. It reached from the tip of her middle finger to about an inch above her wrist. Pulling back her hand, she rubbed it under her other arm, straightened, and latched the door flap. It was too late to make it back to her cabin; she would be caught out on the mountain in the dark.

Ruth checked the supply of firewood against the wall. Several more logs and some kindling. Not a lot left, especially when caught in a snowstorm, she thought, picturing the wood supply back at her cabin, useless to her here. In the morning she would have to try to reach her place. The important thing was to keep herself warm till then.

The embers in the fire ring yet had heat, and a few ends of logs remained unburned. Ruth used those, along with a small helping of kindling, to revive the fire, holding open the front of her jacket to let in the warmth. Her stomach complained of its emptiness, but she had nothing to give it. At once she remembered the quail Jim had roasted over this very fire ring, the taste of the succulent bird coming back to water her mouth anew. She had been sad when they killed the quail; somehow it felt different than with rabbit. Jim had stopped to apologize and thank the quail. His people once had a proper way of thanks, he said, for the killing of game, but he didn't know it, so this would have to do. Since his death, she'd been killing the little birds herself, and without an apology, in fact, enjoying the sight of their innocent heads gone limp, black topknots lying against the ground. She took perverse pleasure in ripping the feathers from their still-warm bodies. She ate the birds, too, of course—and maybe that was enough—but it was no longer the point of it.

They had used up all Jim's supplies—coffee, flour, and everything else—before they'd left, but she dug around in the food tin and found several dried green sticks of the kind he'd used for tea the first time he brought her here. She packed snow high over the sticks in a small pan and set it on the fire to boil. She also found a jar with tiny black and gray seeds. Chia, he'd once told her, sprinkling some in her hand, good food for hiking. She shook out a pile into her palm, touched her tongue to it, and ground the seeds against her teeth. The flavor was something like a spicy nut. She ate about half the seeds and put away the rest. The tea was slightly bitter and tangy, but she drank it, then added more snow and boiled herself another hot cup of it. Afterward, she put a few more logs on the fire, setting some aside for morning.

Easing a warm stone from the ring, Ruth buried it between the top and bottom blankets, near the foot, then pulled Jim's red kerchief from the snag and tied it around her head for warmth. She considered removing her boots, but decided against it, buttoned her coat collar and got under both blankets, lying directly on the mattress of leaves and debris. It took some time before the stone's heat penetrated and she could stop shivering, but gradually even the duff warmed under her.

For a long while Ruth lay awake; the animal skins overhead prancing and alive in the firelight. It seemed strange to her that she should desire to stay alive now, when only this morning she'd had no interest in it at all—or thought so at the time. She wasn't sure why she was so determined to survive; she told her-self it was to fulfill her promise to kill Stine, though she had not once thought of him since she woke from her unplanned nap. Yet given the alien she believed lodged inside her, it might in-deed be easier to fall asleep in this hut and not wake up. Here would be a good place for her bones to stay, where she and Jim had been. No one would know what happened to her. When they returned, the Olsens would think she went back to El Paso.

But she wouldn't die tonight, she knew, would not just fall asleep and never wake. That would be too easy, and things had never been easy for her. More likely, if she did die, it would be out in the open on the way back tomorrow, trudging through deep snow and losing her way in a changed landscape. Ruth wondered how much snow would fall tonight, but it didn't mat-ter—she would walk down the mountain in the morning. And no amount of snow would stop her.

Morning had brightened the hut when Ruth surfaced from a sleep that had finally come to her like a belated gift. For a few moments she kept still so as not to disturb the warm niche she had made around her. Her comfort extended beyond the physi-cal, the remnants of dream encasing her like a campfire's warmth, furnishing the cold hut with the intensity of her feeling. There was Jim above her, his long hair draping a curtain around their faces. "I love you, Ruth," he whispered, as he had not said before—though she had never doubted it. "And I love you, Jim," she had said, speaking into the lips already touching hers. Now she lay steeped in gratitude, longing, and regret. Gradually, the residue faded and the need to pee overruled her desire to hold on to the emotion. She pulled back the covers and confronted the air, rose and unlatched the flap. She found the snow level risen, but not dramatically, now reaching from her fingertip to halfway to her elbow. The sky was overcast, but no snow was falling.

Ruth walked out into the white expanse, fluff falling away from her feet at each step. When she reached the edge of the lake she turned around and looked back. The hut had become a white lump, the rocks beside it bumps in a pool of cream, the tree branches above the ledge draped with a layer of snow. Below them the wall of rocks with petroglyphs had been framed in white, intensifying their etched patterns. It would have been beautiful to her, Ruth thought, such a short time ago. Now it simply sat there, frozen into fact.

She ate snow, heated water to warm herself, and finished the rest of the chia. Standing at the door of the hut, Ruth looked back at the olla and the blanket. They would be harder to carry back in this storm. But she couldn't countenance the thought of leaving these remnants of her lover to freeze here on the mountain, so she wrapped the olla carefully in Jim's blanket and started down the mountain, the bundle over her shoulder. Her worry about getting lost was well founded, she realized, on the transformed mountainside. Even her ability to estimate the location of Glory Springs by sight had been made impossible by the low cloud cover against the mountain, which allowed her to see only a short distance in front of her—about the space from her cabin to the bend, she thought. All she had to go by was down, but she knew she'd end up somewhere at the bottom—as long as she was careful not to walk off the edge of a snow-covered precipice. But no telling where at the bottom she might arrive, for she had learned from experience that a small step in the wrong direction at the top could land her miles from where she intended— not much to worry about on a warm summer's day, but another matter during a snowstorm.

On the first few ridges she followed, she felt confident of her direction. As she went on, the web of ridges became more confusing. Nothing looked familiar buried under the mounds of snow. Confronted with the maze before her, she tried to remember the reverse direction from the way she came up, whether it was to the right or left, but soon would forget whether she'd chosen the ridge to the right or left the time before. Feet aching with cold, and blanket ends wrapped for warmth around the bare hand that carried the olla, Ruth began choosing direction by which way looked easier to negotiate. She tried tying the blanket and olla around her waist to free her aching arm, but kept bashing into brush and getting hung up, so she untied the blanket and lugged the pot over her shoulder again. For a while she progressed downward smoothly until, just at the point where she became the most confident—after thinking that she recognized a stand of oak beside a certain pile of boulders—she found herself trapped in a cage of scrub oak and manzanita, with no way to go but down a sheer dropoff or back up the way she had come. So she backtracked to the place where she had another choice of direction. After that she tempered her choices with intuition.

When the fog finally thinned, lower on the mountain, and Ruth found herself walking in snow above her ankles instead of halfway up her calf, she still found nothing to recognize about the white ridges visible below or the canyons between them. What she did recognize was the fresh trail made by two deer heading down the side of a draw—but in a direction other than she had planned to go. She stood for a moment considering: she was totally disoriented, without a directional clue except which way was up and which down, and she had begun to doubt even that; she could imagine herself wandering around the huge mountain until nightfall if she chose wrong; a few flakes had begun to fall again, and the window of clearing below was starting to close. Ruth took a deep breath and followed the tracks, hoping the deer knew the way better than she did.

The trail cut diagonally across the steep draw and angled up the ridge on the other side, then over a hogback—not a route Ruth would have otherwise attempted, deer being more skilled climbers than humans, but she found the way surprisingly efficient, at least downhill, and snow was easier to walk on than the loose sand she knew was underneath the snowy sides of the draw. The tracks followed the ridgetop for a long stretch, looping down the side again and back up when the top got too rocky and brush-covered to be passable. The trailblazers' familiarity with the landscape reassured her, and she found herself absorbing some of the confidence that came of the creatures' conversancy. She walked past places where they had stopped to nibble scrub oak leaves on the bottoms of snow-covered branches, leaving in exchange fresh brown pellets melted into the white ice. The scattered flakes had increased to a light snow, but unlike yesterday's it wasn't coming down around her, but blowing by on a slant in the wind that had come up, hindering visibility even more. Ruth hastened along, afraid the deer tracks would fill up, her own feet dragging deep streaks in the snow behind her feet. Her fast pace served to keep her warm, even in wind, except for inside her boots, where each foot had turned to a chunk of wood or ice, and her face, which had gone numb against the falling flakes.

When a steep section of trail led off a ridge onto an expanse of level ground, and she saw the hazy outline of another mountain in front of her, Ruth still didn't realize that she'd reached bottom. Then she tramped across a wide path of white stretching as far as she could see in either direction, which was by then only a few yards. She continued to follow the tracks well past the patch before she recognized its significance, before she turned and backtracked. It was indeed the rut road through the canyon. Relief and a faint joy washed over her; she turned to her left and followed it up canyon, already imagining the blaze of fire she would soon have in her stove, the biscuits she would make to go with the can of beans she would open. She could almost taste them. Blessed, delicious beans, hot in her mouth, her stomach mumbled in a language of its own.

She had traveled a few bends up canyon, preoccupying herself with thoughts of the comfort she would soon have, when she noticed a dilapidated wooden structure to her right, then another beside it, beyond that yet another. She came to a standstill. There were no such structures in her canyon. This was not her canyon, not Rattlesnake at all. She had thought this canyon narrower than she remembered, the walls more sheer, but she couldn't see clearly enough in the snow to be sure. Now she remembered that she had turned left to go up canyon, when she should have turned to the right.

After the initial stun of disappointment had turned to a cold knot of fear, Ruth trudged through the wind and blowing snow to the first structure, which she found to be nothing more than three splintering walls left after the roof and another wall had caved in. The rough-hewn planks had darkened with age. She stopped to eat a handful of snow, then made her way to the next structure. All looked long deserted, the wood old and coming apart, but she hoped there might be something left around to eat, her stomach still fixated on the beans, and a place to warm herself. Maybe she could at least find some clue to tell her where she was. The door of the next shack had been nailed shut with a plank, so she walked around the side and peered in the low window whose pane had long since disappeared. The tiny room was more intact than the last; a pile of old clothing lay heaped in the middle of the floor, the trunk around it split open and fallen away. A fireplace, the rocks partially fallen in, occupied the far corner; in another corner, a kangaroo rat peered out at her from its pile of sticks, then vanished back into its nest.

Ruth hoisted the blanketed olla through the window and climbed over the sill, stepping into the drift of snow that had blown in. The room stank of generations of rodent urine. She squatted to examine the pile of clothing, thinking it might hold a clue as to her whereabouts. But when she took hold of the thinned material, it came apart in her fingers. With her boot, she moved aside the top of the pile, rat pellets dropping and bouncing onto the wooden plank floor. She turned her face to avoid the stench. Underneath, the cloth stayed firmer, and she eased out one of the garments, a woman's dress of dark green velvet, now so fragile she could pull the cloth apart with her fingers. Carefully, she spread the garment out, noting the high-button collar, the puff sleeves at the shoulder, the bustle bucket at the back. A woman's high-button shoe lay beneath the dress, its leather twisted and gnarled with age.

Snow blew sideways outside the window, while gusts whistled through cracks between the planks. Stopping her motion was having its effect; Ruth's teeth had begun to chatter. She felt a shaking coming on so deep she was afraid no fire could ever reach it. Rubbing her hands together, she stomped her feet, but it made them hurt. She tried wiggling her toes inside her boots, but couldn't feel much past the pain of moving them.

She decided to clean the litter of rat pellets and debris from the fireplace, but wasn't sure whether the caved-in side would cause the shack to catch on fire. She didn't care, she decided, if this shack burned, she would move to the next one down, and the next, burning them all as she went to keep herself warm. As Ruth looked for something to scrape with, picking up the shoe to use as a tool, she realized she hadn't thought to bring a match with her from the hut. With that she sank down against the wall and buried her head in her hands. She could feel defeat gathering behind her eyes, but knew if she dared give in to it that might be the end of her. What, then, were her options? Walk out into the storm, not knowing where she was or where she was going, or stay put without fire or food, keeping company with the rat until the storm was over. But she had no idea how long that might be. She was already weak and dizzy with hunger. She couldn't even boil up the shoe, she thought in a burst of black humor, as she'd read sailors did when starved at sea, and she had no desire to tackle the hard lump in front of her. What an odd thing to find here, really, she thought, remnants of some woman's life long ago, the very kind of life she'd been fighting to escape.

As Ruth sat examining the shoe, turning it in her hand while her thoughts rambled, a notion struck her. She remembered John Olsen saying something about the Rose Mine being up the North Fork on the way to the onyx mine—and Kate later telling her that there had once been a small settlement there at the end of the last century, now fallen into ruins. Could that be where she was—up the North Fork that connected with Rattlesnake Canyon?

The idea propelled her to her feet. She might be only a short distance from her own cabin, from fire, hot beans, and her warm bed. Glory Springs was less than two miles from the intersection at the North Fork, though she wasn't sure just how far up the fork the Rose Mine was, since she'd never explored that area. But from what the Olsens had said, it must sit midway to the onyx mine. That would make it two miles from the fork itself— surely not more than four, since she knew the onyx mine itself was only four. So she might be four or five miles from home by road. If this were indeed the Rose Mine.

Yet, four or five miles was a long way in a snowstorm, and she feared for her feet, having book knowledge of the results of frostbite. She stopped pacing and wiggled her toes inside her boots. She could feel them better now, after only a short while out of the snow. That seemed a good sign. If she decided to go on, she should leave now, before the snow made it impossible to walk. But what if she walked down canyon and the road didn't meet up with her own, what if she wasn't where she thought she might be, and only letting hope make her decision for her? Then she'd just have to continue on down canyon, she decided. Wherever she was, down was where the desert was, and where other people lived. The snow on the ground would likely lessen as she lost altitude, as it had when she'd descended the mountain. Fortified by that reasoning, Ruth took hold of her bundle, set it outside the window, and followed it out into the storm. When the first gust of snowy wind blasted her face, for a moment she felt unsure again. But she could see the blank path of the road through the storm, and it felt good to breathe air free of the stench of rat urine, even if the wind and snow froze against her face, so she swallowed her fear and went forward, turning down canyon at the road that she hoped would connect with the way home.

Ruth followed her tracks, which had been nearly smoothed over, around the two bends, then to the place where she'd come into the road, and started down the road in the other direction. The cold that had crept into her when she stopped at the shack was still with her. The rest of her body began to feel the way her feet had, as if her clothes were full of icy bones that she was forcing to act as legs and arms. She couldn't pull the collar of her coat tight enough to keep snow from blowing into the space at her neck between the kerchief and coat. Since she no longer had to negotiate the brush, she stopped and tied the olla blanket around her neck, the pot hanging down her back; it closed the crack at her neck but choked her, and she had to move it down and tie it about her waist, continuing on with the huge mound bulging from her back like a reverse pregnancy.

Not long after, she began feeling drowsy, found her pace slowing as she continued moving hypnotically, feeling as if the blank whiteness had seeped inside and emptied her mind, leaving her feet free to trudge without thought. In this state she nearly missed the road she sought, and it was only when she was forced more awake by fighting her way up the steep wash bank where the North Fork wash intersected Rattlesnake that she realized where she was. Ruth turned around and fought her way up the opposite bank, which had to be the road up Rattlesnake Canyon. Even her flash of elation at the discovery was subdued by her semi-stupor, though the thought that she had less than two miles to go bolstered her stamina and quickened her pace for a while.

She vaguely wondered what time of day it had gotten to be; it had to be sometime in the afternoon, she was sure. Even as she squinted against the glare, she thought the daylight might be dimming, but with the brightness of the growing blizzard, she had no way to tell. Her senses and thinking had been dulled the way a thick layer of snow hushes the shapes of small brush and rocks, turning them to indistinguishable lumps. Nothing around her appeared real, not even herself. It was all less real than a dream, as if she weren't really moving as she walked, but was caught in some kind of snow motion, putting one foot in front of the other but going nowhere into endless white. And she was tired, so tired and numb with cold. Flakes were falling fast and thick, mixing with what the wind whipped up, and twice she walked off the road into small gullies, which were brushless like the rut road, understanding her mistake when she felt the lumps of stones under the snow. If she just had a place to rest until she got her strength back—maybe the blizzard would ease meanwhile—she could go on the rest of the way. Somewhere in the back of her brain, she was opposed to resting and kept herself marching on, but the idea of a respite had taken hold, and her eyes kept watch for some place that might shelter her for a while so she could gain back her failing strength. She had to summon her resolve again and again as she labored, a step at a time, through snow now halfway to her knees, not knowing how much further she could go. Yet somehow each bend inched closer, and she made her way around it, then around another that had seemed an impossible distance. She kept moving, often dizzy, not knowing if any moment she might fall face first into the snow. Then, near the road, she spotted an overhang of rock where a juniper and two pinyons came together and remembered resting there in the shade during the summer. Ruth began walking toward it. If she just sat down for a few minutes to wait out of the storm, she told herself, then she could walk the rest of the way home. It couldn't be more than a bend or so away.

As she eased under the lower pine branch, careful not to bring down the thick clumps of snow on its branches, a doe and large fawn rose up suddenly from under the brush, the shock of it whacking Ruth and her olla into the pinyon branches. Her sudden movement and the deer's quick escape sent a shower of snow down on her head and shoulders. She ducked her face, raising her arms to ward off the plague of ice raining down on her, and stumbled into a branch of the juniper. An avalanche dumped over her, flinging her backward out of the shelter. She landed sitting in a snowdrift, held up by the olla, which served as a pillow to prop up her shoulders against the slant of snow, as if she had arranged herself there to wait out the storm. Which didn't seem like such a bad idea—with snow swirling everywhere and building up fast around her, she had lost the desire to push on, had no strength for such efforts anyway. Besides, she was quite comfortable, really, didn't even feel cold anymore, she realized, closing her eyes and laying her head back into the fluff of snow. Even the flakes falling against her face felt warm and feathery on her skin. She found herself melting into the cushion behind her, soft, like the goose-down quilt on her bed; she couldn't be more content in her drowsiness if she were by the fire in her cabin—and then she saw her woodstove there in front of her, as if by magic, and held out her hands to warm them. She felt herself drawn toward a deepening state of rest. Yet something was still holding her back, a voice, faint at first, then louder, saying clearly: "Get up, Ruth."

She opened her eyes. Jim was leaning over her, that curtain of hair blocking the rest of the world from her view. "Come with me," he said, straightening and stretching out his hand. His smile was a patch of blue in the gray sky. She took hold and pulled herself up. As he led her back out to the road, she marveled that the snow had disappeared and she felt the sun's warmth on her body as they walked. It was easier to walk without the snow. Jim was just ahead of her now and she hurried after him. When her cabin came into view not far around the bend, Ruth was startled to see it covered with snow on such a day, but when she looked around, she saw that the good weather was confined to a small spot around them. In amazement she tried to call out to tell Jim, but her words had been hollowed of sound and blew away in the wind. She followed his figure across the clearing in front of her cabin, anxious to catch up and wrap her arms around his warm body.

The cabin door was shut when she reached it. Thinking he must have gone inside, she dug out her key and clicked open the padlock. Inside was dark and cold. She latched the door and looked around but didn't see him anywhere. Yet there was her bed with its down comforter. She untied the olla and set it beside her pillow, then pulled back the comforter. "The fire, Ruth, light the fire." Jim was standing by the stove. She saw the matches as she came toward him, so she opened the firebox and struck the match to the wood she had laid in, stumbling backward against her chair and falling into it as the flame leapt up from the open burner. She couldn't take her eyes off the hot orange glow, its blaze hypnotizing her and driving all else from her mind. She forgot even Jim, who stood behind her chair with his hands on her shoulders.

Ruth became aware that she was shaking violently. She scooted her chair closer, holding her hands above the hot metal. The heat sent unbearable pain into her fingers, and she had to move them back. Her wet clothes sogged against her skin, keeping the fire from reaching her, so she got up and took off her coat. The shirts underneath were wet also. She looked around to see if Jim was watching, but he wasn't there, so she peeled away the shirts, along with her boots and pants, then rushed to her dresser to rummage for her flannel nightgown and dry pants and socks, returning quickly to the fire to dress.

She stuck more chunks of wood into the firebox and put her feet up on the bottom rail so the heat could reach them. She looked around again for Jim, then wondered why she should think he'd be there. But he had been there, she remembered, picturing herself following him in. But how could he be? It was impossible. She recalled falling back into the snow, then thinking herself here by the fire, starting to realize her mind was playing tricks on her—but which was the trick? Was she still lying in the snow, then, simply thinking she was here? The odd thought struck her that maybe she had died and now only imagined she was still alive. Nothing around her seemed real. But Jim had seemed real—and he was not. The room she sat in, the woodstove, the darkness at the windowpanes were all obscure, as if underwater. The only thing real was the pains stabbing her fingers and toes as they warmed. When she rubbed, the pain became worse, so she stopped and tried to endure. A word floated to her through the watery air: *frostbite*; she saw it printed on an airy page as if it were the spirit of an expired medical journal, and she tried to read the directions that followed, but they dissolved in front of her eyes. She took in a breath at the intense pain that squeezed her hands and feet and gritted her teeth to bear it.

Gradually, pain cleared her awareness and she looked down at her hands, but it was too dim in the room to see them clearly, so she rose and struck a match to the lamp on the table. Her white fingers were already blushed with pink—a good sign. She held up a foot, toes still white and bloodless, though they were beginning to tingle. A sizzle hissed from the coffeepot she had left on the back burner, as if to remind her of what she had learned in nurse training, and she took the enamel basin from the table and poured some of the old coffee into it. From the steam rising, Ruth could tell the liquid was too hot, so she mixed in water from her jug till it was barely lukewarm, then took off the dry socks and put the soles of her feet to the surface of the water. Water needles stabbed her toes, but she lowered them and forced her feet to the bottom of the basin. When she could stand it no longer, she lifted her feet, then pushed them back down again, repeating the process several times until she could leave them in the coffee water, making herself add hot liquid as the mixture cooled. She was alive, all right, if agony was any indication.

When her senses came back, Ruth put on her socks, rinsed the coffeepot, and tossed the grounds out into the snow, the dirt of her front yard now only a memory buried beneath white ice. A layer of flakes blew in the door before she could close it. Ignoring the ache that pounded with each step, she walked back to the table and filled the pot with fresh water. When it was on the stove, she opened a can of beans and set that on a burner as well. The world was coming into focus. She could wiggle her toes now, though it hurt badly each time. She'd gone up the mountain and come back. In between was a blur. It could have been the same day, or it could have been a year later.

She drank several cups of coffee, but could eat only a few spoonfuls of the beans—and then she had to force them into her stomach as if she were her own nagging nurse. Her cold bed would have been unbearable if it hadn't been for the heating stones Kate had left in the back of her oven, something Ruth had rolled her eyes over, then forgot about, until last night in the hut, when she saw the campfire stones. She embedded Kate's stones under her covers, finding it slightly less painful to walk, and went back to the fire to sip her last cup of hot coffee. When she closed her eyes, the memory of her dream in the hut came back. Then she saw Jim's back as she followed him home. Why was that more real than anything around her now? It was that vision that gave meaning to the rest of her life. But she couldn't understand what such a thing meant, and the idea slipped away whenever she tried to pin it down. Even building this cabin had been easier than understanding such strangeness. Anyway, she was too tired to think.

Ruth rose and stuffed as much wood as she could into the firebox. After she put on an extra pair of socks, she peed half the slop jar full, then set it in the far corner and got under her down quilt, the hot rocks having made her bed a cocoon of comfort. When she closed her eyes she was glad to find herself back inside the hut. She heard Jim's soft voice as he bent over her and smiled. "Remember, Ruth, our home is a hut on the mountain." She breathed in the smell of him as she felt his lips touch hers.

CHAPTER FIFTEEN

More than anything else when Ruth woke sometime the next day, she wanted a long soak in a hot bath. Her body's assertions had finally pried up her eyelids, leaving her with throbbing feet and hands, hunger, and a need to pee. She woke in confused turmoil, her painful body pulling her back to the assault, and she clung tightly to the edge of sleep as long as she could. Then yesterday's storm came back to her, and the days before, memories so thin and dreamlike that she opened her eyes and pulled her head out from under the comforter to see what was real.

Through the frigid air of the cabin she saw the row of icicles outside the window, where flakes were still coming down, shivered, and pulled the quilt tightly around her neck. Her wet clothing lay heaped near the stove. She pulled her hands from under the quilt and inspected the reddened fingers that hurt to move. So did the rest of her, especially her toes, yet it all seemed to function. Getting out of bed, Ruth tucked in the blankets to save her warmth and danced over the icy cement to the stove, making a detour to the slop jar. Ravenous, she spooned icy beans from last night's open can into her mouth, while stuffing kindling and small chunks into the firebox. She struck a match to the wood, emptied the coffee grounds into the basin, and filled the coffeepot with the last of the water from her jug. She should have listened better to Kate's advice about bringing in more water, she told herself in her shivery race back to the bed.

Her hoarded heat had greatly diminished, though not faded completely, and she concentrated on absorbing its residue to stop her trembling. When she looked up at the windowpanes, the bottoms crusted with ice, her longing for a hot bath began, her body vividly remembering luxurious hours in Aunt Myrtle's porcelain tub. She had never appreciated that comfort more than at this moment when it was entirely out of her reach, had not even understood what a luxury a hot bath really was, out of the question here when she most needed it. Here she would have enough trouble simply keeping herself supplied with water for drinking and kitchen. It took a huge mound of snow to melt into a small amount of water; she imagined her spring would surely be frozen over, and even if it weren't, the distance to it had lengthened with the deep snow. Now she understood the reasons most people chose to live in places with running water and electricity.

When she heard the coffee water sizzle, Ruth fed the fire with larger wood chunks and set a can of stew on to heat. While she waited, she made a batch of biscuit dough, mixing in sugar and a bit of the cinnamon Kate had left, and when her food was ready, she stuffed the stove once more and carried her repast over to the bed, where she consumed every bit of the stew and biscuits, washing down each bite with coffee until only grounds remained in the pot. She savored the sharp tastes she had been denying herself. When every crumb was gone, she sat wanting more, though her stomach would not have held another morsel.

It had stopped mattering whether or not the hunger was hers; her body owned it now.

Her appetite did not diminish in the weeks that followed, though it took nearly three more before she was down to flour—which she still had an entire sack of—and a few cans of beans and a bit of jerky. That she had anything at all was due to the fore-thought of the Olsens, who had stocked her thoroughly. Ruth herself had picked up only minimal supplies on both trips to town, so intent had she been on collecting her mail. And she was not motivated to carry much. She thought she'd be making a trip back soon, never anticipating the ferocity of the storms to come. And come they did, not easing up until a week later, when the snow reached nearly to her hips and approached the bottom of the windowsill, though did not bury the panes as the miners had joked about. It was enough, though, to discourage any thought of making the long walk to Juniper Valley. Once the storms stopped during the second week, the temperature plummeted, making travel even more difficult. And she had learned from her experience on the mountain not to foolishly test the patience of the wilderness, so she stayed put in her cabin and took comfort in a landscape that appeared as alien as her life now felt.

Ruth could not understand what had happened to bring her in from the storm that day. Her memory of it became more vague as the weeks went on, and she rarely thought about it as she brought in loads of wood to dry by the stove and heaped snow into her tub to melt into a water supply. She even treated herself to a hot bath one day—not the long soak she'd dreamed of, but a splash in a few inches of water to get the stink off her body. Afterward she cleaned the tub with a pot of boiling water to purify it again for holding drinking water. What she did find to immerse herself in those housebound days were words, find-ing a snowless road out of the canyon that led directly to Lon-don, Paris, and Moscow, imagining herself in lives and love affairs that had no connection with anything in the life she had known. She began to wake each day anticipating whatever world she had left behind the night before. Sometimes she would look up from a book and be shocked to find herself alone in a snowbound cabin in the wild, rather than in some dusky Old World salon having tea and repartee. Occasionally, she would get up and walk out her front door, standing a few minutes in the cold to remind herself which world was real.

By the time the weather warmed considerably a few weeks later, Ruth's food was running low—she had begun to ration her coffee and count out the cans of beans, noting the single strip of jerky left to her, roasting open some of the pinyon nuts to supplement. The books at first served to distract her from her hunger and her worry about getting some of Cally's herb in time. But as the days wore on, she found herself at the window more often, checking the snow level, and finding reasons to walk outside. After the weather had been warm for a while, she walked down to the spring to see if it was still frozen. Because her spring was on the south-facing slope of the wash, the ice covering the pool had become mushy with the day's sun. By now snow had vanished from the tops of bushes and rocks over most of the south face of the lower mountain. She began considering the trip to town that she had postponed. If the weather held, she might be able walk out in a few days.

The cloud cover returned a day later, along with a few flurries, enough to worry, though not to discourage her completely, and she waited to see how serious it got. Mild flurries continued for the next two days, while she occupied herself with her reading. But with her canned goods diminishing, it became harder to believe in those tenuous worlds of print, and she would end up putting her book down to pace the small floor of the cabin. Ruth waited two more days, then, after a breakfast of biscuits without coffee, decided she would try to make it out for supplies. The morning's flurries had turned more serious, becoming a light snowfall, and wind moaned through the window cracks. If a big storm came in when she had so little food left, she would be in trouble—and she'd be locked in without knowing if Cally had sent the herb or if her uncle had news for her, Ruth thought as she hurried on her layers of clothing. If she could get out of the canyon before the weather got severe, she knew the snow would likely diminish by the time she reached the high desert mesas.

She slid her belt into the scabbard of Jim's hunting knife, noticing she was no longer at the last notch of her belt, and picked up her .22. With a few leftover biscuits in her pocket and a pair of wool socks for gloves, Ruth stepped out into considerable snowfall and started down canyon.

She kept to the south side as she walked, where more snowmelt had occurred. In places the snow level fell to her knees. Even so, movement was slow and laborious, more difficult than in fresh snow that could simply be moved aside or packed underfoot, and she had to jerk her feet up again and again when they broke through the ice crust that had reformed. She was glad she was at least traveling downhill this time.

At the North Fork wash, Ruth spotted movement behind some brush. Branches appeared to be in motion. She stopped, straining to see more clearly through the falling snow. A buck with a huge tree of antlers moved out from the scrub oak clump, turned his head and looked straight at her, unafraid, his coat chocolate against the cream of snow. There was her supply of winter meat. Ruth pulled her hand free of the sock mitten and raised her .22. At the sound of the shot, the animal bounded up the bank of the wash. When she fired again, she thought she saw him flinch, though his pace increased as he fought his way through deep drifts up the far bank. Cocking the .22, Ruth fired again, then cocked once more to get off a final shot before the buck reached the top. But the shell jammed in the chamber, and by the time she turned the rifle on its side and shook the bullet out into the snow, the buck was gone. After putting a new shell in the chamber, she hurried after him.

Small dots of blood interrupted the deer's tracks, which headed down canyon toward the willows. The animal's legs had swept a pair of ruts through the snow as it went, punctuating them with sharp impressions of hooves. The injury didn't appear to be slowing the deer down.

Ruth tramped after her quarry, the deep trail allowing her to move easier in the snow, which now began to come down for real. She didn't have much hope of catching the deer, unless the injury inflicted by her .22 had done more damage than it appeared. A .22 was not the appropriate rifle for shooting such a big animal, she knew, but she had acted out of some kind of desperate impulse. Now she felt obligated to find the creature she had wounded. About half a mile down the road, where willows began to line the wash, the tracks left the road to follow the edge of the small stream, merging with the imprints of other deer who had come to the willows to water. Ruth joined the crowd, continuing down the trail, which was packed and easy to traverse. She moved as softly as she could through the scrunching snow as she approached the deeper thickets, peering through the bare branches of willows in hopes of seeing the buck. The falling snow shushed its sound against the brush around her.

Half hidden behind scrub oak, the buck's dark shape became visible in front of a willow. Surprised that she had overtaken it, and even more so to see it calmly nibbling on oak leaves, she took time for careful aim at the deer's neck. She pulled the trigger and the head dropped from view. After the pop of the rifle, Ruth heard nothing but the faint whisper of falling flakes. Had she been mistaken about the deer's shape, imagined its presence out of need, as she had conjured up Jim when she needed him, her mind already playing tricks and she had not yet gone three miles in this storm? She plowed forward to see.

Discovering the deer's form sunk into the snow was a great relief to her, the red ice around its head proof of her sanity. The kill had saved her from having to walk another nine miles in this growing storm. In her gratitude, Ruth remembered Jim's words. "Thank you, deer," she said, meaning it, as she squatted to pat its shoulder and look down into the one glazed eye. But what happened to the antlers, she wondered, seeing the smooth top of the head between the animal's large collapsed ears. Puzzled, she reached down and ran her hand over the ridge of hide, looking closer at the creature's body. This was not the buck she had chased down the canyon, but a doe, and her belly was hugely swollen. The realization knocked Ruth off her heels into the snow. She stared up at the willow in front of her . . . she must have thought the bare branches were antlers. Gritting her teeth, she reached over and pressed a hand to the bulge at the deer's side. Even through her sock mitten, the heat was intense.

What a bloody cycle she was now part of, she thought, since that first shooting of a rabbit that had disturbed her only a few months ago. But this was such a large and beautiful animal—and she had made such a mess: with a wounded buck off somewhere and now a doe and maybe a fawn dead at her hands, perhaps the same doe who had come to drink with her fawn at Glory Springs last spring. She remembered the way the doe had looked up, startled, when Ruth appeared at the bank, then led her fawn away up the draw. "I'm sorry," Ruth said to the creature whose head and shoulders were now covered with a thin white sheet of snow. "I didn't know." But would it have made a difference, she wondered? What did it matter whether a buck or doe, pregnant or not, when feeding her own child was at stake? "Feeding my own self," Ruth argued aloud, appalled that the idea had occurred to her, "feeding only myself." She did not, would not, care about this cat's-claw root, this boulder stuck inside her; she would certainly use Cally's herb soon to loosen it. What caused such a thought—who inside her thought to protect this obstacle that might be the result of a monster, probably not Jim's at all? Not any Ruth she'd ever known. She would be no doe, subject to forces inside and out of herself, who neither wanted nor did not want the fawn but simply had it, obeying powers she could not understand, much the same way women wound up in knitting circles.

Angered, Ruth got to her feet and took hold of the doe's hind legs, pulling them up against her chest. She turned around and gripped the forelegs like handles, dragging the carcass toward a cottonwood near the edge of the wash, jerking it an inch at a time through the snow. She would not waste time moping. Snow was still coming down steadily, the clouds overhead thick and unbroken. She had shot the doe and that was that; now it was her food, and she had to concentrate on getting it back to her cabin—which wouldn't be easy.

Unbuckling her belt, Ruth used it to lash the hind legs together and, in short jiggling motions, hoisted them up a low branch of the cottonwood, balancing the rear against the trunk of the tree and leaving the deer's head and shoulders on a snow-covered rock to bear most of the weight. Ruth pulled her knife from its scabbard and bled the deer, then made cuts below the ankle bones the way she did with rabbits. The thick skin was tougher to pull down than rabbits' skin, though, which almost melted off beneath the mucous membrane. She had to jerk hard again and again, yanking the hide off in thick strips, all the while fighting against nausea at the meaty sweet smell of blood. She continued until most of the hide up to the ribs draped like a ragged fringed skirt around the deer's front legs and shoulders. She need do only half the deer, she realized, since that was all she could possibly carry. Though the wind had eased some, snowfall was heavy now, collecting on her arms and shoulders, and her memory of that last walk home prompted her to make haste.

For a moment she hesitated, then swallowed and held the knife to the bottom of the belly, slicing straight down the middle of the ballooning flesh. The huge mass of guts sagged outward and down, spilling over onto the raw hide skirt. The sickening sweet smell increased nearly beyond her bearing as she reached her hands into the warm blood to lift out the loops and coils of intestines, ripping away stubbornly attached organs. She averted her eyes from the tangle she was removing, but at the periphery of her vision, she saw, or imagined, a curled shape wrapped in membrane, a small head and dainty hooves. Huge liquid eyes.

Ruth turned to one side, dropping to her knees in time to cover the snow with the contents of her stomach. After the retching eased, she got up from the ice and walked a few feet away from the bloody scene, taking deep gulps of the clean air. When her stomach settled, she scrubbed her bloodied hands with snow and put her makeshift mittens back on. She couldn't allow squeamishness to stop her now. Looking away from the pile of entrails below the carcass, she pushed them to one side with her boot and covered them over with snow.

Knowing it would be struggle enough just to carry half the deer home, Ruth cut through the flesh around the deer just under the rib cage, until the gutted torso hung attached to its skirted half simply by the bony rope of spine. To sever the linked spine bones, she hacked and pried at the seams of the joints, but the attachment would not break. Short of a cleaver, the only way to separate this spine would be to break it the way she snapped the ankles of rabbits—but it would take a giant to snap these big bones. Then another picture flashed into her head, one of boulders and broken planks. She unlatched the belt and let the deer drop, kicking snow off the top of the rock until the stony surface was exposed.

After kicking away snow from two sides of the rock, Ruth dragged the deer over and draped the carcass backward over the stone. Climbing on the slippery meat, she straddled the rock's shape under the spine, one boot on either side, holding on to a branch above her for balance. She made several small jumps. When she felt the spine bend back against itself, Ruth increased her force, and as something began to give, she came down with all her weight. The bones snapped, and she plunged from the rock into the snow, gigantic in her triumph.

Her elated moment of conquest dwindled to ordinary exhaustion on the journey home. Only hunger-induced visions of roasts and steaks kept her from leaving the prized hind end to freeze by the roadside. Though it was too late, she knew now that she would have been better off making the trip into town for provisions, maybe staying with one of the families until the weather eased, then catching a ride back to the canyon's mouth. Perhaps she could have wangled herself a hot bath or two in the process. Surely they would have insisted that she clean up, she thought, remembering the pungent odor of John Olsen when she first encountered him, an odor she later ceased to notice with changes in her own hygiene.

Ruth left the meat outside her door and went in to fire up her stove and put on water to heat, drinking it without the coffee she so craved—which she would have by now if she'd gone into town, she realized. When she had warmed, she dragged the meat inside and cut pieces off the carcass to store in the woodshed, where she could best protect the meat from other predators that might show up once they cleaned up the mess she left at the willows. But she knew that once the pieces froze, they would have little odor to attract animals. If the weather warmed . . . well, she'd figure what to do if it happened.

The section of deer had begun to look more like meat than freshly killed animal, though it was still bloody and raw. The cuts she made looked like none she'd seen in a butcher shop, but they would cook and eat just as well, she suspected. Saving out some steak for dinner, Ruth fried it up to eat with a batch of biscuits. The meat was tough and hard to chew. Its strong taste made her stomach lurch, and she had to keep herself from spitting it out. But she needed to eat it. Something about that taste was familiar. She held a chunk to her nose, closing her eyes and breathing in as she chewed the meat in her mouth. And she began to understand. It was the taste of oak leaves and scraggly pine, of sage and juniper that grew in the rocky canyon, the taste of the canyon and rock itself that she was eating. Her own land, she told herself, though something in her didn't believe the land was hers. She had meant to make the canyon hers, but the canyon was more powerful than she was, she realized, as she looked out the window, where wind was hissing snow against the darkened pane, and it was she that had come to belong to the canyon—becoming simply another one of its creatures, not so different from the deer after all. The idea both frightened and comforted her.

The snow stopped after another foot had fallen. And again, the temperature dropped, then rose after a few cloudless days. During the next two weeks, Ruth broke up her hibernation with routine: after she emptied her slops and fired up the stove to heat the cabin, she would walk to the spring to check how much ice covered the pond. With a pine twig, she would measure the falling snow depth, scratching the promise of her coming libera-tion into the thin bark. On some days she would pluck leaves from various shrubs and boil them in hot water when she re-turned to the cabin, but never found any to her liking except for the long green stalks that Jim had used, so she stayed with those. She continually longed for coffee, dreamed that she drank cups of it at night, when she replaced other missing things she loved;

Jim was a frequent visitor in her sleep. Several times a day she collected snow and icicles to melt for water. In the afternoons she settled in to read and to write in the journal she had begun again, for the first time since Jim died. Her reading had inspired new ways to use the journal, and sometimes she spent most of an afternoon simply perfecting her description of a place or an event. She even wrote of Jim and the days they had together. But she stayed away from the event that most troubled her. To save kerosene, she now ate while it was light, looking forward to the hour when light dimmed and the windowpanes darkened. Then she would warm her comforter with hot rocks and secure herself under it to dream.

On a day the third week after her kill, as she was pulling her measuring stick out of the snow, Ruth thought she heard the sound of voices. She listened closely but heard nothing more, so went on to scratch the snow level into the branch. Each day she'd watched the snow become more subdued by the few hours of sun, and she planned in a few days to make the trip into town. On her way back across the wash, Ruth heard the voices again, and they continued until she climbed the bank to her yard. By then she could see three riders rounding the bend. Heart pounding, she tried to make out who they were. When she couldn't, she bolted into the cabin to get ready.

Both the rifle and shotgun were already loaded, but she checked the chambers to make sure, then put aside a pile of ready ammunition and waited, her door latched. She had seen no big buckskin, but Stine might have gotten rid of it by now; if he had brought back friends thinking he would damage her again, he was dead wrong. This time she was ready for him. Entirely ready, she thought, taking in a breath to steady her shaking hands.

The riders' conversation was constant as they came closer, Ruth staring out of the window for her first view. The fact that they were not creeping up on her lessened the tightness in her bowel, though her fingers still shook as they gripped the trigger of the shotgun pointed at the glass windowpane. Delayed hate and horror took hold of her. When the first up the bank turned out to be Larry Hudson, and the second Jake Tunstall, followed by another familiar neighbor—a tall, thin man whose name Ruth didn't remember—she was almost as disappointed as she was relieved, having already pictured herself blowing a huge hole in Stine's gut. When she heard her name called, Ruth put down the shotgun and sagged into a chair, burying her face in her hands for a moment. Then she took a deep breath and walked to the door. It seemed a strange thing to be opening her door to company; confused, she reached up to adjust her kerchief, then dropped her hand and undid the latch. Swinging the door open, she stood looking at the three apparitions who were dismounting at the side of her house.

"It appears you've survived the winter storms just fine," Larry Hudson said, pulling his hands from gloves as he and Jake walked toward her. Their neighbor led the horses over toward a juniper by the bank. "A lot of folk were worried about you. Afraid we'd find you either starved or froze to death."

"I can take care of myself," Ruth said, though the quaver in her voice caused the men to sharpen their focus on her. They were the first words she had spoken aloud in weeks, except sometimes to herself. Her voice sounded weak and unnatural even to her. "Anyway, I appreciate your concern. Come on in and warm yourselves. I'll get a good fire going."

The two men stomped snow from their feet and followed her inside. "I'm sorry I can't offer you coffee," she said, as she fed sticks into the firebox, "but I've been out for weeks."

"Maybe we can do something about that," Hudson told her, as his neighbor came in carrying two sets of saddlebags over his arm. The man took them over to her table, shedding them on the floor next to the wall, then crouched to dig inside the pouches. "You don't think we'd come all this way up here empty-handed, do you?" Hudson said when the neighbor began setting dry and canned goods on her table. About halfway through his unpacking a coffee can appeared.

"I don't know what to say," Ruth said at the sight of the coffee. She picked up the can and held it to her. "And look at the sugar. And oatmeal. How can I thank you for this?"

"Just being neighborly," he said, "that's all. Told Olsen I'd bring them up. He was in town a couple weeks ago when the last storm hit, him and that big Swede. Saw them at Baxter's store."

"Folks were already talking about stocking you up then," Jake Tunstall said. "Nobody'd seen you since that first big snow hit."

"Got these for you, too." The tall neighbor held out her mail. Besides the check, there was an envelope from her aunt and a package from Cally. Ruth restrained herself from ripping both open at once and flung them into the drawer of the writing table.

"I'll get the water on for coffee," she said.

"This looks like venison," Hudson mused, examining the meat Ruth had set out by the stove to defrost. "Where'd you get venison?"

Ruth dipped water from the snowmelt tub into the coffeepot. "I shot it," she said. "Got tired of beans, and I'd run out of everything but flour, anyway." She stood to place the pot on the stove. "Now I'm tired of venison, since that's about all I've got, so I'm sure glad to see corned beef and stew again. But the deer saved me."

"I only see a twenty-two and a shotgun," Tunstall said, glancing over at the rifles leaning next to the window. "Seems puny for bagging deer."

"I got a close shot with the twenty-two down by the willows."

"Must be a dead eye. Pretty impressive for a woman," the neighbor man said, hunkering down by the stove.

"Not surprising for Ruth, I don't think," Hudson told him, holding his hands out over the stove.

"You're welcome to take some back with you," Ruth said. "Why don't you? It would help me repay you. I've been having to pack it in snow on the north side the last couple days till the night freeze comes." She opened the drawer of her writing table. "Meanwhile, I'll reimburse you for the cost of the supplies."

Hudson shook his head. "Olsen had Baxter's intended, Lily Rose, start a tab for you in the store. Said you can pay them when you get to town."

Their engagement came as no surprise. Ruth was almost glad

of it. "That won't be long if the weather holds," she said, turning to set out cups for the coffee. "Is there more news?"

"Jack Rider ran his Studebaker in a ditch, broke his arm. Marie Hardesty took sick again with the weather. Another pneumonia, the second since the stillborn," the neighbor said.

"Things are tightening up after the crash, but nothing like the hard times hitting the cities," Hudson told her. "That's about it."

Ruth measured out the coffee and dumped it into the boiling water. "What about . . . what about . . . has anything more been learned about Charlie Stine? His whereabouts, I mean?" She stirred the grounds and pulled the pot to the side of the stove. The men were silent.

"Not that I've heard," Hudson said. He looked down at the floor. "We heard about your trouble," he said, laying a hand on her shoulder. "I'm sorry about it. You're a capable woman, Ruth, more than most. Young. You'll get through it." Ruth kept her eyes on the cups; if she looked up, it would all start. She wondered just how much about it they had heard.

"The Indian was a good man, too," he said, removing his hand from her. "I didn't approve, but he was a good man for an Indian."

Ruth looked at him now. "Good for any man," she said. "The best." She took hold of the coffeepot handle, though it burned her hand, held a cup to the spout of the tipped pot, and poured it full. "Charlie Stine was the worst."

"I can agree with you there," Hudson said, taking the cup she offered, "and I hope they catch him. Even that buckskin he rode was mean."

"Reminds me of that one bucked me off every time I climbed on board," Tunstall said, and the conversation lightened while the men drank and refilled their cups. Ruth was glad of it, not really wanting the men to leave so quickly. All three refused her offer of a corned beef and biscuit sandwich, saying they'd brought their own eats, not wanting to use hers up, since another storm could still come in. Hudson did accept a roast of venison when he left, but the others said they greatly preferred beef or chicken.

After their good-byes, Ruth stood out beside Hudson's horse

as he mounted. "Thanks again for everything," she said as he drew up his reins.

"Think nothing of it," he said. "I enjoyed the ride, and especially the visit."

"I did, too," Ruth told him. "Yours are the first faces I've seen in a while."

"Let's hope the storms hold off. March is right around the corner now, just a few weeks off." He tipped his hat and turned his sorrel toward the wash, where the other two men were already descending the bank.

When they were out of sight, Ruth went in and put on a small pot of coffee for herself. She would be sparing with the amount, had spent enough time without, remembering how much excess she had tossed onto the ground each time she made a new pot. She sat at her writing table and opened her aunt's letter, reading through all the innuendos about Cally's behavior and admonitions about the kind of life Ruth must be exposed to in the wild, hoping for the information she'd waited so long for. She found information this time, but it was not at all what she wanted to hear. "Your Uncle Ben says to tell you that he doubts the man you seek has come back to this state. He learned of a Charles Steiner who left Dallas two years ago and is wanted on suspicion of murdering two people, one of them a woman. He was a man fitting the description you gave, especially the unusual color of orange hair. Ben said he has sent this information to the authorities in your area."

"Damn it, damn it, damn it." Ruth clenched her fists and squeezed her eyes tightly shut. Tears were no substitute for rage. She did not know how to rid herself of the rage without killing Stine. The comfort that had come to her with the visit was quickly lost in the light of this news. "Damn it!" This time she yelled it, then quieted, in case the men might still be close enough to hear her shouting, her remaining outlet being to rip up the letter and throw the pieces into the firebox, shoving wood in on top of them. "Wherever you are, you bastard," Ruth said, "I hope you burn in hell."

She untied the string from the parcel Cally had sent, somewhat puzzled by the elongated shape of the package. Pulling apart the wrapping paper, she dug around until her fingers found the dry softness of the herb packet. She was thankful Cally had come through and plucked the folded letter from underneath:

I knew you were too willful to take care of yourself, even after all I taught you. You certainly knew how. Now you tell me that you may be carrying a child belonging either to an Indian or to a man with orange hair who you say raped you. None of this would be the case if you'd come back to El Paso as I told you—or if you'd never left in the first place. I tell you now to come back at once so nothing more happens. You were never meant for nursing and I can surely put you to work, for I need assistance around this place.

As for your problem, I suppose there's no sense in bringing you back in the family way. You wouldn't be much good to me here in such condition. You can see that I've sent the herb you requested. Take it without delay, for it must be used in the very early stages for it to have the proper effect. With the time passed sending it through the mail, it may already be too late. I have sent two packets, each with a strong dose. You will remember how it is used. If something doesn't happen the first time, let a day pass and take the second dose. Be prepared, the nausea is especially bad if you take it twice, much more severe than you had that time here in El Paso. In case neither works, because of the delay, I have included the alternate remedy women have used for ages. Your training and nurses manuals do not cover such a subject, but from what they have told you, you can figure out what to do.

When the letter went on to include a paragraph about Myrtle, Ruth put it down and dug deeper into the package. There to one side she felt something long and hard and tore through the layers of paper until she extracted the object and brought it out into the light. Her puzzlement at the sight of the knitting needle slowly turned to dazed comprehension. She had wished to dig the root of this weed from her body. Now Cally had given her a tool to use. A strange feeling cast itself over Ruth's memories of women she'd seen knitting at every gathering, May, Mrs. Rose, and Martha Hudson. Chills climbed her back at the thought that occurred to her. She shook them off and stood up. She hoped it would not come to that, but with the snow, the delay had been long. Dumping a packet of green-black herb in her coffee cup, Ruth poured in hot water from her pot and began the softening.

CHAPTER SIXTEEN

The excruciating nausea that developed with the second dose of Cally's herbs pinned Ruth firmly to her bed, her head by the edge where she could hang it over and retch into the basin on the floor. For hours, if she dared move, the heaves would continue long after she lay still. She feared she had poisoned herself along with whatever else was in her. In the spring, the Olsens would find her retched to death in her bed. So this was what she had saved herself for. She would have had a far kinder death freezing in the snow, believing she was cozy by her fire. But as the afternoon wore on, any kind of demise began to seem preferable to the state she was in. It was a very long time before she was allowed even the temporary oblivion of sleep.

She woke to find the room bright with moon, her mouth so dry her tongue clung to its roof. The odors that rose from beside her bed nearly set her to retching again, but she turned her head away and waited for her stomach to quiet; it felt like she had taken it out and beaten it like a rug on a clothesline. Holding her breath, she reached under the bed and felt for her canteen, attempted a few small swallows, then cuddled the canteen to her chest and dropped back into sleep. Whenever thirst asserted itself, she unscrewed the cap to quench it.

When morning came, Ruth fought her body to sit up. Every muscle in her sorely protested when she got to her feet and carried the slops out the front door, not even bothering to put on boots. But she could stand no more of its smell. Snow jolted her bare feet, prodding her legs to hurry toward the outhouse. Checking herself there, she found no blood; dejected, she returned to the cabin. The brisk air had revived her body, enabling her to put on boots and go out again to clean the basin and bring in a batch of snow for melting. She would give herself two more days—it was still possible that her release would come. If not, she must resign herself to the other measure. After making a broth from venison and heating water to clean herself, Ruth went back to bed for the night, though the sun had not yet dropped behind the mountain.

The next day flurries returned, but the sun soon came out and tore the clouds apart, scattering them in pieces across the sky. No snow accumulated. She measured again, for the first time since the men had left, and was glad to notch down another couple of inches on the stick. Small patches of dirt could now be seen in places where her old footprints had melted. She replenished her water supply, brought in wood, and tidied her cabin, checking often to see if the remedy had worked. She could not keep her mind free, and gave up any idea of reading. By the end of the day, she was resolved on what she had to do. Pulling out her medical manual, she set it beside her cot, though she did not yet open it.

The following morning was much like the one before it, the

sun borne away often on fast-moving clouds, while wind moaned against the windowpanes and pinyon branches scratched the cabin roof. After coffee and forcing down some oatmeal, Ruth opened the manual and studied the diagrams on female anatomy, which she didn't find terribly helpful—and she did not like the book's impersonal naming and diagramming of the body parts she knew so intimately from experience. But she verified what she was afraid was true—that she would have to pry open the aperture to her womb. Ruth ran her fingers along the long, cool body of the knitting needle on her lap, down to the sharp tip at the end; she could see why it made such a perfect instrument.

It had to be boiled, of course, along with a towel for the blood, which Ruth did and set them in the basin by the bed, along with alcohol and a coffeepot of boiling water. Taking the small vanity mirror from her dresser drawer, she pulled up her nightgown and held the mirror down between her thighs, trying to determine where to put the point of the needle. The sight of her own opening was a shock to her; she had never before had such a perspective. The view repulsed her at first—she didn't want to acknowledge the presence of such a primal place inside her, but she spread her legs and made herself look into the darkened cave between them. Not that she could see far into the fleshy internal folds, even when she contorted her body to bring more light into it. But she could not devise a way to see clearly to the core she knew lurked there. Finally, she found it by feel, with a finger, a bumpy knot at the back. She knew where it was now, and just had to make herself force it open and release its contents.

To be sure she was at the right place, Ruth pressed down on her stomach just below her navel, feeling the push of a soft flesh-covered lump against her fingers. That she was forced to rip such a thing from her own flesh, to risk infection and hemorrhage, filled her with bitterness. Why should she have to further the violence already perpetrated on her? An image of the fawn in the membrane came to her, and Ruth felt a sudden wave of sympathy for whatever creature was growing inside her, caught in such turbulent events. It must have suffered the same nausea she did, found its blood gripped by the hate running through her own. But she shook off such pity; it would not help to get the job done. The creature's root had taken deep hold in her already, spreading its tendrils into her thoughts and feelings. She found it harder each day to separate herself. What would those tendrils do to her once she had cut them from their source?

And what if the thing . . . this being unfolding in her—she shuddered at the thought—were of Jim's and her doing? What difference then? She saw how life worked now, seducing with its pleasures until it was ready to extract the cost. How different the experience—the heat and ecstasy—from the consequence—this oddly pulsating lump of flesh. How corporal and bloody the world was, really, compared to the words and manners people tried to dress it in.

Ruth positioned herself with the knitting needle against the knob on her cervix, recoiling at the prick of the sharp point. She was about to jiggle the needle in when the image of the fawn came back again, that miniature curled body and those unborn eyes. Had she really seen such a thing? Real or not, with that image came the nausea she'd experienced at the doe's evisceration by her own hands. She lay back and waited for her stomach to settle, then sat up again and repositioned the needle, started to ease it in the opening, but the squeamishness returned and her stomach convulsed. She knew of no way to argue with a stomach about to heave. It forced her to wait another day to recover before going through with the procedure. Pulling out the needle, she dropped it into the pot and fell back on her pillow, glad for the reprieve, but determined that it be only a postponement.

That night Ruth dreamed she and Jim were making a pot by the lake. Sun warmed her shoulders, and the air was full of birdsong, as she watched him coil the clay snake around the vessel. The two of them shaped and smoothed the squishy substance until it held firm, happy with the feel of earthy slime again between their fingers. There was a crying somewhere, and Ruth glanced over to see a child with long dark hair beside them. Surprised, she looked up to tell Jim, but she could tell by his smile that he already knew. Yet the crying didn't stop, and now it sounded more like a woman screaming, and when she looked again there was a woman on the ground screaming, then she was that woman struggling to free herself.

Ruth woke thrashing. She lurched to a sit, but the screaming continued. It took her a moment to realize it was not herself screaming but something outside. A mountain lion. The cat sounded very close, closer even than her spring. Throwing her legs over the side of the cot, she slid on her boots, picked up her rifle, walked over, and pulled open her door. As it swung open, the screaming stopped. Snow crunched underfoot as Ruth took a step out into the night. Above the pinyon hung a brilliant moon. She had never seen such a night, where the whole world became a sparkling crust of light, and she stood gawking in awe. Then a movement in the pinyon caught her eye.

Ruth turned her focus toward the dark tree but saw nothing. Then another movement. She took a step back into the shadowed door frame and waited, gun in place, while the big cat dropped gracefully from the tree onto the snow. The cougar stayed still, tail twitching as it studied her, the moon making large green circles of its eyes and golden fleece of its winter coat. Ruth wondered if she had only dreamed she was awake, though the bite of the air reassured her the scene was real. How hard it was, she thought, to tell the difference lately. She felt as if she'd stepped through her door into some world left behind as a child in fairy tales, and if she took one step more, she would be in that world for good. The magic cat had come for her. It would be like walking into the pages of one of her books about other times and places. At the same moment she knew it was a real mountain lion out there, and if she took a step forward it would run away and she would be left standing alone in the cold snow. The real cat hadn't come for her, she knew, but for the venison in the woodshed. It was a creature belonging to the same world as the dead fawn. Ruth had come to Glory Springs wanting a life of freedom that was a part of the moonlit fairy-tale world, but what she had found here was the place where the cat and the fawn lived, a place with blood and suffering that offered another kind of freedom entirely. A pricey freedom that had not magic but mystery surrounding it.

The feline turned and glided away into tree shadow, its soft paws muffling the compression of snow crust, a gilded movement against the moonlit glitter of frozen snow. The cougar continued into the scrub oak on the knoll. When it was out of sight, Ruth went back inside and latched the door against the cold. She built a fire and made herself a small pot of coffee, then sat letting images sort themselves out in her head. She wondered whether the knitting needle could unravel what had been done to the fabric of her life—it could undo yet not touch what had happened. She thought about her dream of Jim and the child, of the screaming woman—and of the way the cat had come to bring them to her with its cries. That was the kind of mystery that interested her, the one she wanted to live with.

CHAPTER SEVENTEEN

Thin patches of snow still clung under shaded thickets and on north-side stretches of road, diminishing as Ruth traveled down canyon, and disappearing completely at the mouth of the canyon. The melt had been slow through most of February, with many days like this one, flurrying, with sun in and out of clouds. Yet another big storm had never developed, and she was grateful for that much. She could have made the trip a week ago, but had waited until she was out of nearly everything, including coffee, before tackling the long walk to Matt's store. Without expecting letters, she had no reason to go in except for her need for provisions—and plenty of reasons to stay away.

By the time she reached the widened stretch of road that ran between Mound Springs and the surrounding rimrock country toward Juniper Valley, the air had warmed, so she peeled off her coat and carried it hanging between her back and knapsack. The clouds that raced across the horizon up canyon dissolved over her head as they encountered the high desert sky. Spring was closer on the mesas than near Rocky Mountain, and Ruth relished the feel of sun seeping into openings in her clothing. Already patches of gray green were breaking through the dirt shoulder along the road, the beginnings of primrose and lupine. The sight lightened her step, and she walked along with the idea of flowers opening in her chest. She had thought such feelings were gone from her. Yet even this celebration she experienced at the sight of emerging leaves was tempered with a new poignancy, knowing the hard winter it took to bring them.

As Ruth walked, she thought about purchasing her own transportation to town, a pony maybe. Better yet, her own vehicle. She had most of two allowance checks saved up, and there would be a third awaiting her at the store. Maybe she would put the word out. When she had gone about half the distance to town, she heard the neigh of a horse somewhere behind her. Ruth checked her desire to step off the road and conceal herself behind a bush. She made sure shells were in the chambers of her shotgun and looked over her shoulder several times until the approaching horse and rider became a bobbing shape behind her.

As soon as she made out the rider to be Johnny Lee, she moved to the side and walked on as if she had no awareness of his approach, careful not to look over even as he rode alongside and slowed his horse to walk at her pace. She sensed he was studying her as they continued to move down opposite sides of the road, hoping he would ride on and not speak to her. The longer he stayed, the less chance of that happening, and sure enough, after some time he began to guide his horse closer. "Want a ride into town, Ruthy?" he asked. She ignored his question and continued on indifferently. "It's a long ways to go," he said, bringing his horse a bit closer. When she still didn't respond, he slid off the sorrel and led it as he walked beside her.

It was all Ruth could do to keep from turning around to

punch him or bash him with the shotgun butt. Finally she said, "Get back on your horse, Johnny Lee, and leave me alone," lacing each word with gall. When he made no move, she turned toward him. "Go on, get out of here," she told him. The contrite expression on his face surprised her.

"I didn't mean nothin' by it, Ruthy. Soon as I said it, I knew I'd done wrong. I . . . I was just mad at you, that's all . . ."

"Stop calling me Ruthy. My name is Ruth."

"I didn't mean no harm to come to you, Ruthy . . . Ruth . . . but when he said how he found you and the Indian naked in the willows . . . well, guess I got jealous and shot off my mouth. There was already talk." She did not answer, and he said, "I got worried, you know, afterwards . . . told Olsen all about it next day at the store. You can ask him."

"You didn't exactly come up to see for yourself if I was all right, did you, if you thought Stine meant me harm," she said, looking straight ahead as she walked.

"I know I didn't," Lee said. "I wish I did. I didn't want to go up there and find you and that Indian together either."

"His name is . . . was Jim."

"Indian Jim, weren't it? Anyway, I'm sorry about your Indian. I wasn't at first, to tell the truth." He fell silent and they continued on for few minutes. "Anyway, Ruthy, I'm glad to see you're looking so good. I was afraid you'd be ruined by it all. But you look pretty as before—even with that red thing on your head you look mighty good to me." Ruth glanced over at him sharply, and he said, "I didn't mean nothin' by that neither. Just wanted you to know you look like the same Ruthy to me."

"That's because you can't see inside me," she said.

"You always were a lot of woman to handle. Too much for me, I guess. But you can't say I didn't try." He pushed back on his hat brim. Ruth turned her face away so he couldn't see her expression softening. "Sometimes I think you're more like us— like a man. Most ladies couldn't go through what you did, do all that homesteadin' and still come out good as new," he said. "You look like a woman an' feel like a woman, but inside you're more like us."

"That's what I used to think, Johnny. But that was because I just didn't know what being a woman was supposed to be like. Maybe no one knows."

"I remember that night you was so mad you punched that Charlie Stine, right in front of everyone."

"I wish I'd shot him instead."

"Well, somebody sure did."

Ruth stopped cold. "What do you mean?"

"That's what I heard last week. He was shot to death in Oklahoma sometime around Christmas."

"Is it true?"

"Frank Thomas was there. Said some troopers were trying to bring him in. He shot one of 'em and they killed him dead."

Ruth suddenly felt removed, like she was floating through the landscape. She watched her feet begin to move again over the ground. Maybe the story wasn't even true, she thought. She'd have her uncle find out for her.

"Let me ride you on to town, Ruthy," Lee said after a few minutes. "Please. I can't leave you out here walkin' all alone. It's a shame."

"Would you worry about leaving me if I were a man?"

"Nope, I guess not."

Ruth tried to meet his grin with a slight one of her own.

They stopped to face each other. Johnny put an awkward arm around her shoulders and gave her a quick brotherly squeeze, then walked to his horse. "Damn," he said as he pulled himself up. "I still wish . . ."

"Don't even let it enter your mind, Johnny," Ruth said, standing at the side of the horse. "Not ever again in your whole life." She raised a hand for him to lift her.

"Aw, I can't help if I think about it once in a while," he said as she settled in behind him.

Ruth didn't lean up against him as they rode. The idea of sex with this good-natured but weak cowboy after Jim made her want to laugh and cry at the same time. Then the thought that she would never replace Jim sobered her. He was not replaceable, ever. As they rode on, the shotgun positioned across her lap, Ruth put a hand on her belly to steady it against the jostling of the horse's gait.

Lee let her off at the general store, going in himself for tobacco to take out to the men at Desert Star Ranch, who were starting the cattle drive back to Mound Springs. She refused his offer to ride her back as far as the canyon's mouth, saying she'd probably find a way. Martha Hudson was in the store when they came in, conversing with Agnes Rose by the counter. Here was a possible ride, though Ruth knew the woman didn't drive herself and was most likely waiting for her husband. Ruth selected her items carefully, knowing she'd be carrying them at least half the way back. She packed her knapsack with as much as it could hold and brought it up to the counter. Martha stood to one side as Ruth walked up, put a hand on Ruth's back as she unloaded her knapsack. "My dear," she said, "I was so sorry to hear of your trouble."

Mrs. Rose tidied the items next to the register. "I'm just minding the front while Lily gets ready," she told Ruth. "We're taking her in to buy her trousseau today. I'll let them know someone's ready for checkout." She disappeared through the door behind the counter.

"I appreciate your concern," Ruth said to Martha Hudson. "Will your husband be taking you home soon?"

"No, dear, Bob and I are taking the Rose women in to San Bernardino for the shopping." She looked out the front store window. "If ever he gets back here." She turned to Ruth. "Oh, dear, you must need a ride back yourself."

"I'll find one," Ruth said, as Larry Hudson walked in the front of the store. "Or I'll walk."

"Ruth," he said, giving her a quick hug. "You're looking better and better."

"I was just telling Ruth it was too bad we aren't heading home. We could drop her off."

"I'll be glad to run you out as far as the mouth of the canyon before we get on the road," Hudson said.

"I don't mind walking," Ruth told him. "But I'm thinking of buying my own vehicle. Have you heard anything about one for sale around here?"

"Don't know for sure," Hudson said. "How about you, Matt?" he asked as the store owner came in to ring up Ruth's groceries. "Ruth here's looking for a car. You know of any for sale?"

Matt gave Ruth a nod, his eyes lingering on her face. "Not right off," he said, "but I'll keep my eyes open, spread the word." He began ringing up the items.

"I owe you for the stuff John Olsen bought, too," Ruth said. "And I'd like to cash my check—two of them if you have enough cash. And get my mail. Should be another check here by now."

Matt stopped to dig through the mail tray. "There is a letter here for you, but it didn't seem to be your usual check. Has a Boston postmark." He handed Ruth a long blue envelope. A glance at the return address confirmed it was from the Stacels, her father's family. Ruth put it in the knapsack.

The back door swung open and Lily flounced into the room, her golden curls bouncing against her shoulders. She blinked at the sight of Ruth, then smiled at her and stood by her mother, who had come in behind. "We're ready," she said.

Matt opened an arm to receive Lily's tiptoed kiss to his cheek. A quick look sparked between them, before Lily followed the Hudsons and her mother to the door. "So nice to see you again, Ruth," she said, bells sounding as the door swung shut behind her. Ruth began repacking her bag.

"I'll run you home, if you like, Ruth," Matt said as he counted out the change on the counter from her cashed checks. "No sense you having to carry this all that way. I can close the store up early in two or three hours. We can go then."

Ruth looked up in surprise. His expression seemed one of honest concern. For a moment she was tempted. "Thanks for the offer," she said finally, "but I really don't mind the walk. If I leave now, I'll be home well before dark." She shrugged her shoulders into the straps, half regretting her decision as she felt its weight on her back. "But you can let me know if you hear of someone with a vehicle for sale," she said, escaping down the aisle. She pulled the door open so forcefully, she could still hear bells rattling all the way across the parking lot.

Her regret grew as she trudged down the road with the knapsack of groceries, though she knew she would refuse again if he asked. Maybe someone would come along. But her hope for a ride dimmed the farther she went. When she reached the intersection at the mouth of the canyon, she took off the pack and sat down to rest her back before starting up the rut road. Thus far, the uphill had been gradual; in the canyon the grade would intensify, was steep enough so that John Olsen coasted his truck all the way down to the intersection. As she rested, Ruth remembered the letter in her knapsack and pulled it out. She read the neat script of the handwriting with increasing astonishment. When she finished, Ruth sat looking around. Everything looked clean and new.

The letter was from a man named Theodore Stacel, who said he was her late father's brother. He told her that her father had placed money in a stock account for her a few months before he was killed, and it was from that account that her allowance had come. He had been planning to remit to her the entire amount this year, since she had turned twenty-one. At the time, the account had prospered, being worth over a hundred thousand dollars, but most had disappeared in the crash of the market. The brother had managed to extract a small portion just before everything slammed shut and fell to the bottom. He enclosed a check for the amount, the last she would ever receive, and said he was sorry it was so little, but he himself had lost a third of his fortune in the event. The check was for $6,764.29. Ruth was a rich woman.

She folded the letter with the check inside and fitted it carefully into her pack, hardly daring to think what it meant to her life. It certainly would make easier what was to come. She was used to having so little to live on, the money would last for a very long time—years. It would give her time to find a way to make her living—perhaps making pots to sell somewhere. And she could actually buy herself her own car, a good one. She saw herself driving over to the Black Canyon Reservation to see where Jim had come from. Then her new elation leveled and sank to bittersweet, knowing that he would not be there to share in her good fortune.

Seeing that the sun was halfway to the horizon, Ruth hoisted her pack and gun and started up the rut road, her mind brimming with fresh possibility. She did not stop to rest her shoulders again until she reached the Olsens' yard at the willows. There she lowered herself onto a rock and looked at the empty stone house, the dirt yard swept clean by winter snows, forlorn without the goats and chickens running everywhere—and especially without John and Kate. She wished they were there so she could tell them her news. It made her happy that they would be back soon, by the middle of March, in about three weeks. They could ride in together to San Bernardino to purchase her a car, and she could put them all up in a nice hotel.

As she rose and put on her pack, Ruth thought she heard a motor. Even when she listened closer, it continued to sound like a motor, and she felt a blast of gladness that it might just be the Olsens returning early—and at the very moment she was passing by. This seemed like a day for miracles, she thought, as she stood in the road to wait for them. Yet the vehicle that came over the knoll was not the Olsens' flatbed but Matt Baxter's Model A. He pulled to a halt in front of her and leaned out the window.

"I couldn't stand to think of you walking all the way up this canyon carrying that heavy load of groceries," he said when she stepped up to his window. "Besides, I wanted to tell you about a way you can get a car for yourself. Get in and I'll explain it on the way up."

Ruth watched his eyes as he spoke, searching for some hint of insincerity, and though she saw none, she was yet uncomfortable with the change in this man, who had been first indifferent then ugly toward her in his jealousy. But perhaps what had happened to her had softened him, or maybe his love for Lily had really changed him the same way hers for Jim had changed her. Maybe the deaths had given them an odd bond. "All right," she said quietly and walked around to the door on the other side.

His idea about the car seemed hastily thought out. It seemed he had been thinking and now had suddenly decided that he needed a larger vehicle than his Model A for small in-between grocery hauls from San Bernardino, so he wouldn't have to use the huge truck for such things. He proposed that he make her a very special kind of deal on the Model A if she was interested, though he wouldn't go into detail. Nor did she respond, not wanting to reveal why she now had less need for a deal.

When they drove up in front of her cabin, Matt seemed surprised at the sight of it, as if he had pictured her living in her tent through all these winter months, though he must surely have heard about the house-raising. He followed her to the door, remained standing in front of it to inspect the walls as she set her knapsack on the table and leaned the gun against the wall. She realized she would have immediately invited anyone else who had given her a ride to come inside. "Come on in, Matt," she said. "I'll put on a pot for coffee before you go."

"Who did the rock work?" he asked, settling into the chair by the stove as she filled the coffeepot with water from her container.

"Me, mostly. Took most of the summer. Then folks came and put up the rest."

"So I heard."

"It was a bad day to schedule a raising, I know," Ruth said, setting the pot on the burner. "But I knew nothing about their coming until everyone showed up at the bend. It was Martha Hudson who told me that day about May." She laid kindling into the fire box and struck a match to it.

"The last time I was here you were cooking on a campfire. A stove must make things a lot easier for you."

Ruth pulled the coffee can from the knapsack and set it on the table. "It took some getting used to. When the weather was still warm I cooked outside. But I was sure glad of the stove when winter came on."

"No other woman I know would want to live like you do. I'll never understand what you like about being up here without conveniences."

"Conveniences aren't everything. If I were somewhere with conveniences, I wouldn't have the rest of what's here."

"And whatever might that be, Ruth? There's not a soul around for miles."

"No people, you mean. But there are other kinds of souls. Sometimes I think this whole place has a soul of its own."

"Strange talk, even from you. Lily's nothing like you at all. I've missed you, Ruth," he said, rising. He paced across to the window and looked out toward Rocky Mountain. "You don't know how many times I've thought of how it used to be between us."

"What kind of price are you proposing for your car?" Ruth asked quickly.

He turned toward her. "I think about you each day that goes by. It can't really be over between us, can it? I don't want it to be."

"You made a choice a long time ago, Matt, and it was the right one. I'm glad of it now. Your bride is out buying her trousseau as we speak. It's too late for us. Far too late."

Matt walked over and placed a hand on her shoulder. "Not if we come to some kind of understanding, Ruth. You take the car. And I can come up and see you once in a while. It can be like before."

Ruth shrugged his hand off and stepped to one side. "I'm not interested in that kind of a deal," she said. "If that's what you're offering, you might as well leave."

Matt was silent for a moment, and when he spoke again, there was a familiar edge to his voice. "I wonder what you did up here alone all winter?" he asked, looking around at her bed. "Or maybe you weren't alone."

"I asked you to leave, Matt."

"I noticed how you rode up with that cowboy today . . . and I know what he told the boys at the Lone Star." Matt reached out with one hand and tried to turn her toward him, but she resisted. "I heard those stories about you naked with that Indian."

"How dare you! You have no right to accuse me. What I do is no business of yours." Ruth kept her eyes locked on the coffee she was now returning to the can. "Get out, Matt. Now."

But he wasn't listening. "Oh, I remember how you are, all right. I'll never forget that day on the fender of my car." He shook his head and drew in a breath. "All those times we had. . . . I haven't been able to think of anything else since I saw you in the store today."

"You're getting married, Matt. That's what you'd best be thinking about." Ruth marched to the cabin door and swung it open.

"What difference does that make? I was married before. My wife was dying and it didn't stand in your way then."

"Well, it makes a difference to me now. I was stupid then." She stepped outside and turned back toward him. "This makes the fourth time I've asked you to leave. This time it's a demand."

He walked halfway to the door, stopping beside her bed. "You were ready enough to give in before, remember? And why not? You've given it to everyone else on the desert."

"I didn't give anything away that I didn't take back for myself," she said. "That's the kind of woman I was. But that was before Jim. Jim changed all that."

"Then," he said, "who's going to keep a woman like you satisfied way up here in the wilderness?" He crossed the distance between them and stood facing her, his breath hot vomit in her face. "It's not over between us, Ruth. I know what kind of woman you are." His eyes glazed over with a hostile lust not so different from Stine's, and for once she was comforted by the fact that Matt was a coward. "What happened up here that day, huh, Ruth," he hissed, "really? Too many men in your bed at one time and someone got jealous? Well, just don't forget your buck's gone for good now."

For a moment Ruth considered going for her rifle and requiting her need for revenge on this poor substitute for the real villain. Then her arms sagged to her sides along with her rage. "You make me sick, Matt Baxter. The whole of you isn't worth as much as any single hair on Jim's body," she said. "I can't stand to think I ever wanted you. I wish Lily could see you now and know what a prize she's getting. You're a pitiful excuse for a man." She looked up into the shallow face beneath all that buttery hair she'd once adored, a rock calm coming over her.

"Here's what, Matt," she said. "You get in your car and drive back to town. If you ever even look funny at me again, I'll make sure your wife knows about it."

"Who would believe you? You a . . ."

"I'll make sure she does believe me. Make no mistake about that. And here's what else. When I come into the store—since yours in the only place around here a person can buy groceries—you act like nothing ever happened between us. Not before, not now. You treat me with respect, because you know what will happen if you don't. Now, get out of here."

Ruth stepped back inside and latched the door, free even from the words he sent after her: "Bitch," she heard him shout, then, "Whore," before his car engine caught and his wheels spun up a whorl of dust as he made his exit.

CHAPTER EIGHTEEN

Ruth gazed absentmindedly out the window, pen poised on a page in the journal she'd been filling daily since the letter came three weeks ago. Her eyes fell on light specks whirling through the air outside. If someone had asked her, she would have said the specks were part of the flurries that had persisted long after snow melted from the ground and daily winds ripped holes in clouds, leaving fragments afloat in large lakes of sunlight. The fact that the flecks were not drifting, but exercising some kind of control, finally occurred to her, and she leaned her forehead against the pane to see more clearly. These were not escaping flakes, she soon realized, but tiny insects, spreading wings and circling. She shed the red-and-black blanket from her shoulders and walked outside to inspect this unexpected awakening. She couldn't quite make them out, but the shapes indicated several kinds of insects swarming in the patches of sunlight. She leaned back against the stone wall and savored the warmth on her face. A faint tickle on her skin caused her to look down; a ladybug preened for a moment on her forearm, then peeled back its shell, opened wings, and whirred away.

Ruth watched the bug's flight, remembering the beaded trees and rocks Jim had shown her on the mountain, the delight she had felt at that moment—and other moments in this place, as when she stood a spring ago, elated amid the flowers, her new life a shining beacon in front of her, her biggest worry a boulder where she didn't want it to be. Some boulders were harder to bury than others. Squatting to retrieve a shard from the ground next to her cabin, Ruth took it up into her palm and studied the patterns on its surface. Without thinking, she sank down and spread out her arms over the ground. Its texture was airy from melted snow, like a sponge thirsty for the warmth of sun. The earth seemed to have endless capacity to soak up tears and blood before it gave birth again to lupine and bluebells, she thought, yet lay her wet cheek against the pebbly surface as if it were a lover's chest. This place had claimed the whole of her now; she could feel it in the marrow of her bones.

Would she ever be done with this crying? she wondered, but allowed her moisture to saturate the dirt under her face. Then something caused her to open her eyes. She blinked once or twice to see more clearly through her watery vision; it was odd, even so, to imagine she saw tiny pebble-size rocks hopping. She squeezed her eyes shut again, then swiped tears with her shoulder and looked more closely, her elbows on the ground, chin propped on her palms. It was unmistakable. The pebbles really were moving about, making barely discernible hops. The sight was so strange that she forgot all about her pain and laughed out loud. Small rocks rising.

But how could that be? Rocks were immobile, had no capacity themselves for life, even if everything about her had sprung from rock. Yet here they were, like tiny chips of boulder come back to life. Close up, she began to make sense of that movement; these were not rocks she watched, but camouflaged creatures, cleverly designed to appear as rock, the way imagination shapes words so they seem solid.

Ruth watched the insects a few moments more, then turned over on her back and opened her arms to the sky. A small cloud was forming in the blue patch overhead. It stayed to stretch out arms and legs, a long mane of hair sweeping away from its face. Ruth smiled as it changed shape and moved on.

She sat up, feeling the now familiar flutter of wings in her abdomen, as if she had a butterfly inside her. Yet she had written in her journal only last week that if the child were born with light skin and orange hair, she would hack it up like the cat's-claw root, and bury it, as she had the boulder—or stake it out for the coyotes. But already such a thing was impossible for her. Something powerful had taken hold, melting away the Ruth she knew like sun disperses snow, then reshaping her like an olla. All her life she had seen the ways of Myrtle and Cally as the choices open to her, other women appearing to be variations of those extremes—the persnickety busybody or the bitter bohemian. For a short time she had been drawn to the promises of flapperhood, but like Cally's defiance, it turned out to be empty and going nowhere. Ruth had come to this canyon to escape those extremes, to make her way like a man was allowed to do.

But now she knew she was strong enough to walk between the extremes and be another kind of woman entirely. She wasn't yet sure what that was, but it didn't worry her. The canyon would teach her. All she had in mind at the moment was climbing the mountain again to see the ladybugs, digging up clay from the spring to make pots a lot like the ones made here long ago. This year she would plant a decent garden. Buy goats and chickens from the Olsens. She was glad Kate would soon be back and they would sit down together and talk over coffee. A child she hadn't planned would be born, and even if its skin were dark and hair black, as she believed it would be, it would not be Jim come back. But she would not blink when people looked askance at her. She knew lupines and bluebells would soon grow again, another doe bring her fawn to water at the spring. Ruth was, after all, akin to them, the child in her an embodiment of the power she sensed in rock. She would do her part in its rising.